EVOLUTION OF THE "PATIENT CARE TECHNICIAN TEXTBOOK" PUBLISHED

Increasing demand for patient care technicians and lack of all in one compiled educational resources led to the development of the patient care technician textbook. This book has been created after an extensive search of patient care technician profession and keeping in mind the new trends and procedures required for the on job tasks. Our author K.M.Farooq has over 39 years of experience in the healthcare field and especially in patient care area. His expertise and input have served as a valuable resource which provided a unique touch to this project. After many years of working on this project, the book is ready, and we are proud to present our book "PATIENT CARE TECHNICIAN TEXTBOOK: THEORY AND CLINICAL APPROACH". The authors have tried to keep the book concise and to the point. The knowledge in this book has been provided for individuals planning to pursue a patient care technician or associate profession at a postsecondary or college level. The language used in the book is simplistic and somewhat easy to comprehend for individuals to understand the concepts of patient care. Checking your state, local and federal scope of practice for patient care technician is recommended and advised. Finally, the authors would like to thank everyone who has contributed in making this project possible.

PATIENT CARE TECHNICIAN TEXTBOOK: THEORY & CLINICAL APPROACH 2ND EDITION

NOTICE:

PATIENT CARE TECHNICIAN TEXTBOOK
THEORY & CLINICAL APPROACH
Author: Khan, Sultan K.M.Farooq & Faisal Farooq, et al.
ISBN: 978-1-4951-0799-3
COPYRIGHT © OPRET Education

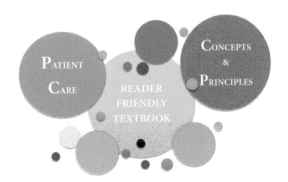

OPRET Education: "An easy learning experience".

PATIENT CARE FOUNDATION PRECAP: START TO END

YELLOW ZONE: CHAPTERS

Chapter 1: Introduction to Patient Care

Chapter 2: Infection Control & Standard Precautions

Chapter 3: Legal Issues in Healthcare

Chapter 4: Introduction to Human Anatomy & Physiology

Chapter 5: Medical Conditions, Diseases & Disorders

Chapter 6: Physical Assessment and Examination

Chapter 7: Patient Positioning and Bed Mobility

Chapter 8: Range Of Motion

Chapter 9: Therapeutic Exercises

Chapter 10: Gait

Chapter 11: Assistive Devices

Chapter 12: Orthosis and Prosthesis

Chapter 13: Transfer Techniques

Chapter 14: Wound care and pressure sores

Chapter 15: Wheelchair Management

Chapter 16: Patient Care Skills Competency Skills

BLUE ZONE: SPECIAL TOPICS

Topic 1: Postural Imbalance

Topic 2: Confusion & Dementia

Topic 3: Nutrition & Meal

Topic 4: Measurement of Intake and Output

Topic 5: Ostomy and its Care

Topic 6: Draping Techniques

Topic 7: Aphasia & its Types

Topic 8: CPR and AED

Topic 9: Patient Defense Mechanism

Topic 10: Admission Discharge & Transfer

Topic 11: Activities of Daily Life

Topic 12: Levels of Need

Topic 13: Aging and Its Changes

Topic 14: End of Life Care

Topic 15: Fall In Elderly

Topic 16: Relaxation Exercises

Topic 17: Gait Belt and Its Uses

Topic 18: Breathing Exercises

Topic 19: Professions in Therapeutic Services

Topic 20: Psychological Disorders

Topic 21: Personality Disorders

Topic 22: Death and Dying

Topic 23: Restraints & Incident Reports

Topic 24: Urine Specimen Collection

Topic 25: Stool and Sputum Specimen Collection

Topic 26: Safety Data Sheet (SDS)

Topic 27: Postmortem Care

Topic 28: Communication

RED ZONE: COMPETENCY SKILLS

- Indirect Care
- Hand Washing
- For Giving a Bed Bath & Back Rubs
- Make an Occupied Bed
- Assist With Range Of Motion Exercises
- Undressing and Dressing Patients
- Take/Record Height
- Take/Record Weight
- Assisting With Applying and Removing Prosthesis
- Assisting With Applying Ace (Elastic) Bandages
- Assisting With Applying Ted's (Elastic Stockings)
- Assisting With Applying Binders
- Urine Output Measurement
- Collect / Test Urine Specimen
- Collecting a Stool Specimen
- Perineal Care (Female)
- Perineal Care (Male)
- Catheter Care (Female and Male)
- Gait Belt and Transfer Belt Use: Ambulation
- Lifting a Client Using a Mechanical Lift (Hoyers)
- Positioning On Side (Turning Client Towards You)
- Change Non-Sterile (Clean) Dressing
- Assisting Patients in Using Bed Pan
- Feeding Patients
- Foot Care
- Denture Care
- Mouth Care
- Hand and Nail Care
- Hot Compresses Application
- Applying Cold Compresses
- Care of a Non-Infected Decubitus Ulcer
- Demonstrating Skill to a Patient
- Vital Signs (Temperature)
- Vital Signs (Pulse)
- Vital Signs (Respiration)
- Vital Signs (Blood Pressure)
- Using an Autoclave
- Pulmonary Function Test
- How to turn patient (supine to prone, prone to supine)
- Perform manual muscle testing
- General steps in performing therapeutic exercises
- Gait Walking (2 point, 3 point, 4 point, Swing through & Swing to)
- Prosthesis and orthosis care
- Wheelchair measurement illustration
- Ostomy
- Draping patient (upper and lower body) Illustrations
- CPR
- AED
- Putting on a sling
- Transfer techniques

TABLE OF CONTENT

Chapter 4: Introduction to Human Anatomy & Physiology

Chapter 5: Medical Conditions, Diseases & Disorders (Brief Description)

SECTION 2

Chapter 6: Physical Assessment and Examination

Chapter 7: Patient Positioning and Bed Mobility Techniques

Patient Positioning

Bed Mobility Techniques

Chapter 8: Range Of Motion

Chapter 9: Therapeutic Exercises

SECTION 3

Chapter 10: Gait

Chapter 11: Assistive Devices

Chapter 12: Orthosis and Prosthesis

Chapter 13: Transfer Techniques

SECTION 4
Chapter 14: Wound care and pressure sores

SECTION 5: SPECIAL TOPICS PART I

SECTION 6: SPECIAL TOPICS PART II

SECTION 7: SPECIAL TOPICS PART III

SECTION 8: SPECIAL TOPICS PART IV

IN THIS BOOK: OVER 60 COMPETENCY SKILLS

Competency Skill: Indirect Care (General Overview)

Competency Skill: Hand Washing

Competency Skill: For Giving a Bed Bath & Back Rubs

Competency Skill: Make an Occupied Bed

Competency Skill: Assist With Range Of Motion Exercises

Competency Skill: Undressing and Dressing Patients

Competency Skill: Take/Record Height

Competency Skill: Take/Record Weight

Competency Skill: Assisting With Applying and Removing Prosthesis or Orthosis

Competency Skill: Assisting With Applying Ace (Elastic) Bandages

Competency Skill: Assisting With Applying Ted's (Elastic Stockings)

Competency Skill: Assisting With Applying Binders

Competency Skill: Urine Output Measurement

Competency Skill: Collect / Test Urine Specimen

Competency Skill: Collecting a Stool Specimen

Competency Skill: Perineal Care (Female)

Competency Skill: Perineal Care (Male)

Competency Skill: Catheter Care (Female and Male)

Competency Skill: Gait Belt and Transfer Belt Use: Ambulation

Competency Skill: Lifting a Patient Using a Mechanical Lift (Hoyers)

Competency Skill: Positioning On Side (Turning Patient Towards You)

Competency Skill: Change Non-Sterile (Clean) Dressing

Competency Skill: Assisting Patients in Using Bed Pan

Competency Skill: Feeding Patients

Competency Skill: Foot Care

Competency Skill: Denture Care

Competency Skill: Mouth Care

Competency Skill: Hand and Nail Care

Competency Skill: Hot Compresses Application

Competency Skill: Applying Cold Compresses

Competency Skill: Care of a Non-Infected Decubitus Ulcer

Competency Skill: Demonstrating Skill to a Patient

Competency Skill: Vital Signs (Temperature)

Competency Skill: Vital Signs (Pulse)

Competency Skill: Vital Signs (Respiration)

Competency Skill: Vital Signs (Blood Pressure)

Competency Skill: Using an Autoclave

Competency Skill: Pulmonary Function Test

Competency Skill: How to Turn Patient (Supine to Prone, Prone to Supine)

Competency Skill: Perform Manual Muscle Testing

Competency Skill: General Steps in Performing Therapeutic Exercises

Competency Skill: Gait Walking (2 Point, 3 Point, 4 Point, Swing Through & Swing To)

Competency Skill: Prosthesis and Orthosis Care

Competency Skill: Transfer Techniques Illustrations

- ✓ Bed to wheelchair
- ✓ Wheelchair to chair
- ✓ Chair to wheelchair
- ✓ Wheelchair to floor
- ✓ Wheelchair to bed
- ✓ Floor to Bed
- ✓ Floor to wheelchair
- ✓ Floor to wheelchair (independent)
- ✓ Wheelchair to floor (independent)
- ✓ Sit to stand
- ✓ Stand to sit

Competency Skill: Wheelchair Measurement Illustration

Competency Skill: Ostomy

Competency Skill: Draping Patient (Upper and Lower Body) Illustrations

Competency Skill: CPR

Competency Skill: AED

Competency Skill: Putting On a Sling

Competency Skill: Abdominal Thrust

Competency Skill: 4 Step ADL Performance

Competency Skill: Steps in Performing Post Mortem Care

Competency Skill: Dressing a Patient Illustration

Competency Skill: Undressing a Patient Illustration

15

SECTION 1

CHAPTER 1: INTRODUCTION TO PATIENT CARE

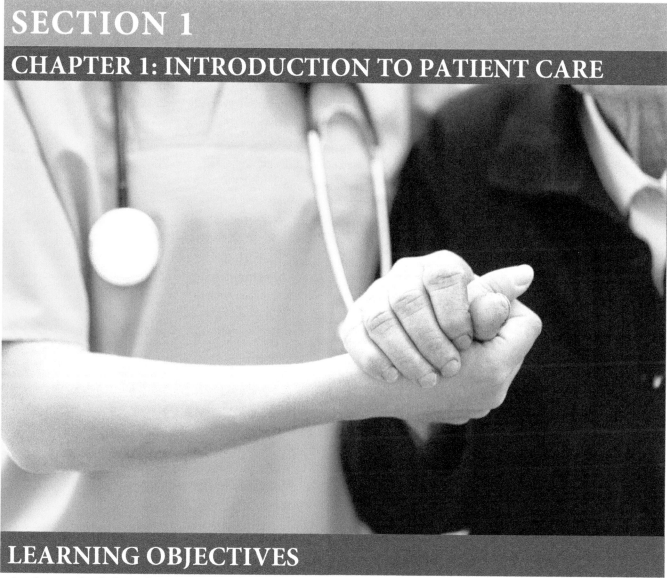

LEARNING OBJECTIVES

At the end of this chapter the student will be able to describe:

1. Functional performance of an individual.
2. The concept of patient care.
3. Causes and risk factors of immobility.
4. The goal of patient care for residents or patients.
5. Patient care skills overview.
6. Regulatory compliance: long-term care facility.
7. Types of Healthcare Facilities and Varying Levels of Care.
8. Medicare & Medicaid.

INTRODUCTION TO PATIENT CARE
FUNCTIONAL PERFORMANCE OF AN INDIVIDUAL

The resident is a term used for patients in a long-term facility or nursing homes. Functional performance of an individual reduces as a result of injury, condition onset, or debilitating pre-existing conditions. Functional performance can also reduce as a result of non-use leading to misuse atrophy. In a healthcare setting, the patients or the residents activities of daily life or living (ADLs) performance usually are based on how the caregivers take care of the patient or resident. Caregivers should ensure that proper assistance is given to the patients or residents. Providing too much assistance can result in dependency and providing too less of assistance can cause discouragement and demotivation. Care should be taken to avoid the patient or resident from being dependent on activities which can be performed by themselves. Patient or resident needs must be addressed by performing an appropriate evaluation by a qualified healthcare professional. Nurses play a very crucial role in performing patient care skills. One should understand that patient care is an ongoing process, and it needs a team effort to achieve the desired results. Assistants and technicians can play an important role in assisting the nurse in performing patient care activities as designated by the nurse. Functional performance decline can be stopped by performing proper patient care skills. This will not only decrease the level of dependency but will also lead to positive effects on the patient's or resident's functional performance level. The increase in the degree of dependency of patients or residents can result in an increase in the demand for caregivers.

CONCEPT OF PATIENT CARE

Patients or residents problem associated with immobility can cause an increase in caregiving activities by nurses, assistants, and technicians. These patients or residents may require more assistance. Patient care skills should be implemented for these patient's or residents. Performing patient care activities can decrease the level of dependency and also slow down other problems that can arise as a result of patients or residents being immobile. Few complications that can arise as a result of immobility of the patients or residents are muscle contractures, osteoporosis, pressure ulcer (bed sores), muscle stiffness, muscle tightness, muscle wasting (atrophy), deep vein thrombosis, and more.

Some of the common causes and risk factors of immobility are as follows:

Musculature, joint, and skeleton problems:-

1. Arthritis
2. Osteoporosis
3. Fractures (especially hip & femur)
4. Podiatric problems

Neurological problems:-

1. Stroke
2. Parkinson's disease
3. Cerebellar dysfunction
4. Neuropathies

Heart, lung, and circulation problems:-

1. Chronic coronary heart disease
2. Chronic obstructive lung disease
3. Severe heart failure
4. Peripheral vascular disease

Cognitive, psychological and sensory problems:-

1. Dementia
2. Depression
3. Fear and anxiety (e.g. fear from instability and falling)
4. Pain
5. Impaired vision

Environmental causes:-

1. Forced immobilization (restraint use)
2. Inadequate aids for mobility

Others

1. General weakness after prolonged bed rest
2. Malnutrition
3. Drug side effects
4. Severe illness of any type

Patient care skills include restoring and maintaining physical functions and helping the resident by achieving the highest level of functional performance. The goal of this should be to focus on what activities can be done by the resident to maximize the level of performance. The performance of different activities under the plan of patient care skills can help residents prevent the complication that could result from immobility and increased dependence. Walking with appropriate assistance can decrease the risk of deep vein thrombosis. Performing range of motion activities can prevent or reduce the possibility of muscle tightness or contractures.

GOAL OF PATIENT CARE FOR RESIDENTS

- Promote required mobility.
- Increase in muscle strength.
- Maintain muscle strength.
- Help prevent contracture and tightness.
- Decrease level of dependence while performing activities.
- Decrease risk factors for decubitus ulcer (bed sores).
- Increase in the sense of satisfaction and self-esteem.
- Increase in skills performance due to increase muscle coordination.
- Improvement in the quality of life
- Improvement in quality of self-care.

PATIENT CARE SKILLS TO BE PERFORMED ON THE RESIDENTS ARE:

1. Range of Motion – Passive
2. Range of Motion – Active
3. Splint or Brace Assistance
4. Bed Mobility
5. Transfer
6. Walking/Ambulation
7. Bladder/Bowel Training
8. Dressing or Grooming
9. Eating or Swallowing
10. Amputation or Prosthesis Care
11. Communication

RANGE OF MOTION EXERCISES (ROM)

1. Passive ROM (PROM)
2. Active ROM (AROM)
3. Active-Assist ROM (AAROM)

For Range of Motion (Passive): The person performing the range of motion moves the patient's joint through the available range of motion.

For Range of Motion (Active): The patient can actively move his or her own joint through the available range of motion.

For Range of Motion (Active Assisted): The patient can actively move his or her own joint through the available range of motion and may require assistance from another person.

SPLINT OR BRACE ASSISTANCE – (2 TYPES):

1. Staff provides verbal and physical guidance and direction that teaches the patient or resident on how to apply, manipulate and care for the brace/splint;

2. Staff has a scheduled program of:
   a) Applying and removing a splint/brace,
   b) Observing the resident's skin for circulation,
   c) Observing the resident's correct position of the body part (limb).

BED MOBILITY

Bed mobility activities are used to improve or maintain the patient's or resident's self-performance in:
-Moving to and from a lying position.
-Turning from supine to side or side to prone.
-Self-positioning in bed.

WALKING/AMBULATION

Walking-activity to improve or maintain self-performance in walking with or without assistive devices.

TRAINING AND SKILLS PRACTICE TRANSFER TRAINING

This activity is used to improve or maintain the patient's or resident's self-performance in moving between surfaces or planes with or without assistive devices.

DRESSING/GROOMING ACTIVITY

Dressing/Grooming activity is used to improve or maintain the patient's or resident's self-performance in:
1. Dressing/undressing
2. Bathing and washing
3. Other personal hygiene tasks:
   - Shaving
   - Brushing hair
   - Brushing teeth
   - Applying makeup

EATING/SWALLOWING ACTIVITY

Eating or swallowing-activity is used to improve or maintain self-performance in:
1. Feeding one's self with food and fluids.
2. Activities used to improve or maintain patient's or resident's ability to ingest nutrition and hydration by mouth.

COMMUNICATION ACTIVITY

Communication activity is used to improve or maintain patient's or resident's self-performance in:

- Self-performance in newly acquired functional communication skills or
- Assisting the patient or resident in using residual communication and adaptive services.

AMPUTATION/PROSTHESIS CARE

Amputation/Prosthesis Care-activity is used to improve or maintain the patient's or resident's self-performance in putting on and removing a prosthesis, caring for the prosthesis, and providing appropriate hygiene at the site where the prosthesis attaches to the body.

REGULATORY COMPLIANCE

42 CFR PART 483, SUBPART B - REQUIREMENTS FOR LONG TERM CARE FACILITIES
Regulations Impact Every Aspect of Nursing Home Care. A decline in resident functioning is not permitted unless they are medically unavoidable. If the resident has a chronic disease or degenerative condition, the facility is expected to slow and delay the deterioration as much as possible.

§ 483.15 Quality of life.

A facility must care for its residents in a manner and in an environment that promote maintenance or enhancement of each resident's quality of life.

(a) Dignity. The facility must promote care for residents in a manner and in an environment that maintain or enhances each resident's dignity and respect in full recognition of his or her individuality.

(b) Self-determination and participation. The resident has the right to—

1) Choose activities, schedules, and health care consistent with his or her interests, assessments, and plans of care;
2) Interact with members of the community both inside and outside the facility; and
3) Make choices about aspects of his or her life in the facility that are significant to the resident.

(c) Participation in resident and family groups.

1) A resident has the right to organize and participate in resident groups in the facility;
2) A resident's family has the right to meet in the facility with the families of other residents in the facility;
3) The facility must provide a resident or family group, if one exists, with private space;
4) Staff or visitors may attend meetings at the group's invitation;

5) The facility must provide a designated staff person responsible for providing assistance and responding to written requests that result from group meetings;
6) When a resident or family group exists, the facility must listen to the views and act upon the grievances and recommendations of residents and families concerning proposed policy and operational decisions affecting resident care and life in the facility.

(d) Participation in other activities. A resident has the right to participate in social, religious, and community activities that do not interfere with the rights of other residents in the facility.

(e) Accommodation of needs. A resident has the right to—

1) Reside and receive services in the facility with reasonable accommodation of individual needs and preferences, except when the health or safety of the individual or other residents would be endangered; and
2) Receive notice before the resident's room or roommate in the facility is changed.

(f) Activities.

1) The facility must provide for an ongoing program of activities designed to meet, in accordance with the comprehensive assessment, the interests and the physical, mental, and psychosocial well-being of each resident.
2) The activities program must be directed by a qualified professional who—

(i) Is a qualified therapeutic recreation specialist or an activities professional who—
   A. Is licensed or registered, if applicable, by the State in which practicing; and
   B. Is eligible for certification as a therapeutic recreation specialist or as activities professional by a recognized accrediting body on or after October 1, 1990; or

(ii) Has 2 years of experience in a social or recreational program within the last 5 years, 1 of which was full-time in a patient activities program in a health care setting; or

(iii) Is a qualified occupational therapist or occupational therapy assistant; or

(iv) Has completed a training course approved by the State.

(g) Social Services.

1) The facility must provide medically-related social services to attain or maintain the highest practicable physical, mental, and psychosocial well-being of each resident.

2) A facility with more than 120 beds must employ a qualified social worker on a full-time basis.

3) Qualifications of a social worker. A qualified social worker is an individual with—

    i.   A bachelor's degree in social work or a bachelor's degree in a human services field including but not limited to sociology, special education, rehabilitation counseling, and psychology; and

    ii.   One year of supervised social work experience in a health care setting working directly with individuals.

(h) Environment. The facility must provide—

1) A safe, clean, comfortable, and homelike environment, allowing the resident to use his or her personal belongings to the extent possible;

2) Housekeeping and maintenance services necessary to maintain a sanitary, orderly, and comfortable interior;

3) Clean bed and bath linens that are in good condition;

4) Private closet space in each resident room, as specified in § 483.70(d)(2)(iv) of this part;

5) Adequate and comfortable lighting levels in all areas;

6) Comfortable and safe temperature levels. Facilities initially certified after October 1, 1990 must maintain a temperature range of 71-81 °F; and

7) For the maintenance of comfortable sound levels.

[56 FR 48871, Sept. 26, 1991, as amended at 57 FR 43924, Sept. 23, 1992]

§ 483.25 Quality of care.

Each resident must receive, and the facility must provide the necessary care and services to attain or maintain the highest practicable physical, mental, and psychosocial well-being, in accordance with the comprehensive assessment and plan of care.

(a) Activities of daily living. Based on the comprehensive assessment of a resident, the facility must ensure that—

A resident's abilities in activities of daily living do not diminish unless circumstances of the individual's clinical condition demonstrate that diminution was unavoidable. This includes the resident's ability to—

- Bathe, dress, and groom;
- Transfer and ambulate;
- Toilet;
- Eat; and
- Use speech, language, or other functional communication systems.

A resident is given the appropriate treatment and services to maintain or improve his or her abilities specified in paragraph (a)(1) of this section; and

A resident who is unable to carry out activities of daily living receives the necessary services to maintain good nutrition, grooming, and personal and oral hygiene.

(b) Vision and hearing. To ensure that residents receive proper treatment and assistive devices to maintain vision and hearing abilities, the facility must, if necessary, assist the resident—

1) In making appointments, and

2) By arranging for transportation to and from the office of a practitioner specializing in the treatment of vision or hearing impairment or the office of a professional specializing in the provision of vision or hearing assistive devices.

(c) Pressure sores. Based on the comprehensive assessment of a resident, the facility must ensure that—

1) A resident who enters the facility without pressure sores does not develop pressure sores unless the individual's clinical condition demonstrates that they were unavoidable; and

2) A resident having pressure sores receives necessary treatment and services to promote healing, prevent infection and prevent new sores from developing.

(d) Urinary Incontinence. Based on the resident's comprehensive assessment, the facility must ensure that—

1) A resident who enters the facility without an indwelling catheter is not catheterized unless the resident's clinical condition demonstrates that catheterization was necessary; and

2) A resident who is incontinent of bladder receives appropriate treatment and services to prevent urinary tract infections and to restore as much normal bladder function as possible.

(e) Range of motion. Based on the comprehensive assessment of a resident, the facility must ensure that—

(1) A resident who enters the facility without a limited range of motion does not experience reduction in range of motion unless the resident's clinical condition demonstrates that a reduction in range of motion is unavoidable; and

(2) A resident with a limited range of motion receives appropriate treatment and services to increase the range of motion and/or to prevent further decrease in range of motion.

(f) Mental and Psychosocial functioning. Based on the comprehensive assessment of a resident, the facility must ensure that—

(1) A resident who displays mental or psychosocial adjustment difficulty, receives appropriate treatment and services to correct the assessed problem, and

(2) A resident whose assessment did not reveal a mental or psychosocial adjustment difficulty does not display a pattern of decreased social interaction and/or increased withdrawn, angry, or depressive behaviors, unless the resident's clinical condition demonstrates that such a pattern was unavoidable.

(g) Naso-gastric tubes. Based on the comprehensive assessment of a resident, the facility must ensure that—

(1) A resident who has been able to eat enough alone or with assistance is not fed by naso-gastric tube unless the resident's clinical condition demonstrates that use of a naso-gastric tube was unavoidable; and

(2) A resident who is fed by a naso-gastric or gastrostomy tube receives the appropriate treatment and services to prevent aspiration pneumonia, diarrhea, vomiting, dehydration, metabolic abnormalities, and nasal-pharyngeal ulcers and to restore, if possible, normal eating skills.

(h) Accidents. The facility must ensure that—

(1) The resident environment remains as free of accident hazards as is possible; and

(2) Each resident receives adequate supervision and assistance devices to prevent accidents.

(i) Nutrition. Based on a resident's comprehensive assessment, the facility must ensure that a resident—

(1) Maintains acceptable parameters of nutritional status, such as body weight and protein levels, unless the resident's clinical condition demonstrates that this is not possible; and

(2) Receives a therapeutic diet when there is a nutritional problem.

(j) Hydration. The facility must provide each resident with sufficient fluid intake to maintain proper hydration and health.

(k) Special needs. The facility must ensure that residents receive proper treatment and care for the following special services:

1) Injections;
2) Parenteral and enteral fluids;
3) Colostomy, ureterostomy, or ileostomy care;
4) Tracheostomy care;
5) Tracheal suctioning;
6) Respiratory care;
7) Foot care; and
8) Prostheses.

(l) Unnecessary drugs—

(1) General. Each resident's drug regimen must be free from unnecessary drugs. An unnecessary drug is any drug when used:

    i. In excessive dose (including duplicate drug therapy); or

    ii. For excessive duration; or

    iii. Without adequate monitoring; or

    iv. Without adequate indications for its use; or

    v. In the presence of adverse consequences which indicate the dose should be reduced or discontinued; or

    vi. Any combinations of the reasons above.

(2) Antipsychotic Drugs. Based on a comprehensive assessment of a resident, the facility must ensure that—

    i. Residents who have not used antipsychotic drugs are not given these drugs unless antipsychotic drug therapy is necessary to treat a specific condition as diagnosed and documented in the clinical record; and

    ii. Residents who use antipsychotic drugs receive gradual dose reductions, and behavioral interventions, unless clinically contraindicated, in an effort to discontinue these drugs.

(m) Medication Errors. The facility must ensure that—

(1) It is free of medication error rates of five percent or greater; and

(2) Residents are free of any significant medication errors.

(n) Influenza and pneumococcal immunizations—

(1) Influenza. The facility must develop policies and procedures that ensure that—

i. Before offering the influenza immunization, each resident or the resident's legal representative receives education regarding the benefits and potential side effects of the immunization;

ii. Each resident is offered an influenza immunization October 1 through March 31 annually, unless the immunization is medically contraindicated or the resident has already been immunized during this time period;

iii. The resident or the resident's legal representative has the opportunity to refuse immunization; and

iv. The resident's medical record includes documentation that indicates, at a minimum, the following:

A. That the resident or resident's legal representative was provided education regarding the benefits and potential side effects of influenza immunization; and

B. That the resident either received the influenza immunization or did not receive the influenza immunization due to medical contraindications or refusal.

(2) Pneumococcal disease. The facility must develop policies and procedures that ensure that—

i. Before offering the pneumococcal immunization, each resident or the resident's legal representative receives education regarding the benefits and potential side effects of the immunization;

ii. Each resident is offered a pneumococcal immunization, unless the immunization is medically contraindicated or the resident has already been immunized;

iii. The resident or the resident's legal representative has the opportunity to refuse immunization; and

iv. The resident's medical record includes documentation that indicates, at a minimum, the following:

A. That the resident or resident's legal representative was provided education regarding the benefits and potential side

effects of pneumococcal immunization; and

B. That the resident either received the pneumococcal immunization or did not receive the pneumococcal immunization due to medical contraindication or refusal.

V. Exception. As an alternative, based on an assessment and practitioner recommendation, a second pneumococcal immunization may be given after 5 years following the first pneumococcal immunization, unless medically contraindicated or the resident or the resident's legal representative refuses the second immunization.

[56 FR 48873, Sept. 26, 1991, as amended at 57 FR 43925, Sept. 23, 1992; 70 FR 58851, Oct. 7, 2005]

TYPES OF HEALTHCARE FACILITIES
LONG-TERM CARE FACILITY

Long term care setting provides a supervised nursing care for 24 hours or more. Another name used for long-term care facilities are Convalescent Care Facility, Skilled Nursing Facility or Extended Care Facilities. These facilities provides general nursing care to those residents who are:

* unable to take care of daily living needs or
* chronically ill or physically challenged.

These facilities also assist residents in performing Activities of Daily Living (ADL), the services are provided to make the resident independent.

HOME HEALTH CARE

* Home Care: provides personal care assistance, also sometimes assist with household activities.
* Home Health Care: provide skilled services for the short term as prescribed.
* Home Maker: assist with more household activities.

ASSISTED LIVING

As the name itself suggest "Assisted Living" is a type of facility in which an individual can get assistance in different areas, like assistance with personal care, laundry, medication, meals etc.

PATIENT CARE TECHNICIAN TEXTBOOK: THEORY & CLINICAL APPROACH

ADULT DAY CENTER OR ADULT DAY CARE

A type of facility that provides care for an individual during the day time, duties may range from personal care assistance to skilled care (therapeutic services). These facilities provide supervision during day time and giving the caregiver or family the time to work, take rest or some other activities while the individual is in the adult day care.

WHAT ARE THE VARYING LEVELS OF CARE?

ACUTE (HOSPITAL) CARE

A type of care usually short-term in nature, and provided at a hospital (inpatient or outpatient) or doctor's office or short term facility. The primary goal of acute care is to provide recovery by bringing the individual back to their normal health status.

SUB-ACUTE CARE

A type of care provided to individuals who need post-acute care. Sub-acute care much concentrated as compared to the traditional nursing facility care (long-term care facilities) and less concentrated than acute care.

HOSPICE CARE

A type of care provided to terminally ill individuals with a life expectancy of six months or less. Hospice care focuses mainly towards the spiritual, mental, emotional and physical comfort of the patients. It also provides support for families of the terminally ill individual.

PALLIATIVE CARE

A type of care that provides specialized medical care for individuals with symptoms, discomfort and stress of serious illness. The focus is to provide relief of symptoms, discomfort, and stress of a serious illness. The goal is to improve the quality of life for the patient and family.

REHABILITATION CARE

A type of care provided to restore the function of the individual using specialized skills like physical therapy, occupational therapy, respiratory therapy, speech therapy, etc.

Professions in Therapeutic Services will be discussed in **section 8 topic 19.**

Centers for Medicare and Medicaid Services (CMS)

The Centers for Medicare and Medicaid Services (CMS), a component of the Department of Health and Human Services (HHS), administers Medicare and Medicaid.

What is Medicare?

A health insurance plan for individuals who are 65 or older. This insurance plan is also provided to a younger individual with disabilities and end-stage renal disease.

Medicare has 4 parts:

PART A (covers inpatient services)

PART B (covers outpatient services)

PART C (covers advantage plan)

PART D (covers prescription drugs)

What is Medicaid?

A health insurance plan for low income individuals and special circumstances (for example pregnant women). Eligibility is categorical.

References:

- Center for Medicare & Medicare
- 42 C.F.R. Title 42: Public Health: PART 483—REQUIREMENTS FOR STATES AND LONG TERM CARE FACILITIES §483.15 Quality of life & §483.25 Quality of care.

CHAPTER 1
END OF CHAPTER REVIEW QUESTIONS

CRITICAL THINKING

5 POINTS EACH QUESTION
50 POINTS TOTAL

1. Explain about the functional performance of an individual?

2. List common causes and risk factors of immobility.

3. What are the goals of patient care?

4. Explain in brief; the patient care approach?

5. List and explain any 3 patient care skills performed on patients or residents.

6. What are the types of range of motion exercises?

7. Explain quality of life as per the regulatory compliance?

8. Explain quality of care as per the regulatory compliance?

9. Explain the types of healthcare facilities.

10. Explain the varying levels of care.

SECTION 1

CHAPTER 2: INFECTION CONTROL & STANDARD PRECAUTIONS

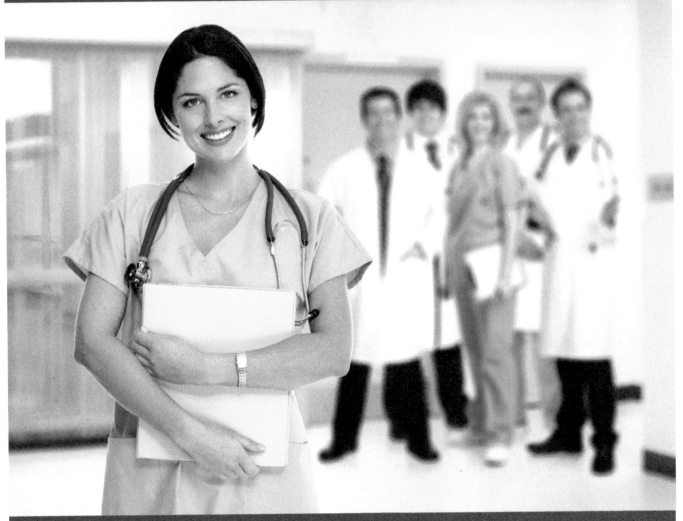

LEARNING OBJECTIVES

At the end of this chapter the student will be able to describe:

- Occupational Safety and Health Administration (OSHA)
- What type of hazards do healthcare workers face?
- Healthcare safety hazards
- Latex allergy and prevention
- Chain of infection
- Mode of transmission
- Identifying infectious patients
- Breaking the chain of infection
- Hand hygiene
- Personal protective equipment
- Standard precautions
- What are blood borne pathogens?

OCCUPATIONAL SAFETY AND HEALTH ADMINISTRATION (OSHA)

The Occupational Safety and Health Act (OSH Act) allows Occupational Safety and Health Administration (OSHA) to issue workplace health and safety regulations. These regulations include limits on chemical exposure, employee access to information, requirements for the use of personal protective equipment, and requirements for safety procedures.

OSHA's mission is to "assure safe and healthful working conditions for working men and women by setting and enforcing standards and by providing training, outreach, education, and assistance".

WHAT TYPES OF HAZARDS DO WORKERS FACE?

Healthcare workers face a number of serious safety and health hazards. This includes bloodborne pathogens, biological hazards, potential chemicals, drug exposures, waste anesthetic gas exposures, respiratory hazards, ergonomic hazards from lifting and repetitive tasks, laser hazards, workplace violence, hazards associated with laboratories, radioactive material, and x-ray hazards. Some of the potential chemical exposures include formaldehyde (used for preservation of specimens for pathology) ethylene oxide, glutaraldehyde, peracetic acid (used for sterilization) and numerous other chemicals used in healthcare laboratories.

HEALTHCARE SAFETY HAZARDS

- Biological Hazards
- Physical Hazards
- Sharps Hazard
- Chemical Hazards
- Electrical Hazards
- Fire or Explosive Hazards

PROCEDURE TO FOLLOW POST-EXPOSURE TO BLOOD

- Wash the area with water or antiseptic.
- Report to the employer.
- Document the injury.
- The employer must provide medical evaluation and follow-up.

LATEX

Latex Allergy: is a medical term used for a range of allergic reactions to the proteins present in natural rubber latex. Latex allergy generally develops after repeated exposure to the products containing natural rubber latex. When latex-containing medical devices or supplies come in contact with mucous membranes, the mucous membranes may absorb latex proteins. The immune system of some susceptible individuals produces antibodies that react immunologically with latex antigenic proteins.

Latex Sensitivity: Natural rubber latex can also cause irritant contact dermatitis, this is a less severe form of reaction that does not involve the immune system. Contact dermatitis may cause dry, itchy, irritated areas on the skin, most commonly on the hands. Latex-gloves induced dermatitis increases the chance of hospital-acquired infections (nosocomial infection).

Irritant Contact Dermatitis	Allergic Contact Dermatitis	Hypersensitivity
Reactions	Reactions	Reactions
Red, dry, itchy irritated areas	Itchy, red rash, small blisters	Hives, swelling, runny nose, nausea, abdominal cramps, dizziness, low blood pressure, bronchospasm, anaphylaxis (shock)

Table 2.1

WHAT IS CONTACT DERMATITIS?

Occupationally related contact dermatitis can develop from frequent and repeated use of hand hygiene products, exposure to chemicals and glove use. Contact dermatitis is classified as either irritant or allergic. Irritant contact dermatitis is common, nonallergic and develops as a dry, itchy, irritated areas on the skin around the area of contact. By comparison, allergic contact dermatitis (type IV hypersensitivity) can result from exposure to accelerators and other chemicals used in the manufacture of rubber gloves as well as from exposure to other chemicals found in a practice setting. Allergic contact dermatitis often manifests as a rash beginning hours after contact and, like irritant dermatitis, is usually confined to the areas of contact.

WHAT IS LATEX ALLERGY?

Latex allergy (type I hypersensitivity to latex proteins) can be a more serious systemic allergic reaction. It usually begins within minutes of exposure but can sometimes occur hours later. It produces varied symptoms, which commonly include a runny nose, sneezing, itchy eyes, scratchy throat, hives, and itchy burning sensations. However, it can involve more severe symptoms including asthma marked by breathing difficulty, coughing spells and wheezing; cardiovascular and gastrointestinal ailments; and in rare cases, anaphylaxis and death.

RECOMMENDED POWDER-FREE GLOVES

When powdered gloves are worn, more latex protein reaches the skin. When gloves are put on or removed, particles of latex protein powder become aerosolized and can be inhaled, contacting mucous membranes. As a result, allergic health care personnel and patients can experience symptoms related to cutaneous, respiratory, and conjunctival exposure. Dental health care personnel can become sensitized to latex proteins after repeated exposure. Work areas where only powder-free, low-allergen (i.e. reduced-protein) gloves are used show low or undetectable amounts of allergies of such type.

PREVENTING LATEX REACTIONS

- Screen all patients for latex allergy.
- Be aware of some common predisposing conditions (e.g., spina bifida, urogenital anomalies or allergies to avocados, kiwis, nuts or bananas).
- Be familiar with different types of hypersensitivity (immediate and delayed) and the risks that these pose to patients and staff.
- Patients with a history of latex allergy may be at risk.
- Provide an alternative treatment area free of materials containing latex.
- Ensure a latex-safe environment or one in which no personnel use latex gloves and no patient contact occurs with other latex devices, materials and products. Remove all latex-containing products from the patient's vicinity.

- Adequately cover/isolate any latex-containing devices that cannot be removed from the treatment environment.
- Be aware that latent allergens in the ambient air can cause respiratory and or anaphylactic symptoms in people with latex hypersensitivity.
- Frequently change ventilation filters and vacuum bags used in latex-contaminated areas.
- Be aware that allergic reaction can be provoked from indirect contact as well as direct contact. Hand hygiene, is, therefore, an essential component.
- If latex-related complications occur during or after the procedure, manage the reaction and seek emergency assistance as indicated. Follow current medical emergency response recommendations for management of anaphylaxis.

INFECTION CONTROL

- Infection control addresses factors related to the spread of infection within the health-care setting (whether patient-to-patient, from patients to staff, from staff to patients or among staff members).
- Including prevention (via hand hygiene/hand washing, cleaning/disinfection/sterilization/vaccination and surveillance).
- Monitoring/investigation of demonstrated or suspected spread of infection within a particular health-care setting (surveillance and outbreak investigation) and management (interruption of outbreaks).

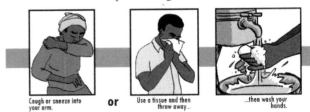

Protect Others. Protect Yourself.

Cover your cough or sneeze.

Cough or sneeze into your arm. **or** Use a tissue and then throw away... ...then wash your hands.

Stop the spread of TB, colds, and influenza.

CHAIN OF INFECTION

A process that begins when an agent leaves its reservoir or host through a portal of exit, than is conveyed by some mode of transmission and enters through an appropriate portal of entry to infect a susceptible host.

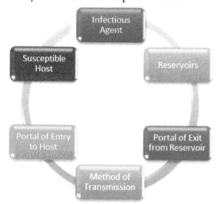

Chain of Infection Illustration 2.1

MODES OF TRANSMISSION

An infectious agent may be transmitted from its natural reservoir to a susceptible host directly or indirectly.

DIRECT

Direct contact occurs through skin-to-skin contact, kissing and sexual intercourse. Direct contact also refers to contact with soil or vegetation harboring infectious organisms. Thus, infectious mononucleosis ("kissing disease") and gonorrhea are spread from person to person by direct contact. Hookworm is spread by direct contact with contaminated soil.

Droplet spread refers to spray with relatively large, short-range aerosols produced by sneezing, coughing or even talking. Droplet spread is classified as direct because transmission is by direct spray over a few feet before the droplets fall to the ground. Pertussis and meningococcal infection are examples of diseases transmitted from an infectious patient to a susceptible host by droplet spread.

INDIRECT

Airborne transmission occurs when infectious agents are carried by dust or droplet nuclei suspended in the air. Airborne dust includes material that has settled on surfaces and become re-suspended by air currents as well as infectious particles wind-blown from the soil. Droplet nuclei are dried residue of fewer than 5 microns in size. In contrast to droplets that fall to the ground within a few feet, droplet nuclei may remain suspended in the air for long periods of time and may be blown over great distances.

Vehicles that may indirectly transmit an infectious agent include food, water, biologic products (blood) and fomites (inanimate objects such as handkerchiefs, bedding or surgical scalpels).

A vehicle may passively carry a pathogen, as food or water may carry hepatitis A virus. Alternatively, the vehicle may provide an environment in which the agent grows, multiplies or produces toxin

Vectors such as mosquitoes, flies, and ticks may carry an infectious agent through purely mechanical means or may support growth or changes in the agent. Examples of mechanical transmission are flies carrying Shigella on their appendages and flies carrying Yersinia pestis, the causative agent of plague. In contrast to biologic transmission, the causative agent of malaria or guinea worm disease undergoes maturation in an intermediate host before it can be transmitted to humans.

IDENTIFYING POTENTIALLY INFECTIOUS PATIENTS

- Facility staff shall remain alert for any patient arriving with symptoms of an active infection (e.g., diarrhea, rash, respiratory symptoms, draining wounds or skin lesions).
- If the patient calls ahead:
  - If possible have patients with symptoms of active infection come at a time when the facility is less crowded.
  - Alert registration staff ahead of time to place the patient in a private exam room upon arrival if available and follow the procedures pertinent to the route of transmission as specified by the facility.
  - If the purpose of the visit is non-urgent, patients are encouraged to reschedule the appointment until symptoms have resolved.

CONTACT PRECAUTIONS

- Applies to patients with any of the following conditions and/or diseases:
  - The presence of stool incontinence (may include patients with norovirus, rotavirus or clostridium

difficile), draining wounds, uncontrolled secretions, pressure ulcers, or presence of ostomy tubes and/or bags of draining body fluids.
- Presence of generalized rash or exanthems (rash).
- Prioritize having the patient in an exam room if they have stool incontinence, uncontrolled secretions, draining wounds and/or skin lesions that cannot be covered.
- Perform hand hygiene prior to wearing gloves and before touching the patient.
- Personal Protective Equipment (PPE) use:
    - Wear gloves when touching the patient and the patient's immediate environment or belongings.
    - Wear a gown if substantial contact with the patient is anticipated.
- Perform hand hygiene after removal of PPE, use soap and water when hands are visibly soiled (e.g., blood, body fluids), or after caring for patients with known or suspected infectious diarrhea (e.g., Clostridium difficile, norovirus).
- Clean and disinfect the exam room accordingly.
- Instruct patients with known or suspected infectious diarrhea to use a separate bathroom, if possible clean and disinfect the bathroom before it can be used again.

DROPLET PRECAUTIONS

- Applies to patients known or suspected to be infected with a pathogen that can be transmitted by droplet route, these includes but are not limited to:
    - Respiratory viruses (influenza, parainfluenza virus, adenovirus, respiratory syncytial virus, and human metapneumovirus).
    - Bordetella pertussis.
    - For the first 24 hours of therapy (Neisseria meningitides, group A streptococcus), Place the patient in an exam room (with door closed) as soon as possible (prioritize patients who have excessive cough and sputum production); if an exam room is not available, the patient is provided a facemask and placed in a separate area as far from other patients as possible while awaiting care.
- Personal Protective Equipment's (PPE) use:

- Wear a facemask, such as a procedure or surgical mask, for close contact with the patient; the facemask should be donned upon entering the exam room.
- If substantial spraying of respiratory fluids is anticipated: gloves, gown and goggles (or a face shield in place of goggles) should be worn.
- Perform hand hygiene before and after touching the patient and after contact with respiratory secretions and/or contaminated objects/materials. Note: use soap and water when hands are visibly soiled (e.g. with blood and body fluids).
- Instruct patient to wear a facemask when exiting the exam room; avoid coming into close contact with other patients and practice respiratory hygiene and cough etiquette.
- Clean and disinfect the exam room accordingly.

AIRBORNE PRECAUTIONS

- Applies to patients known or suspected to be infected with a pathogen that can be transmitted by airborne route; these include, but are not limited to:
    - Tuberculosis
    - Measles
    - Chickenpox (until lesions are crusted over)
    - Localized (in immunocompromised patient) or disseminated herpes zoster (until lesions are crusted over)
- Have patient enter through a separate entrance to the facility (e.g. dedicated isolation entrance). If possible, avoid the reception and registration area.
- Place the patient immediately in an **airborne infection isolation room** (AIIR).
- If an AIIR is not available:
    - Provide a facemask (e.g. procedure or surgical mask) to the patient and place the patient immediately in an exam room with the door closed.
    - Instruct the patient to keep the facemask on while in the exam room. Change the mask if it becomes wet.
    - Initiate protocol to transfer patient to a healthcare facility that has the recommended infection-control capacity to manage the patient properly.

- PPE use:
  - Wear a fit-tested N-95 or higher-level disposable respirator. If available, don the respirator before entering the room and remove after exiting room.
  - If substantial spraying of respiratory fluids is anticipated: gloves, gown, and goggles (or a face shield in place of goggles) should be worn.
- Perform hand hygiene before and after touching the patient and after contact with respiratory secretions and/or body fluids and contaminated objects/materials. Use soap and water when hands are visibly soiled (e.g., blood, body fluids).
- Instruct patient to wear a facemask when exiting the exam room, avoid coming into close contact with other patients, and practice respiratory hygiene and cough etiquette.
  - Once the patient leaves, the exam room should remain vacant for generally one hour before anyone enters. However, the adequate wait time may vary depending on the ventilation rate of the room and should be determined accordingly.
- If staff must enter the room during the wait time, they are required to use respiratory protection.

Respiratory Hygiene and Cough Etiquette

To prevent the transmission of respiratory infections in the facility, the following infection prevention measures are implemented for all potentially infected persons at the point of entry and continuing throughout the duration of the visit. This applies to any individual (e.g., patients and accompanying family members, caregivers, and visitors) with signs and symptoms of respiratory illness, including cough, congestion, rhinorrhea, or increased production of respiratory secretions.

1. Identifying Persons with Potential Respiratory Infection

- Facility staff remains alert for any persons arriving with symptoms of a respiratory infection.
- Signs are posted at the reception area instructing patients and accompanying persons to:
- Self-report symptoms of a respiratory infection during registration.

- Practice respiratory hygiene and cough etiquette (a technique described below) and wear facemask as needed.

2. Availability of Supplies:

The following supplies are provided in the reception area and other common waiting areas:

- Facemasks, tissues, and no-touch waste receptacles for disposing of used tissues.
- Dispensers of alcohol-based hand rub.

3. Respiratory Hygiene and Cough Etiquette:

All persons with signs and symptoms of a respiratory infection (including facility staff) are instructed to:

- Cover the mouth and nose with a tissue when coughing or sneezing.
- Dispose of the used tissue in the nearest waste receptacle.
- Perform hand hygiene after contact with respiratory secretions and contaminated objects/materials.

4. Masking and Separation of Persons with Respiratory Symptoms

If patient calls ahead:

- Have patients with symptoms of a respiratory infection come at a time when the facility is less crowded or through a separate entrance, if available.
- If the purpose of the visit is non-urgent, patients are encouraged to reschedule the appointment until symptoms have resolved.
- Upon entry to the facility, patients are to be instructed to don a facemask (e.g., procedure or surgical mask).
- Alert registration staff ahead of time to place the patient in an exam room with a closed door upon arrival.

If identified after arrival:

- Provide facemasks to all persons (including persons accompanying patients) who are coughing and have symptoms of a respiratory infection.
- Place the coughing patient in an exam room with a closed door as soon as possible (if suspicious for airborne transmission, refer to Airborne Precautions, if an exam room is not available, the

patient should sit as far from other patients as possible in the waiting room.

- Accompanying persons who have symptoms of a respiratory infection should not enter patient-care areas and are encouraged to wait outside the facility.

5. Healthcare Personnel Responsibilities

- Healthcare personnel observe Droplet Precautions, in addition to Standard Precautions, when examining and caring for patients with signs and symptoms of a respiratory infection (if suspicious for an infectious agent spread by airborne route, refer to Airborne Precautions.
- These precautions are maintained until it is determined that the cause of the symptoms is not an infectious agent that requires Droplet or Airborne Precautions.
- All healthcare personnel are aware of facility sick leave policies, including staff who are not directly employed by the facility but provide essential daily services.
- Healthcare personnel with a respiratory infection avoid direct patient contact; if this is not possible, then a facemask should be worn while providing patient care and frequent hand hygiene should be reinforced.
- Healthcare personnel are up-to-date with all recommended vaccinations, including annual influenza vaccine.

BREAKING THE CHAIN OF INFECTION

    a. Using effective hand hygiene.
    b. Using personal protective equipment (PPE).
    c. Isolating patients with infectious diseases.
    d. Follow standard precautions.

HAND HYGIENE

- Clean hands are the single most important factor in preventing the spread of pathogens in healthcare settings.
- Hand hygiene reduces the incidence of healthcare-associated infections.
- Centers for Disease Control and Prevention (CDC) estimates that each year nearly 2 million patients in the United States get infected in hospitals, and about 90,000 of these patients die as a result of their infection.

- Widespread use of hand hygiene products that improve adherence to recommended hand hygiene practices will promote patient safety and prevent infections.
- There is substantial evidence that hand hygiene reduces the incidence of infections.
- In more recent studies healthcare-associated infection rates were lower when antiseptic hand washing was performed by personnel and went down when adherence to recommended hand hygiene practices improved.
- Healthcare workers have reported several factors that may negatively impact their adherence to recommended practices including:

    a. Hand washing agents cause irritation and dryness.
    b. Inconvenient sink location.
    c. Lack of soap and paper towels.
    d. Lack of time to perform hand hygiene.
    e. Understaffing or overcrowding.

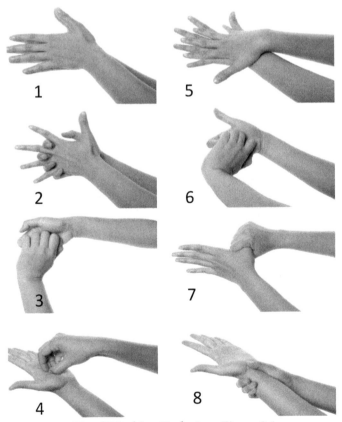

Hand Washing Technique Figure 2.1

- Lack of knowledge of guidelines/protocols, forgetfulness, and disagreement with the recommendations are also self-reported factors for poor adherence with hand hygiene.
- Hand hygiene is a general term that applies to either handwashing, antiseptic handwash, alcohol-based handrub, or surgical hand hygiene/antisepsis.
- Hand washing refers to washing hands with plain soap and water. Hand washing with soap and water remains a sensible strategy for hand hygiene in non-healthcare settings and is recommended by CDC and other experts.
  a. Antiseptic handwash refers to washing hands with water and soap or other detergents containing an antiseptic agent.
  b. Alcohol-based handrub refers to the alcohol-containing preparation applied to the hands to reduce the number of viable microorganisms.
  c. Surgical hand hygiene/antisepsis refers to an antiseptic handwash or antiseptic handrub performed preoperatively by surgical personnel to eliminate transient and reduce resident hand flora. Antiseptic detergent preparations often have persistent antimicrobial activity.
  d. Healthcare workers should wash hands with soap and water when hands are visibly dirty, contaminated or soiled. Use an alcohol-based hand-rub when hands are not visibly soiled to reduce bacterial counts.

HAND HYGIENE: BEFORE & AFTER

- Inserting urinary catheters, peripheral vascular catheters or other invasive devices that do not require surgery.
- Before and after direct patient contact.
- After completing tasks at one patient's station before moving to another station.
- Before procedures, such as administering intravenous medications.
- Before and after contact with vascular access.
- Before and after dressing changes.
- After contact with items/surfaces at patient stations.
- Contact with a patient's skin.

- Contact with body fluids or excretions, non-intact skin and wound dressings.
- Removing gloves.

PRODUCTS USED FOR HAND HYGIENE

- Plain soap is appropriate at reducing bacterial counts, but antimicrobial soap is better and alcohol-based handrubs are the most recommended.
- Alcohol-based handrubs are less damaging to the skin than soap and water.
- The skin's water content decreases for those that use soap and water (resulting in dryer skin) as compared with those who use an alcohol-based handrub.
- Rapid access to hand hygiene materials could help improve adherence.
- Alcohol-based handrubs may be a better option than traditional hand washing with plain soap and water or antiseptic handwash because they require less time, act faster, and irritate hands less often.

HANDRUBS

- Apply to the palm of one hand, rub hands together covering all surfaces until dry.
- Application volume: based on instructions provided by the manufacturer.

HANDWASHING

- Wet hands with water, apply soap, rub hands together for at least 15 seconds.
- Rinse and dry with a disposable towel.
- Use towel to turn off faucet.
- When an antimicrobial soap is used, the hands and forearms should be scrubbed for the length of time recommended by the product's manufacturer, usually 2-6 minutes. Longer scrub times (e.g. 10 minutes) are usually not necessary.
- When an alcohol-based handrub with persistent activity is used, follow the manufacturer's instructions on the amount of product to use. Pre-wash hands and forearms with a non-antimicrobial soap and allow them to dry completely. After application of the alcohol-based product as recommended, allow hands

and forearms to dry thoroughly before donning sterile gloves.

FINGERNAILS AND ARTIFICIAL NAILS

- Natural nail tips should be kept to ¼ inch in length.
- Artificial nails should not be worn when having direct contact with high-risk patients.

PERSONAL PROTECTIVE EQUIPMENT (PPE)

- "Specialized clothing or equipment worn by an employee for protection against infectious materials" (OSHA)
- OSHA issues workplace health and safety regulations. Regarding PPE, employers must:
  - Provide appropriate PPE for employees.
  - Ensure that PPE is disposed or if reusable, that PPE is cleaned, laundered, repaired and stored after use.
- OSHA also specifies circumstances for which PPE is indicated.
- CDC recommends when, what and how to use PPE.

TYPES & FUNCTIONS OF PPE

Types	Functions
Gloves	protect hands
Gowns/Aprons	protect skin and/or clothing
Masks	protect mouth/nose
Respirators	protect respiratory tract from airborne infectious agents
Goggles	protect eyes
Face shields	protect face, mouth, nose, and eyes

Types & Functions of PPE Table 2.2

SELECTING PPE

When you are selecting PPE, consider the following:

- Type of procedure to be performed.
- Amount of exposure.
- Durability and appropriateness of the PPE for the task.
- Fit (appropriate size).

GLOVES

- Wearing gloves reduces the risk of healthcare workers acquiring infections from patients, prevents flora from being transmitted from healthcare workers to patients, and reduces contamination of the hands of healthcare workers by flora that can be transmitted from one patient to another.
- Gloves should be used when Healthcare Workers (**HCWs**) have contact with blood or other body fluids.
- Gloves should be removed after caring for a patient.
- The same pair of gloves should not be worn for the care of more than one patient.
- Gloves should not be washed or reused.
- Following application of alcohol-based handrubs, hands should be rubbed together until all the alcohol has evaporated. In other words, "**Let It Dry**".
- Alcohol-based handrubs should be stored away from high temperatures or flames in accordance with the National Fire Protection Agency recommendations.

ALCOHOL-BASED RUBS

What benefits do they provide?

a. Requires less time.
b. Is more effective than standard handwashing with soap.
c. More accessible than sinks.
d. Reduces bacterial counts on hands.
e. Improves skin condition.

INSTRUCTION ON GLOVES

Most patient care activities require the use of a single pair of nonsterile gloves made of either latex, nitrile, or vinyl. However, because of allergy concerns, some facilities have eliminated or limited latex products, including gloves, and now use gloves made of nitrile or other material. Vinyl gloves are also frequently available and work well if there is limited patient contact. However, some gloves do not provide a proper fit on the hand, especially around the wrist, and therefore should not be used if extensive contact is likely to take place during patient care.

Gloves should fit the user's hands comfortably. They should not be too loose or too tight. They should not tear or damage easily. Gloves are sometimes worn for several hours and need to stand up to the task.

Type of gloves:

- ✓ **Glove material**: Vinyl, latex, nitrile or others.
- ✓ **Sterile or nonsterile**: Sterile surgical gloves are worn by surgeons and other healthcare personnel who perform invasive patient procedures. During some surgical procedures, two pairs of gloves may be worn, whereas the nonsterile gloves are worn for patient care activities as recommended.

DO'S AND DON'TS OF GLOVE USE.

1. Work from clean to dirty. This is a basic principle of infection control. In this instance, it refers to touching clean body sites or surfaces before touching the heavily contaminated areas.
2. Limit opportunities for "touch contamination" - protect yourself, others and environmental surfaces. Avoid touching any surfaces with gloves once the gloves have been in contact with a patient as this could result in a touch contamination. Surfaces, such as light switches, door and cabinet knobs can become contaminated if touched by soiled gloves.
3. Change gloves as needed. If gloves become torn or heavily soiled and additional patient care tasks must be performed, change the gloves before starting the next task. Always change gloves after use on each patient, and discard them in the nearest appropriate waste container. Patient care gloves should never be washed and used again. Washing gloves do not necessarily make them safe for reuse. It may not be possible to eliminate all microorganisms and washing can make the gloves more prone to tearing or leaking.

GOWNS OR APRONS

3 factors influence the selection of a gown or apron as PPE.

First is the purpose of use. Isolation gowns are generally the preferred PPE for clothing, but aprons occasionally are used where limited contamination is anticipated. If contamination of the arms can be anticipated, a gown should be selected. Gowns should fully cover the torso, fit comfortably over the body, and have long sleeves that fit snuggly at the wrist.

Second are the material properties of the gown. Isolation gowns are made either of cotton or a spun synthetic material that dictates whether they can be laundered and reused or disposed. If fluid penetration is likely, a fluid-resistant gown should be used.

The last factor is concerned with patient risks. Clean gowns are generally used for isolation. Sterile gowns are only necessary for performing invasive procedures, such as inserting a central line. In this case, a sterile gown would serve purposes of patient and healthcare worker protection.

PPE FOR FACE

1. Masks – protect nose and mouth

   Masks should fully cover the nose and mouth and prevent fluid penetration. Masks should fit snuggly over the nose and mouth. For this reason, masks that have a flexible nose piece and can be secured to the head with string ties or elastic are preferable.

2. Goggles – protect eyes

   Goggles provide barrier and protection for the eyes. Personal prescription lenses do not provide optimal eye protection and should not be used as a substitute for goggles.

3. Face shield – protect face

   Use face shield when skin protection, in addition to mouth, nose, and eye protection is needed. For example, when irrigating a wound or suctioning copious secretions, a face shield can be used as a substitute to wearing a mask or goggles. The face shield should cover the forehead, extend below the chin, and wrap around the side of the face.

PPE DONNING ORDER

1. Gown first
2. Mask or respirator
3. Goggles or face shield
4. Gloves

USING PPE:-

1. Keep gloved hands away from the face.
2. Avoid touching or adjusting other PPE.
3. Remove gloves if they become torn; perform hand hygiene before donning new gloves.
4. Limit surfaces and items touched.

SEQUENCE FOR PUTTING ON PERSONAL PROTECTIVE EQUIPMENT (PPE)

The type of PPE used will vary based on the level of precautions required, such as standard and contact, droplet or airborne infection isolation precautions. The procedure for putting on and removing PPE should be tailored to the specific type of PPE.

1. GOWN

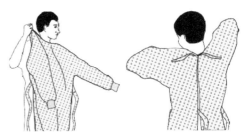

- Fully cover torso from neck to knees, arms to end of wrists, and wrap around the back
- Fasten in back of neck and waist

2. MASK OR RESPIRATOR

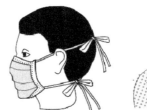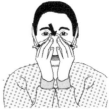

- Secure ties or elastic bands at middle of head and neck
- Fit flexible band to nose bridge
- Fit snug to face and below chin
- Fit-check respirator

3. GOGGLES OR FACE SHIELD

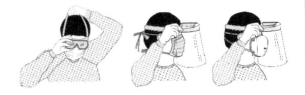

- Place over face and eyes and adjust to fit

4. GLOVES

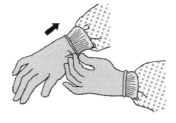

- Extend to cover wrist of isolation gown

USE SAFE WORK PRACTICES TO PROTECT YOURSELF AND LIMIT THE SPREAD OF CONTAMINATION

- Keep hands away from face
- Limit surfaces touched
- Change gloves when torn or heavily contaminated
- Perform hand hygiene

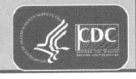

Reference: Centers for Disease Control and Prevention

HOW TO SAFELY REMOVE PERSONAL PROTECTIVE EQUIPMENT (PPE) EXAMPLE 1

There are a variety of ways to safely remove PPE without contaminating your clothing, skin, or mucous membranes with potentially infectious materials. Here is one example. **Remove all PPE before exiting the patient room** except a respirator, if worn. Remove the respirator **after** leaving the patient room and closing the door. Remove PPE in the following sequence:

1. GLOVES

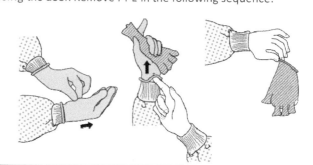

- Outside of gloves are contaminated!
- If your hands get contaminated during glove removal, immediately wash your hands or use an alcohol-based hand sanitizer
- Using a gloved hand, grasp the palm area of the other gloved hand and peel off first glove
- Hold removed glove in gloved hand
- Slide fingers of ungloved hand under remaining glove at wrist and peel off second glove over first glove
- Discard gloves in a waste container

2. GOGGLES OR FACE SHIELD

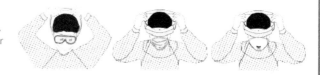

- Outside of goggles or face shield are contaminated!
- If your hands get contaminated during goggle or face shield removal, immediately wash your hands or use an alcohol-based hand sanitizer
- Remove goggles or face shield from the back by lifting head band or ear pieces
- If the item is reusable, place in designated receptacle for reprocessing. Otherwise, discard in a waste container

3. GOWN

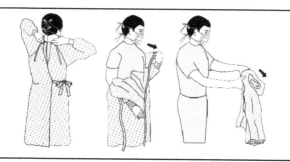

- Gown front and sleeves are contaminated!
- If your hands get contaminated during gown removal, immediately wash your hands or use an alcohol-based hand sanitizer
- Unfasten gown ties, taking care that sleeves don't contact your body when reaching for ties
- Pull gown away from neck and shoulders, touching inside of gown only
- Turn gown inside out
- Fold or roll into a bundle and discard in a waste container

4. MASK OR RESPIRATOR

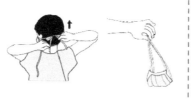
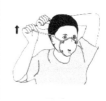

- Front of mask/respirator is contaminated — DO NOT TOUCH!
- If your hands get contaminated during mask/respirator removal, immediately wash your hands or use an alcohol-based hand sanitizer
- Grasp bottom ties or elastics of the mask/respirator, then the ones at the top, and remove without touching the front
- Discard in a waste container

5. WASH HANDS OR USE AN ALCOHOL-BASED HAND SANITIZER IMMEDIATELY AFTER REMOVING ALL PPE

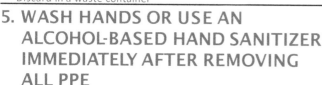
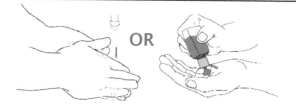

PERFORM HAND HYGIENE BETWEEN STEPS IF HANDS BECOME CONTAMINATED AND IMMEDIATELY AFTER REMOVING ALL PPE

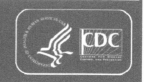

Reference: Centers for Disease Control and Prevention

CS250672-E

HOW TO SAFELY REMOVE PERSONAL PROTECTIVE EQUIPMENT (PPE) EXAMPLE 2

Here is another way to safely remove PPE without contaminating your clothing, skin, or mucous membranes with potentially infectious materials. **Remove all PPE before exiting the patient room** except a respirator, if worn. Remove the respirator **after** leaving the patient room and closing the door. Remove PPE in the following sequence:

1. GOWN AND GLOVES

- Gown front and sleeves and the outside of gloves are contaminated!
- If your hands get contaminated during gown or glove removal, immediately wash your hands or use an alcohol-based hand sanitizer
- Grasp the gown in the front and pull away from your body so that the ties break, touching outside of gown only with gloved hands
- While removing the gown, fold or roll the gown inside-out into a bundle
- As you are removing the gown, peel off your gloves at the same time, only touching the inside of the gloves and gown with your bare hands. Place the gown and gloves into a waste container

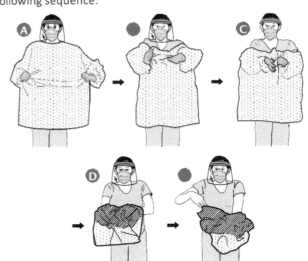

2. GOGGLES OR FACE SHIELD

- Outside of goggles or face shield are contaminated!
- If your hands get contaminated during goggle or face shield removal, immediately wash your hands or use an alcohol-based hand sanitizer
- Remove goggles or face shield from the back by lifting head band and without touching the front of the goggles or face shield
- If the item is reusable, place in designated receptacle for reprocessing. Otherwise, discard in a waste container

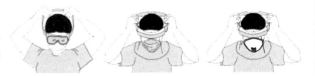

3. MASK OR RESPIRATOR

- Front of mask/respirator is contaminated — DO NOT TOUCH!
- If your hands get contaminated during mask/respirator removal, immediately wash your hands or use an alcohol-based hand sanitizer
- Grasp bottom ties or elastics of the mask/respirator, then the ones at the top, and remove without touching the front
- Discard in a waste container

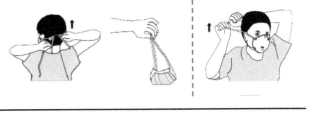

4. WASH HANDS OR USE AN ALCOHOL-BASED HAND SANITIZER IMMEDIATELY AFTER REMOVING ALL PPE

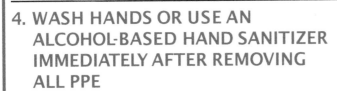

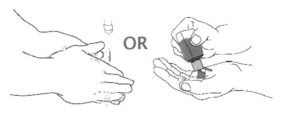

OR

PERFORM HAND HYGIENE BETWEEN STEPS IF HANDS BECOME CONTAMINATED AND IMMEDIATELY AFTER REMOVING ALL PPE

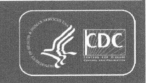

Reference: Centers for Disease Control and Prevention

CS250672-E

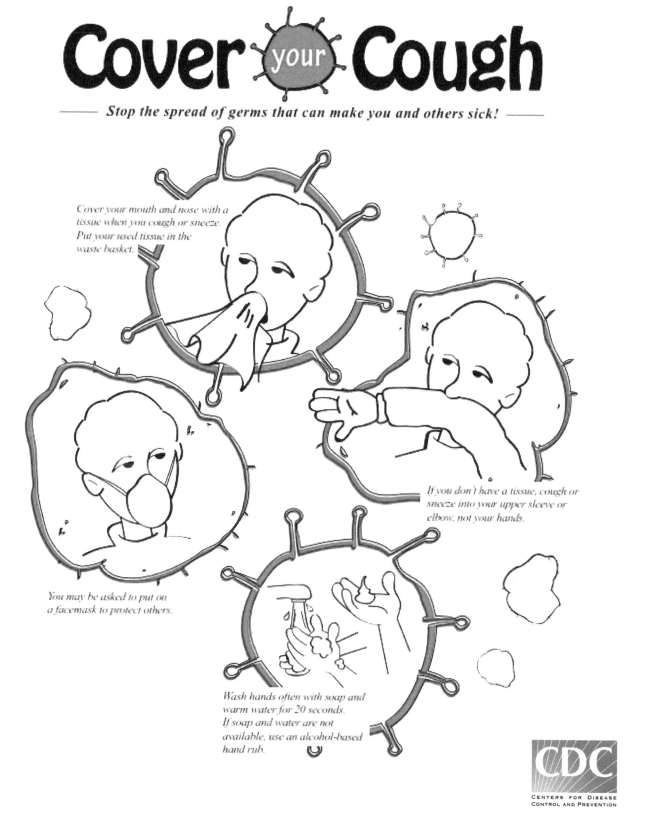

Reference: Centers for Disease Control and Prevention

AIRBORNE PRECAUTIONS

2007 Guideline for Isolation Precautions: Preventing Transmission of Infectious Agents in Healthcare Settings

V.D.	**Airborne Precautions**
V.D.1.	Use Airborne Precautions as recommended in Appendix A for patients known or suspected to be infected with infectious agents transmitted person-to-person by the airborne route (e.g., M tuberculosis, measles, chickenpox, disseminated herpes zoster.
V.D.2.	**Patient placement**
V.D.2.a.	In *acute care hospitals and long-term care settings*, place patients who require Airborne Precautions in an AIIR that has been constructed in accordance with current guidelines.
V.D.2.a.i.	Provide at least six (existing facility) or 12 (new construction/renovation) air changes per hour.
V.D.2.a.ii.	Direct exhaust of air to the outside. If it is not possible to exhaust air from an AIIR directly to the outside, the air may be returned to the air-handling system or adjacent spaces if all air is directed through HEPA filters.
V.D.2.a.iii	Whenever an AIIR is in use for a patient on Airborne Precautions, monitor air pressure daily with visual indicators (e.g., smoke tubes, flutter strips), regardless of the presence of differential pressure sensing devices (e.g., manometers).
V.D.2.a.iv.	Keep the AIIR door closed when not required for entry and exit.
V.D.2.b.	When an AIIR is not available, transfer the patient to a facility that has an available AIIR.
V.D.2.c.	In the event of an outbreak or exposure involving large numbers of patients who require Airborne Precautions:
	✓ Consult infection control professionals before patient placement to determine the safety of alternative room that do not meet engineering requirements for an AIIR.
	✓ Place together (cohort) patients who are presumed to have the same infection(based on clinical presentation and diagnosis when known) in areas of the facility that are away from other patients, especially patients who are at increased risk for infection (e.g., immunocompromised patients).
	✓ Use temporary portable solutions (e.g., exhaust fan) to create a negative pressure environment in the converted area of the facility. Discharge air directly to the outside, away from people and air intakes, or direct all the air through HEPA filters before it is introduced to other air spaces.
V.D.2.d.	In *ambulatory settings*:
V.D.2.d.i.	Develop systems (e.g., triage, signage) to identify patients with known or suspected infections that require Airborne Precautions upon entry into ambulatory settings.
V.D.2.d.ii.	Place the patient in an AIIR as soon as possible. If an AIIR is not available, place a surgical mask on the patient and place him/her in an examination room. Once the patient leaves, the room should remain vacant for the appropriate time, generally one hour, to allow for a full exchange of air.
V.D.2.d.iii.	Instruct patients with a known or suspected airborne infection to wear a surgical mask and observe Respiratory Hygiene/Cough Etiquette. Once in an AIIR, the mask may be removed; the mask should remain on if the patient is not in an AIIR.
V.D.3.	**Personnel restrictions**
	Restrict susceptible healthcare personnel from entering the rooms of patients known or suspected to have measles (rubella), varicella (chickenpox), disseminated zoster, or smallpox if other immune healthcare personnel are available.
V.D.4.	**Use of PPE (Personal Protective Equipment)**
V.D.4.a.	Wear a fit-tested NIOSH-approved N95 or higher level respirator for respiratory protection when entering the room or home of a patient when the following diseases are suspected or confirmed:
	✓ Infectious pulmonary or laryngeal tuberculosis or when infectious tuberculosis skin lesions are present and procedures that would aerosolize viable organisms (e.g., irrigation, incision and drainage, whirlpool treatments) are performed.
	✓ Smallpox (vaccinated and unvaccinated). Respiratory protection is recommended for all healthcare personnel, including those with a documented "take" after smallpox vaccination due to the risk of a genetically engineered virus against which the vaccine may not provide protection, or of exposure to a very large viral load (e.g., from high-risk aerosol-generating procedures, immunocompromised patients, hemorrhagic or flat smallpox.
V.D.4.b.	No recommendation is made regarding the use of PPE by healthcare personnel who are presumed to be immune to measles (rubella) or varicella-zoster based on history of disease, vaccine, or serologic testing when caring for an individual with known or suspected measles, chickenpox or disseminated zoster, due to difficulties in establishing definite immunity. Unresolved issue
V.D.4.c.	No recommendation is made regarding the type of personal protective equipment (i.e., surgical mask or respiratory protection with a N95 or higher respirator) to be worn by susceptible healthcare personnel who must have contact with patients with known or suspected measles, chickenpox or disseminated herpes zoster. *Unresolved issue*
V.D.5.	**Patient transport**
V.D.5.a.	In *acute care hospitals and long-term care and other residential settings*, limit transport and movement of patients outside of the room to medically-necessary purposes.
V.D.5.b.	If transport or movement outside an AIIR is necessary, instruct patients to wear a surgical mask, if possible, and observe Respiratory Hygiene/Cough Etiquette.
V.D.5.c.	For patients with skin lesions associated with varicella or smallpox or draining skin lesions caused by *M. tuberculosis*, cover the affected areas to prevent aerosolization or contact with the infectious agent in skin lesions.
V.D.5.d.	Healthcare personnel transporting patients who are on Airborne Precautions do not need to wear a mask or respirator during transport if the patient is wearing a mask and infectious skin lesions are covered.
V.D.6.	**Exposure management**
	Immunize or provide the appropriate immune globulin to susceptible persons as soon as possible following unprotected contact (i.e., exposed) to a patient with measles, varicella or smallpox:
	✓ Administer measles vaccine to exposed susceptible persons within 72 hours after the exposure or administer immune globulin within six days of the exposure event for high-risk persons in whom vaccine is contraindicated.
	✓ Administer varicella vaccine to exposed susceptible persons within 120 hours after the exposure or administer varicella immune globulin (VZIG or alternative product), when available, within 96 hours for high-risk persons in whom vaccine is contraindicated (e.g., immunocompromised patients, pregnant women, newborns whose mother's varicella onset was <5 days before or within 48 hours after delivery).
	✓ Administer smallpox vaccine to exposed susceptible persons within 4 days after exposure.
V.D.7.	Discontinue Airborne Precautions according to pathogen-specific recommendations in Appendix A.
V.D.8.	Consult CDC's "Guidelines for Preventing the Transmission of *Mycobacterium tuberculosis* in Health-Care Settings, 2005" and the "Guideline for Environmental Infection Control in Health-Care Facilities" for additional guidance on environment strategies for preventing transmission of tuberculosis in healthcare settings. The environmental recommendations in these guidelines may be applied to patients with other infections that require Airborne Precautions.

CONTACT PRECAUTIONS

2007 Guideline for Isolation Precautions: Preventing Transmission of Infectious Agents in Healthcare Settings

V.B.	**Contact Precautions**
V.B.1.	Use Contact Precautions as recommended in Appendix A for patients with known or suspected infections or evidence of syndromes that represent an increased risk for contact transmission. For specific recommendations for use of Contact Precautions for colonization or infection with MDROs. MDRO guideline at http://www.cdc.gov/hicpac/mdro/mdro_toc.html
V.B.2.	**Patient placement**
V.B.2.a.	In acute care hospitals, place patients who require Contact Precautions in a single-patient room when available. When single-patient rooms are in short supply, apply the following principles for making decisions on patient placement:

    ✓ Prioritize patients with conditions that may facilitate transmission (e.g., uncontained drainage, stool incontinence) for single-patient room placement.

    ✓ Place together in the same room (cohort) patients who are infected or colonized with the same pathogen and are suitable roommates

    ✓ If it becomes necessary to place a patient who requires Contact Precautions in a room with a patient who is not infected or colonized with the same infectious agent:

    ✓ Avoid placing patients on Contact Precautions in the same room with patients who have conditions that may increase the risk of adverse outcome from infection or that may facilitate transmission (e.g., those who are immunocompromised, have open wounds, or have anticipated prolonged lengths of stay).

    ✓ Ensure that patients are physically separated (i.e., >3 feet apart) from each other. Draw the privacy curtain between beds to minimize opportunities for direct contact.)

    ✓ Change protective attire and perform hand hygiene between contact with patients in the same room, regardless of whether one or both patients are on Contact Precautions.

V.B.2.b.	In long-term care and other residential settings, make decisions regarding patient placement on a case-by-case basis, balancing infection risks to other patients in the room, the presence of risk factors that increase the likelihood of transmission, and the potential adverse psychological impact on the infected or colonized patient.
V.B.2.c.	In ambulatory settings, place patients who require Contact Precautions in an examination room or cubicle as soon as possible.
V.B.3.	**Use of personal protective equipment**
V.B.3.a.	**Gloves** Wear gloves whenever touching the patient's intact skin or surfaces and articles in close proximity to the patient (e.g., medical equipment, bed rails). Don gloves upon entry into the room or cubicle.
V.B.3.b.	**Gowns**
V.B.3.b.i.	Wear a gown whenever anticipating that clothing will have direct contact with the patient or potentially contaminated environmental surfaces or equipment in close proximity to the patient. Don gown upon entry into the room or cubicle. Remove gown and observe hand hygiene before leaving the patient-care environment.
V.B.3.b.ii.	After gown removal, ensure that clothing and skin do not contact potentially contaminated environmental surfaces that could result in possible transfer of microorganism to other patients or environmental surfaces.
V.B.4.	**Patient transport**
V.B.4.a.	In acute care hospitals and long-term care and other residential settings, limit transport and movement of patients outside of the room to medically-necessary purposes.
V.B.4.b.	When transport or movement in any healthcare setting is necessary, ensure that infected or colonized areas of the patient's body are contained and covered.
V.B.4.c.	Remove and dispose of contaminated PPE and perform hand hygiene prior to transporting patients on Contact Precautions.
V.B.4.d.	Don clean PPE to handle the patient at the transport destination.
V.B.5.	**Patient-care equipment and instruments/devices**
V.B.5.a.	Handle patient-care equipment and instruments/devices according to Standard Precautions.
V.B.5.b.	In acute care hospitals and long-term care and other residential settings, use disposable noncritical patient-care equipment (e.g., blood pressure cuffs) or implement patient-dedicated use of such equipment. If common use of equipment for multiple patients is unavoidable, clean and disinfect such equipment before use on another patient.
V.B.5.c.	In home care settings
V.B.5.c.i.	Limit the amount of non-disposable patient-care equipment brought into the home of patients on Contact Precautions. Whenever possible, leave patient-care equipment in the home until discharge from home care services.
V.B.5.c.ii.	If noncritical patient-care equipment (e.g., stethoscope) cannot remain in the home, clean and disinfect items before taking them from the home using a low- to intermediate-level disinfectant. Alternatively, place contaminated reusable items in a plastic bag for transport and subsequent cleaning and disinfection.
V.B.5.d.	In ambulatory settings, place contaminated reusable noncritical patient-care equipment in a plastic bag for transport to a soiled utility area for reprocessing.
V.B.6.	**Environmental measures** Ensure that rooms of patients on Contact Precautions are prioritized for frequent cleaning and disinfection (e.g., at least daily) with a focus on frequently-touched surfaces (e.g., bed rails, overbed table, bedside commode, lavatory surfaces in patient bathrooms, doorknobs) and equipment in the immediate vicinity of the patient.
V.B.7.	Discontinue Contact Precautions after signs and symptoms of the infection have resolved or according to pathogen-specific recommendations in Appendix A.

DROPLET PRECAUTIONS
2007 Guideline for Isolation Precautions:
Preventing Transmission of Infectious Agents in Healthcare Settings

V.C.	Droplet Precautions

V.C.1. Use Droplet Precautions as recommended in Appendix A for patients known or suspected to be infected with pathogens transmitted by respiratory droplets (i.e., large-particle droplets >5µ in size) that are generated by a patient who is coughing, sneezing or talking.

V.C.2.	Patient placement

V.C.2.a. In acute care hospitals, place patients who require Droplet Precautions in a single-patient room when available. When single-patient rooms are in short supply, apply the following principles for making decisions on patient placement:

- Prioritize patients who have excessive cough and sputum production for single-patient room placement
- Place together in the same room (cohort) patients who are infected the same pathogen and are suitable roommates.
- If it becomes necessary to place patients who require Droplet Precautions in a room with a patient who does not have the same infection:
  - ✓ Avoid placing patients on Droplet Precautions in the same room with patients who have conditions that may increase the risk of adverse outcome from infection or that may facilitate transmission (e.g., those who are immunocompromised, have or have anticipated prolonged lengths of stay).
  - ✓ Ensure that patients are physically separated (i.e., >3 feet apart) from each other. Draw the privacy curtain between beds to minimize opportunities for close contact.
  - ✓ Change protective attire and perform hand hygiene between contact with patients in the same room, regardless of whether one patient or both patients are on Droplet Precautions.

V.C.2.b. In *long-term care and other residential settings*, make decisions regarding patient placement on a case-by-case basis after considering infection risks to other patients in the room and available alternatives.

V.C.2.c. In *ambulatory settings*, place patients who require Droplet Precautions in an examination room or cubicle as soon as possible. Instruct patients to follow recommendations for Respiratory Hygiene/Cough Etiquette.

V.C.3.	Use of personal protective equipment

V.C.3.a. Don a mask upon entry into the patient room or cubicle.

V.C.3.b. No recommendation for routinely wearing eye protection (e.g., goggle or face shield), in addition to a mask, for close contact with patients who require Droplet Precautions. *Unresolved issue*

V.C.3.c. For patients with suspected or proven SARS, avian influenza or pandemic influenza, refer to the following websites for the most current recommendations (www.cdc.gov/ncidod/sars/ ; www.cdc.gov/flu/avian/ ; www.pandemicflu.gov/)

V.C.4.	Patient transport

V.C.4.a. In *acute care hospitals and long-term care and other residential settings*, limit transport and movement of patients outside of the room to medically-necessary purposes.

V.C.4.b. If transport or movement in any healthcare setting is necessary, instruct patient to wear a mask and follow Respiratory Hygiene/Cough Etiquette www.cdc.gov/flu/professionals/infectioncontrol/resphygiene.htm).

V.C.4.c. No mask is required for persons transporting patients on Droplet Precautions.

V.C.4.d. Discontinue Droplet Precautions after signs and symptoms have resolved or according to pathogen-specific recommendations in Appendix A.

REMOVING PPE

To remove PPE safely, you must first be able to identify what sites are considered "clean" and what are "contaminated." In general, the outside front and sleeves of the isolation gown and outside front of the goggles, mask, respirator, and face shield are considered "contaminated," regardless of whether there is visible soil. Also, the outside of the gloves are contaminated shield.

Order of removing PPE:

1. Gloves
2. Face shield or goggles
3. Gown
4. Mask or respirator

Remove your PPE:

1. At the doorway, before leaving the patient room.
2. Remove respirator outside the room, after the door, has been closed.

Removing Glove Instructions:

First, using one gloved hand, grasp the outside of the opposite glove near the wrist.

Second, pull and peel the glove away from the hand. The glove should now be turned inside-out, with the contaminated side now on the inside. Hold the removed glove in the opposite gloved hand.

Third, slide one or two fingers of the ungloved hand under the wrist of the remaining glove.

Fourth, peel glove off from the inside, creating a bag for both gloves.

Finally, discard in a waste container.

Hand hygiene is the cornerstone of preventing infection transmission. You should perform hand hygiene immediately after removing PPE. If your hands become visibly contaminated during PPE removal, wash hands before continuing to remove PPE. Wash your hands thoroughly with soap and warm water or, if hands are not visibly contaminated, use an alcohol-based hand rub.

PPE DONNING & REMOVING

- Don before contact with the patient, generally before entering the room.
- Use carefully – do not spread contamination.
- Remove and discard carefully, either at the doorway or immediately outside the patient room; remove respirator outside the room.
- Immediately perform hand hygiene.

STANDARD PRECAUTIONS

Standard Precautions is an outgrowth of Universal Precautions. Universal Precautions was first recommended in 1987 to prevent the transmission of bloodborne pathogens to healthcare personnel. In 1996, the application of the concept was expanded and renamed "Standard Precautions". Standard Precautions is intended to prevent the transmission of common infectious agents to healthcare personnel, patients and visitors in any healthcare setting.

During care for patients, one should assume that an infectious agent could be present in the patient's blood or body fluids, including all secretions and excretions, except tears and sweat. Therefore, appropriate precautions, including use of PPE, must be taken. Whether PPE is needed, and if so, which type, is determined by the type of clinical interaction with the patient and the degree of blood and body fluid contact that can be reasonably anticipated and by whether the patient has been placed in isolation precautions (such as Contact or Droplet Precautions or Airborne Infection Isolation).

STANDARD PRECAUTIONS INCLUDE:

Gloves – Use when touching blood, body fluids, secretions, excretions and contaminated items; for touching mucous membranes and non-intact skin.

Gowns – Use during procedures and patient care activities. When contact of clothing/exposed skin with blood/body fluids, secretions or excretions is anticipated.

Mask and goggles or a face shield – Use during patient-care activities likely to generate splashes or sprays of blood, body fluids, secretions or excretions.

Note: For Contact Precautions – Gown and gloves are used for contact with the patient or to create an environment of care. (e.g., medical equipment, environmental surfaces)

- In some instances, these are required for entering patient's environment;
  - **For Droplet Precautions:** Use surgical masks within 3 feet of the patient.
  - **For Airborne Infection Isolation:** Use particulate respirator.

Guideline for isolation precautions: preventing transmission of infectious agents in healthcare settings
RECOMMENDATIONS

IV. Standard Precautions

Assume that every person is potentially infected or colonized with an organism that could be transmitted in the healthcare setting and apply the following infection control practices during the delivery of health care.

IV.A. Hand Hygiene

IV.A.1. During the delivery of healthcare, avoid unnecessary touching of surfaces in close proximity to the patient to prevent both contamination of clean hands from environmental surfaces and transmission of pathogens from contaminated hands to surfaces.

IV.A.2. When hands are visibly dirty, contaminated with proteinaceous material, or visibly soiled with blood or body fluids, wash hands with either a nonantimicrobial soap and water or an antimicrobial soap and water.

IV.A.3. If hands are not visibly soiled, or after removing visible material with nonantimicrobial soap and water, decontaminate hands in the clinical situations described in IV.A.2.a-f. The preferred method of hand decontamination is with an alcohol-based hand rub. Alternatively, hands may be washed with an antimicrobial soap and water. Frequent use of alcohol-based hand rub immediately following handwashing with nonantimicrobial soap may increase the frequency of dermatitis. Perform hand hygiene:

IV.A.3.a.

Before having direct contact with patients.

IV.A.3.b.

After contact with blood, body fluids or excretions, mucous membranes, nonintact skin, or wound dressings.

IV.A.3.c.

After contact with a patient's intact skin (e.g., when taking a pulse or blood pressure or lifting a patient).

IV.A.3.d.

If hands will be moving from a contaminated-body site to a clean-body site during patient care.

IV.A.3.e.

After contact with inanimate objects (including medical equipment) in the immediate vicinity of the patient.

IV.A.3.f.

After removing gloves.

IV.A.4. Wash hands with non-antimicrobial soap and water or with antimicrobial soap and water if contact with spores (e.g., C. difficile or Bacillus anthracis) is likely to have occurred. The physical action of washing and rinsing hands under such circumstances is recommended because alcohols, chlorhexidine, iodophors, and other antiseptic agents have poor activity against spores.

IV.A.5. Do not wear artificial fingernails or extenders if duties include direct contact with patients at high risk for infection and associated adverse outcomes (e.g., those in ICUs or operating rooms).

IV.A.5.a.

Develop an organizational policy on the wearing of non-natural nails by healthcare personnel who have direct contact with patients outside of the groups specified above 984. Category II

IV.B. Personal protective equipment (PPE)

IV.B.1. Observe the following principles of use:

IV.B.1.a.

Wear PPE, as described in IV.B.2-4, when the nature of the anticipated patient interaction indicates that contact with blood or body fluids may occur.

IV.B.1.b.

Prevent contamination of clothing and skin during the process of removing PPE.

IV.B.1.c.

Before leaving the patient's room or cubicle, remove and discard PPE.

IV.B.2. Gloves

IV.B.2.a.

Wear gloves when it can be reasonably anticipated that contact with blood or other potentially infectious materials, mucous membranes, nonintact skin, or potentially contaminated intact skin (e.g., of a patient incontinent of stool or urine) could occur.

IV.B.2.b.

Wear gloves with fit and durability appropriate to the task.

IV.B.2.b.i. Wear disposable medical examination gloves for providing direct patient care.

IV.B.2.b.ii. Wear disposable medical examination gloves or reusable utility gloves for cleaning the environment or medical equipment.

IV.B.2.c.

Remove gloves after contact with a patient and/or the surrounding environment (including medical equipment) using proper technique to prevent hand contamination. Do not wear the same pair of gloves for the care of more than one patient. Do not wash gloves for the purpose of reuse since this practice has been associated with transmission of pathogens.

IV.B.2.d.

Change gloves during patient care if the hands will move from a contaminated body-site (e.g., perineal area) to a clean body-site (e.g., face).

IV.B.3. Gowns

IV.B.3.a.

Wear a gown, that is appropriate to the task, to protect skin and prevent soiling or contamination of clothing during procedures and patient-care activities when contact with blood, body fluids, secretions, or excretions is anticipated.

IV.B.3.a.i. Wear a gown for direct patient contact if the patient has uncontained secretions or excretions.

IV.B.3.a.ii. Remove gown and perform hand hygiene before leaving the patient's environment.

IV.B.3.b.

Do not reuse gowns, even for repeated contacts with the same patient.

IV.B.3.c.

Routine donning of gowns upon entrance into a high-risk unit (e.g., ICU, NICU, HSCT unit) is not indicated.

IV.B.4. Mouth, nose, eye protection

IV.B.4.a.

Use PPE to protect the mucous membranes of the eyes, nose and mouth during procedures and patient-care activities that are likely to generate splashes or sprays of blood, body fluids, secretions and excretions. Select masks, goggles, face shields, and combinations of each according to the need anticipated by the task performed.

IV.B.5. During aerosol-generating procedures (e.g., bronchoscopy, suctioning of the respiratory tract [if not using in-line suction catheters], endotracheal intubation) in patients who are not suspected of being infected with an agent for which respiratory protection is otherwise recommended (e.g., M. tuberculosis, SARS or hemorrhagic fever viruses), wear one of the following: a face shield that fully covers the front and sides of the face, a mask with attached shield, or a mask and goggles (in addition to gloves and gown).

IV.C. Respiratory Hygiene/Cough Etiquette

IV.C.1. Educate healthcare personnel on the importance of source control measures to contain respiratory secretions to prevent droplet and fomite transmission of respiratory pathogens, especially during seasonal outbreaks of viral respiratory tract infections (e.g., influenza, RSV, adenovirus, parainfluenza virus) in communities.

IV.C.2. Implement the following measures to contain respiratory secretions in patients and accompanying individuals who have signs and symptoms of a respiratory infection, beginning at the point of initial encounter in a healthcare setting (e.g., triage, reception and waiting areas in emergency departments, outpatient clinics and physician offices).

IV.C.2.a.

Post signs at entrances and in strategic places (e.g., elevators, cafeterias) within ambulatory and inpatient settings with instructions to patients and other persons with symptoms of a respiratory infection to cover their mouths/noses when coughing or sneezing, use and dispose of tissues, and perform hand hygiene after hands have been in contact with respiratory secretions.

IV.C.2.b.

Provide tissues and no-touch receptacles (e.g., foot-pedal operated lid or open, plastic-lined waste basket) for disposal of tissues.

IV.C.2.c.

Provide resources and instructions for performing hand hygiene in or near waiting areas in ambulatory and inpatient settings; provide conveniently-located dispensers of alcohol-based hand rubs and, where sinks are available, supplies for handwashing.

IV.C.2.d.

During periods of increased prevalence of respiratory infections in the community (e.g., as indicated by increased school absenteeism, increased number of patients seeking care for a respiratory infection), offer masks to coughing patients and other symptomatic persons (e.g., persons who accompany ill patients) upon entry into the facility or medical office and encourage them to maintain special separation, ideally a distance of at least 3 feet, from others in common waiting areas.

> **IV.C.2.d.i.** Some facilities may find it logistically easier to institute this recommendation year-round as a standard of practice.

IV.D. Patient placement

IV.D.1. Include the potential for transmission of infectious agents in patient-placement decisions. Place patients who pose a risk for transmission to others (e.g., uncontained secretions, excretions or wound drainage; infants with suspected viral respiratory or gastrointestinal infections) in a single-patient room when available

IV.D.2. Determine patient placement based on the following principles:
- Route(s) of transmission of the known or suspected infectious agent
- Risk factors for transmission in the infected patient
- Risk factors for adverse outcomes resulting from an healthcare-associated infection (HAI) in other patients in the area or room being considered for patient- placement
- Availability of single-patient rooms

- Patient options for room-sharing (e.g., cohorting patients with the same infection) Category II

IV.E. Patient-care equipment and instruments/devices

IV.E.1. Establish policies and procedures for containing, transporting, and handling patient-care equipment and instruments/devices that may be contaminated with blood or body fluids.

IV.E.2. Remove organic material from critical and semi-critical instrument/devices, using recommended cleaning agents before high level disinfection and sterilization to enable effective disinfection and sterilization processes.

IV.E.3. Wear PPE (e.g., gloves, gown), according to the level of anticipated contamination, when handling patient-care equipment and instruments/devices that is visibly soiled or may have been in contact with blood or body fluids.

IV.F. Care of the environment

IV.F.1. Establish policies and procedures for routine and targeted cleaning of environmental surfaces as indicated by the level of patient contact and degree of soiling.

IV.F.2. Clean and disinfect surfaces that are likely to be contaminated with pathogens, including those that are in close proximity to the patient (e.g., bed rails, over bed tables) and frequently-touched surfaces in the patient care environment (e.g., door knobs, surfaces in and surrounding toilets in patients' rooms) on a more frequent schedule compared to that for other surfaces (e.g., horizontal surfaces in waiting rooms).

IV.F.3. Use EPA-registered disinfectants that have microbiocidal (i.e., killing) activity against the pathogens most likely to contaminate the patient-care environment. Use in accordance with manufacturer's instructions.

IV.F.3.a.

Review the efficacy of in-use disinfectants when evidence of continuing transmission of an infectious agent (e.g., rotavirus, C. difficile, norovirus) may indicate resistance to the in-use product and change to a more effective disinfectant as indicated.

IV.F.4. In facilities that provide health care to pediatric patients or have waiting areas with child play toys (e.g., obstetric/gynecology offices and clinics), establish policies and procedures for cleaning and disinfecting toys at regular intervals.

Use the following principles in developing this policy and procedures:

- Select play toys that can be easily cleaned and disinfected
- Do not permit use of stuffed furry toys if they will be shared
- Clean and disinfect large stationary toys (e.g., climbing equipment) at least weekly and whenever visibly soiled
- If toys are likely to be mouthed, rinse with water after disinfection; alternatively wash in a dishwasher
- When a toy requires cleaning and disinfection, do so immediately or store in a designated labeled container separate from toys that are clean and ready for use.

IV.F.5.   Include multi-use electronic equipment in policies and procedures for preventing contamination and for cleaning and disinfection, especially those items that are used by patients, those used during delivery of patient care, and mobile devices that are moved in and out of patient rooms frequently (e.g., daily).

IV.F.5.a.

No recommendation for use of removable protective covers or washable keyboards. Unresolved issue

IV.G. Textiles and laundry

IV.G.1. Handle used textiles and fabrics with minimum agitation to avoid contamination of air, surfaces and persons.

IV.G.2. If laundry chutes are used, ensure that they are properly designed, maintained, and used in a manner to minimize dispersion of aerosols from contaminated laundry.

IV.H. Safe injection practices

The following recommendations apply to the use of needles, cannulas that replace needles, and, where applicable intravenous delivery systems.

IV.H.1. Use aseptic technique to avoid contamination of sterile injection equipment.

IV.H.2. Do not administer medications from a syringe to multiple patients, even if the needle or cannula on the syringe is changed. Needles, cannulae and syringes are sterile, single-use items; they should not be reused for another patient nor to access a medication or solution that might be used for a subsequent patient.

IV.H.3. Use fluid infusion and administration sets (i.e., intravenous bags, tubing and connectors) for one patient only and dispose appropriately after use. Consider a syringe or needle/cannula contaminated once it has been used to enter or connect to a patient's intravenous infusion bag or administration set.

IV.H.4. Use single-dose vials for parenteral medications whenever possible.

IV.H.5. Do not administer medications from single-dose vials or ampules to multiple patients or combine leftover contents for later use.

IV.H.6. If multidose vials must be used, both the needle or cannula and syringe used to access the multidose vial must be sterile.

IV.H.7. Do not keep multidose vials in the immediate patient treatment area and store in accordance with the manufacturer's recommendations; discard if sterility is compromised or questionable.

IV.H.8. Do not use bags or bottles of intravenous solution as a common source of supply for multiple patients.

IV.I. Infection control practices for special lumbar puncture procedures

Wear a surgical mask when placing a catheter or injecting material into the spinal canal or subdural space (i.e., during myelograms, lumbar puncture and spinal or epidural anesthesia. Worker safety adhere to federal and state requirements for protection of healthcare personnel from exposure to bloodborne pathogens.

WHAT ARE BLOODBORNE PATHOGENS?

Bloodborne pathogens are infectious micro-organisms in human blood that can cause disease in humans. These pathogens include, but are not limited to, hepatitis B (HBV), hepatitis C (HCV) and human immunodeficiency virus (HIV). Needlesticks and other sharps-related injuries may expose workers to bloodborne pathogens. Workers in many occupations, including first aid team members, housekeeping personnel in some industries, nurses and other healthcare personnel, may be at risk of exposure to bloodborne pathogens.

WHAT CAN BE DONE TO CONTROL EXPOSURE OF BLOODBORNE PATHOGENS?

In order to reduce or eliminate the hazards of occupational exposure to bloodborne pathogens, an employer must implement an exposure control plan for the worksite with details on employee protection measures. The plan must also describe how an employer will use a combination of engineering and work practice controls, ensure the use of personal protective clothing and equipment, provide training, medical surveillance, hepatitis B vaccinations, and signs and labels among other provisions. Engineering controls are the primary means of eliminating or minimizing employee exposure and include the use of safer medical devices, such as needleless devices, shielded needle devices, and plastic capillary tubes.

POST EXPOSURE TO BLOODBORNE PATHOGENS

If a healthcare worker gets stuck by a needle or other sharps or gets blood or other potentially infectious materials into their eyes, nose, mouth, or on broken skin, immediately flood the exposed area with water and clean any wound with soap and water or a skin disinfectant, if available. Report this immediately to your employer and seek immediate medical attention.

BLOODBORNE PATHOGEN STANDARD
Requires employers to:

- **Establish an exposure control plan.** This is a written plan to eliminate or minimize occupational exposures. The employer must prepare an exposure determination that contains a list of job classifications in which workers have occupational exposure, along with a list of the tasks and procedures performed by those workers that result in their exposure.

- **Employers must update the plan annually** to reflect changes in tasks, procedures, positions that affect occupational exposure, and also technological changes that eliminate or reduce occupational exposure. In addition, employers must annually document in the plan that they have considered and begun using appropriate, commercially available, effective safer medical devices designed to eliminate or minimize occupational exposure. Employers must also document that they have solicited input from frontline workers in identifying, evaluating and selecting effective engineering and work practice controls.

- **Implement the use of universal precautions** (treating all human blood and **Other Potentially Infectious Materials (OPIM)** as if known to be infectious for bloodborne pathogens).

- **Identify and use engineering controls**. These are devices that isolate or remove the bloodborne pathogens hazard from the workplace. They include sharps disposal containers, self-sheathing needles, and safer medical devices, such as sharps with engineered sharps injury protection and needleless systems.

- **Identify and ensure the use of work practice controls**. These are practices that reduce the possibility of exposure by changing the way a task is performed, such as appropriate practices for handling and disposing of contaminated sharps, handling specimens, handling laundry, and cleaning contaminated surfaces and items.

- **Provide personal protective equipment (PPE),** such as gloves, gowns, eye protection, and masks. Employers must clean, repair, and replace these equipment's as required. Provision, maintenance, repair and replacement are at no cost to the worker.

- **Make available hepatitis B vaccinations** to all workers with occupational exposure. The vaccination must be offered after the worker has received the required bloodborne pathogens training and within 10 days of initial assignment to a job with occupational exposure.

- **Maintain worker medical and training records.** The employer also must maintain a sharps injury log.

- **Make available post-exposure evaluation and follow-up** to any occupationally exposed worker who experiences an exposure incident. An exposure incident to a specific eye, mouth, other mucous membrane, non-intact skin, or parenteral contact with blood or **other potentially infectious materials (OPIM)**.

- **Medical evaluation and follow-up must be at no cost** to the worker and includes:
  1. Documenting the route(s) of exposure.
  2. Circumstances under which the exposure incident occurred.
  3. Identifying and testing the source individual for HBV and HIV infection.
  4. Collecting and testing the exposed worker's blood.

- **Use labels and signs to communicate hazards.** Warning labels must be affixed to containers of regulated waste:
  1. Containers of contaminated reusable sharps.
  2. Refrigerators and freezers containing blood or OPIM.
  3. Other containers used to store, transport, or ship blood or OPIM.
  4. Contaminated equipment that is being shipped or serviced and
  5. Bags or containers of contaminated laundry, except as provided in the standard. Facilities may use red bags or red containers instead of labels.

- **Provide information and training to workers.** Employers must ensure that their workers receive regular training that covers all elements of the standard including, but not limited to:
  1. Information on bloodborne pathogens and diseases.
  2. Methods used to control occupational exposure.
  3. Hepatitis B vaccine.
  4. Medical evaluation.
  5. Post-exposure follow-up procedures.

- **Employers must offer this training on initial assignment**, at least annually after that, and when new or modified tasks or procedures affect a worker's occupational exposure. The training must be presented at an educational level and in a language that workers understand.

Sterilization is a process that destroys or eliminates all forms of microbial life and can be carried out via physical or chemical methods. Steam under pressure, dry heat, hydrogen peroxide gas plasma, and liquid chemicals are some sterilizing agents used in healthcare facilities. When chemicals are used for destroying all forms of microbiological lives, they can be called as chemical sterilants.

METHODS OF STERILIZATION

- **Steam** is the preferred method for sterilizing critical medical and surgical instruments that are not damaged by heat, steam, pressure, or moisture.
- **Cool steam- or heat-sterilized** items before they are handled or used in the operative setting.
- Follow the sterilization times, temperatures, and other operating parameters (e.g., gas concentration, humidity) recommended by the manufacturers of the instruments, the sterilizer, and the container or wrap used, and that are consistent with guidelines published by government agencies and professional organizations.
- **Use low-temperature sterilization** technologies (e.g., EtO, hydrogen peroxide gas plasma) for reprocessing critical patient-care equipment that is heat or moisture sensitive.
- Completely aerate surgical and medical items that have been sterilized in the EtO sterilizer (e.g., polyvinylchloride tubing requires 12 hours at 50°C, 8 hours at 60°C) before using these items in patient care.
- **Sterilization using the peracetic acid immersion system** can be used to sterilize heat-sensitive immersible medical and surgical items.
- **Critical items that have been sterilized by the peracetic acid immersion** process must be used immediately (i.e., items are not completely protected from contamination, making long-term storage unacceptable).
- **Dry-heat sterilization** (e.g., 340oF for 60 minutes) can be used to sterilize items (e.g., powders, oils) that can sustain high temperatures.

- Comply with the sterilizer manufacturer's instructions regarding the sterilizer cycle parameters (e.g., time, temperature, concentration).
- Because narrow-lumen devices provide a challenge to all low-temperature sterilization technologies, and direct contact is necessary for the sterilant to be effective, ensure that the sterilant has direct contact with contaminated surfaces (e.g., scopes processed in peracetic acid must be connected to channel irrigators).

Disinfection is a process that eliminates many or all pathogenic microorganisms, except some bacterial spores. In health-care settings, most of the objects are disinfected by liquid chemicals or wet pasteurization.

Some Chemical Disinfectants are:-
- ✓ Alcohol
- ✓ Chlorine and Chlorine Compounds
- ✓ Formaldehyde
- ✓ Glutaraldehyde
- ✓ Hydrogen Peroxide
- ✓ Iodophors
- ✓ Ortho-phthalaldehyde (OPA)
- ✓ Peracetic Acid
- ✓ Peracetic Acid and Hydrogen Peroxide
- ✓ Phenolics
- ✓ Quaternary Ammonium Compounds

Factors that affect the effectiveness of both disinfection and sterilization include
1. Prior cleaning of the object
2. Type and the level of microbial contamination
3. Concentration of and exposure time to the germicide
4. Physical nature of the object
5. Presence of biofilms
6. Temperature and pH of the disinfection process
7. Relative humidity of the sterilization process.

Cleaning is the process of removing visible soil from objects and surfaces. This can be accomplished manually or mechanically using water with detergents or enzymatic products. Cleaning is an essential part of the process before high-level disinfection and sterilization is performed, because soiling that remains on the surface of the instrument can interfere with the effectiveness of the processes.

DISINFECTION AND STERILIZATION GUIDELINE
Disinfection and sterilization are essential for making sure that medical instruments do not transmit infectious pathogens from patient to patient. Sterilization of all patient-care items may not be necessary. Health-care facility policy must specifically identify, whether an item should be cleaned, disinfected, or sterilized.

Reference:
1. Centers for Disease Control and Prevention: http://www.cdc.gov/
2. Siegel JD, Rhinehart E, Jackson M, Chiarello L, and the Healthcare Infection Control Practices Advisory Committee, 2007 Guideline for Isolation Precautions: Preventing Transmission of Infectious Agents in Healthcare Settings http://www.cdc.gov/ncidod/dhqp/pdf/isolation2007.pdf
3. Occupational safety and health administration https://www.osha.gov
4. "Allergy to Latex Rubber". American Dental Association.

CHAPTER 2
END OF CHAPTER REVIEW QUESTIONS

Question Set 1: Match the Following
20 points (2 points each)

Answers	Column A	Column B
	Gloves	A. may indirectly transmit an infectious agent include food, water, biologic products (blood), and fomites (inanimate objects such as handkerchiefs, bedding, or surgical scalpels).
	Sterilization	B. hives, swelling, runny nose, nausea, abdominal cramps, dizziness, low blood pressure, bronchospasm, anaphylaxis (shock).
	Gowns	C. red, dry, itchy irritated areas.
	OSHA	D. are used when touching blood, body fluids, secretions, excretions, and contaminated items; for touching mucous membranes and non-intact skin.
	Contact dermatitis	E. refers to the alcohol-containing preparation applied to the hands to reduce the number of viable microorganisms.
	Irritant Contact Dermatitis Reactions (Latex Reaction)	F. workplace health and safety regulations.
	Alcohol-based handrub	G. is a process that destroys or eliminates all forms of microbial life and can be carried out via physical or chemical methods.
	Allergic Contact Dermatitis Reactions (Latex Reaction)	H. causes dry, itchy, irritated areas on the skin, most often on the hands.
	Vehicle mode of infection transmission	I. are used during procedures and patient care activities. When contact of clothing/exposed skin with blood/body fluids, secretions, or excretions is anticipated.
	Hypersensitivity Reactions (Latex Reaction)	J. itchy, red rash, small blisters.

Question Set 2: Essay Questions
48 points (6 points each)

1. What are bloodborne pathogens & what can be done to control exposure to bloodborne pathogens?
2. What are PPE? Explain types and procedure for donning and removing PPE?
3. Explain the chain of infection and various ways to break the chain of infection?
4. Explain in brief contact dermatitis?
5. Outline the cleaning up procedure for blood spills using bleach solution?
6. Explain in brief about standard precautions?

7. In brief, explain the hand hygiene procedure?
8. Explain the direct and indirect mode of transmission of infectious agents?

Question Set 3: Fill in the Blanks   10 points (2 points each)

1. Latex allergy generally develops after repeated exposure to products containing _____.

2. Latex allergy produces varied symptoms, which commonly include _____ nose, sneezing, _____ eyes,

   _____ throat, hives, and _____ burning sensations.

3. Chain of infection is a process that begins when an _____ leaves its _____ or host through a portal of _____,

   and is conveyed by some mode of _____, then enters through an appropriate portal of _____ to infect

   a susceptible _____.

4. Droplet spread refers to spray with relatively large, short-range _____ produced by _____,

   _____, or even _____.

5. Bloodborne pathogens are _____ microorganisms in human blood that can cause disease in humans.

Question Set 4: Multiple Choice   12 points (2 points each)

1. Latex allergy produces varied symptoms, which commonly include all the following except:
   _____a)   runny nose
   _____b)   sneezing
   _____c)   radiating pain
   _____d)   scratchy throat

2. Breaking the chain of infection can be done by all of the following except:
   _____a)   Using effective hand hygiene.
   _____b)   Using PPE (Personal Protective Equipment).
   _____c)   Isolating patients with infectious diseases.
   _____d)   Using HIPAA recommendations.

3. All of the followings are benefits of using alcohol-based rubs except:
   _____a)   Require less time.
   _____b)   Are less effective for standard handwashing than soap.
   _____c)   Reduce bacterial counts on hands.
   _____d)   Improve skin condition.

4. All of the following are Personal Protective Equipment except:
   _____a)   Gloves
   _____b)   Gowns
   _____c)   Sterile Pack

_____d)   Mask

5.   The correct order of donning personal protective equipment:
     _____a)   Mask or respirator, Gown first, Goggles or Face Shield, Gloves
     _____b)   Goggles or Face Shield, Gown first, Mask or Respirator, Gloves
     _____c)   Gown first, Mask or Respirator, Goggles or Face Shield, Gloves
     _____d)   Gloves, Gown first, Mask or Respirator, Goggles or Face Shield

6.   The correct order of removing personal protective equipment:
     _____a)   Gloves, Face shield or goggles, Gown, Mask or respirator
     _____b)   Gown, Gloves, Face shield or goggles, Mask or respirator
     _____c)   Mask or respirator, Gloves, Face shield or goggles, Gown
     _____d)   Gloves, Mask or respirator, Face shield or goggles, Gown

Question Set 5: True or False (T/F)   10 Points (1 Point Each) Circle Answers

1.   Infection control addresses factors related to the spread of infections within the health-care setting.
     Answer: TRUE OR FALSE

2.   OSHA addresses factors related to monitoring/investigation of demonstrated or suspected spread of infection within a particular health-care setting (surveillance and outbreak investigation), and management (interruption of outbreaks).
     Answer: TRUE OR FALSE

3.   Modes of transmission is a process that begins when an agent leaves its reservoir or host through a portal of exit, and is conveyed by some mode of transmission, then enters through an appropriate portal of entry to infect a susceptible host.
     Answer: TRUE OR FALSE

4.   Vector transmission occurs when infectious agents are carried by dust or droplet nuclei suspended in air.
     Answer: TRUE OR FALSE

5.   Droplet precautions apply to patients known or suspected to be infected with a pathogen that can be transmitted by droplet route; these include, but are not limited to respiratory viruses and bordetella pertussis.
     Answer: TRUE OR FALSE

6.   Plain soap is good at reducing bacterial counts, but antimicrobial soap is better and alcohol-based handrubs are the best.
     Answer: TRUE OR FALSE

7.   Artificial nails can be worn when having direct contact with high-risk patients.
     Answer: TRUE OR FALSE

8.   Standard Precautions is intended to prevent the transmission of common infectious agents to healthcare personnel, patients and visitors in any healthcare setting.
     Answer: TRUE OR FALSE

9.   Vectors such as mosquitoes, flies, and ticks may carry an infectious agent through purely mechanical means or may support growth or changes in the agent.
     Answer: TRUE OR FALSE

10. Infection control addresses factors related to the spread of infections within the health-care setting (whether patient-to-patient, from patients to staff, from staff to patients or among staff).
     Answer: TRUE OR FALSE

SECTION 1

CHAPTER 3: LEGAL ISSUES IN HEALTHCARE

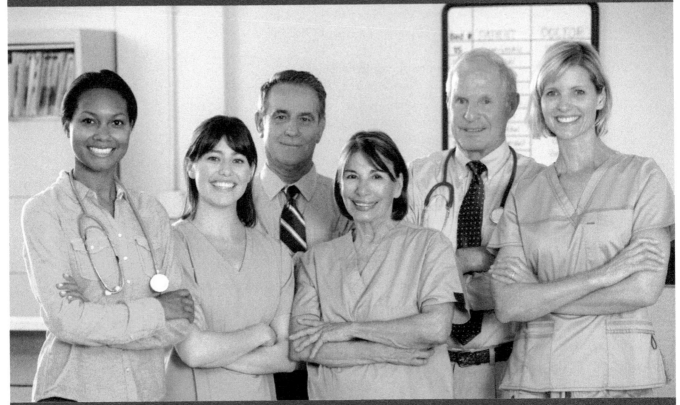

LEARNING OBJECTIVES

At the end of this chapter the student will be able to describe in brief:

Types of Laws (Civil and Criminal), with their brief descriptions, tort law

Negligence vs malpractice

What is Standard of care?

Basic elements of negligence (duty, breach of duty, direct cause and damage)

Types of damages

    1. Special damage

    2. General damage

    3. Punitive damage

Sources of laws

Consents and its types

Patient abuse and types of abuse

Patients' rights

Patient self-determining act (PSDA), living will, advance directives and false imprisonment

Restraints (physical and chemical)

Scope of Practice, Good Samaritan Law (GSL) and Uniform Anatomical Gift Act (UAGA)

Americans with Disabilities Act (ADA)

LEGAL ISSUES IN HEALTHCARE

Each facility has their own policies and procedures to ensure that procedures are performed as safely and correctly as possible. A standard of care should always be followed when performing a procedure. Make sure that you follow the established standard of care.

LAWS

CIVIL LAW

Deals with enforcement of all public rights (non-criminal laws). Example Tort law

TORT LAW

Torts are wrongdoings as a result of unreasonable actions of others. This may cause injury or damage to the person on whom the unreasonable action is being performed. As a result of which the injured person may take a civil action against the person or party performing the unreasonable action.

There are basically three types of torts:
1. Intentional torts
2. Negligence
3. Strict liability

Intentional Torts: action are intended to harm

- **Assault**: Threatening or causing bodily injury to another person, it may be a crime or a tort.
- **Battery**: Touching a patient without his or her consent is termed as a battery, it can either be a civil or criminal offense.
- **Defamation**: In general is a written or oral statement which causes harm to the reputation of a person or third party.
- **Slander**: A defamatory statement presented in an oral or spoken format.
- **Libel**: A defamatory statement presented in a published or written format.
- **Fraud**: Intentionally hiding the truth for unlawful gains.
- **Invasion of privacy**: Health Insurance Portability and Accountability Act of 1996 (HIPAA): Title II of HIPAA (Administrative Simplification) consists of the privacy and security rule. The main purpose of these rules is to keep a patient's health information confidential and secure.

Negligence
Unintentional Tort: actions are unintentional

Negligence: Legal cause of action resulting from a failure to exercise the care that a reasonable person would exercise in like, same or similar circumstances. Types of negligence:
- **Comparative negligence**: Both parties are involved and the compensation depends on the contribution of the negligence, the jury decides the percentage of fault and the compensation has to be paid based on the percentage/proportion of the fault.
- **Contributory negligence**: Cases in which the plaintiffs own negligence lead to the injury.

Strict Liability:

Liability regardless of fault.

Malpractice: A substandard delivery of care by the healthcare provider causing injury to the patient.

NEGLIGENCE VS MALPRACTICE

Medical negligence occurs when a medical professional fails to do something that should have been done.

Medical malpractice means that a medical professional performed their job in a way that deviated from the accepted medical standards of care, causing injury or death. Medical malpractice is a type of negligence.

WHAT IS STANDARD OF CARE?

A standard of care can be explained as *"what would have another professional done under similar situation or circumstances"*.

BASIC ELEMENTS OF NEGLIGENCE

Duty:

Is what one person owes to another. In this element, it must be proven that the defendant owed a duty to the plaintiff. A duty should first be established to prove that the defendant owed a duty to the plaintiff.

Breach of Duty:

Once established that the defendant owed a duty to the plaintiff, it must be proved that the defendant breached that duty. To prove that there was a breach of duty, the plaintiff must show that the defendant violated the standard of care or acted negligently.

Direct Cause:

The breach of duty was a direct cause of injury to the plaintiff.

Damage:

The last element in which plaintiff's injury is reviewed and compensation is sought.

TYPES OF DAMAGES

- **Special Damages** – Dollar values for damages or injury suffered by the individual (i.e. medical bills and lost wages).
- **General Damages** – No dollar value can be applied (i.e. example pain and suffering cannot be valued).
- **Punitive Damages** – Are to punish the defendant for the negligence rather than to compensate the plaintiff.

CRIMINAL LAW

The body of law that defines and governs the actions that constitute crimes.

Felony

Severe Crime, Prison for more than 1 year.

Misdemeanors

Less Severe Crime, Prison for less than 1 year.

SOURCES OF LAWS

Common Law

Law that is derived from judicial decisions instead of from statutes.

Statutory Law

Law that comes from the state and federal legislatures Statutory law consists of the laws passed by the legislature.

Administrative Law

Created by the administrative agencies for carrying out their duties and responsibilities. Administrative agencies are established to perform a specific function; they can be state or federal agencies.

CONSENT

Informed Consent

A process in which the permission is granted from the patient prior to the start of a healthcare procedure.

Expressed Consent

A type of consent in which the person expresses the permission in written or spoken words before the onset of a healthcare procedure.

Implied Consent:

A type of consent in which the permission is not expressed but rather inferred by the person's action, signs, and facts.

PATIENT ABUSE

Is any action or failure to act, which can result in physical, mental or emotional pain or injury to the patient.

- **Physical abuse**. Causes harm to a patient. Examples include pinching, punching, kicking, slapping, burning, bruising, pushing, shoving.
- **Sexual abuse**. Forcing a patient, using physical or verbal threats to indulge or participate in a sexual acts.
- **Psychosocial or mental abuse**. An act of emotionally harming a patient using threats, humiliation, intimidation, isolation, insult or threatening to stop the treatment.
- **Verbal abuse**. An act of oral (yelling, calling out names, swearing, teasing) or written (insulting language) words, pictures (inappropriate pictures), or gestures that threatens, embarrasses or insults the patient.
- **Involuntary seclusion**. Involuntary isolation or separation of the patient from others.
- **Substance abuse**. Use of any drug which is illegal or lethal and can cause harm to the patient.

Abuse by others

If you find a patient being abused by anyone, report the findings to the appropriate authority. Sometimes even the patient would not know that an abuse is taking place on them. **REMEMBER: IT MUST BE REPORTED.**

PATIENTS' RIGHTS

Type of Patient Right	Purpose
The right to give or withhold authorization of disclosures	The patient generally has the right to control who has access to confidential information except as otherwise provided by law. The patient needs to give specific authorization or permission to allow a third party to have access to confidential information.
The right to maintain privacy	Only those persons directly involved in the care of the patient's health problem should have access to private information. Health care workers should protect information revealed during provider health care worker encounters, including all written or electronic records of these encounters.
The right to have autonomy	Autonomy is the right of a patient to determine what will be done with his or her body, personal belongings, and personal information; this concept applies to any adult person who is mentally competent. Sometimes the right to autonomy can be overridden in the interest of protecting others who may be harmed by the patient's decisions.
The right to be given information	The patient has a right to information about his or her medical diagnosis, treatment regimen, and progress. This allows the patient to make appropriate, informed decisions about his or her health care.

Patients have the right to:

- get the best possible care
- know their rights
- refuse treatments
- refuse restraints
- review medical records
- privacy and confidentiality
- know about their health status (transfer & discharge)
- to have their visitors
- to attend support group activities

The patient-health care worker relationship is the basis for

1. Sharing information.
2. Communicating beliefs and feelings that affect care.
3. Building trust between the patient and health care worker.

Three ways to earn a patient's trust include

1. Respecting the patient's autonomy, the right of a patient to determine what will be done with his or her body, belongings, and personal information.
2. Freely providing complete and accurate information.
3. Rigorously maintaining confidentiality.

PATIENT CONFIDENTIALITY

HOW TO PROTECT

ANY SITUATION

- Confirm the patient's identity at the first encounter.
- Never discuss the patient's case with anyone without the patient's permission (including family and friends during off-duty hours).
- Never leave hard copies of forms or records where unauthorized persons may access them.
- Use only secure routes to send patient information (for example, official mail) and always mark this information confidential.
- When using an interpreter, ensure that the interpreter understands the importance of patient confidentiality.

WHEN IN AN OFFICE, CLINIC, OR INSTITUTION

- Conduct patient interviews in private rooms or areas.
- Never discuss cases or use patients' names in a public area.
- If a staff member or health care worker requests patient information, establish his or her authority to do so before disclosing anything.
- Keep records that contain patient names and other identifying information in closed, locked files.

- Restrict access to electronic databases to designated staff.
- Carefully protect computer passwords or keys; never give them to unauthorized persons.
- Carefully safeguard computer screens.
- Keep computers in a locked or restricted area; physically or electronically lock the hard disk.
- Keep printouts of electronic information in a restricted or locked area; printouts that are no longer needed should be destroyed.

WHEN IN THE FIELD

- Be discreet when making patient visits.
- Conduct patient interviews in private; never discuss the case in a public place.
- Do not leave sensitive or confidential information in messages for the patient on a door; but if a message must be left on the door, it should be left in a sealed envelope, marked confidential, and addressed to a specific person.
- Do not leave sensitive or confidential information on an answering machine that other people can access.
- Do not leave sensitive or confidential information with a neighbor or friend, and be careful not to disclose the patient's condition when gathering information on his or her whereabouts.

The Patient Self Determination Act (PSDA)

The Patient Self-Determination Act (PSDA), enacted in 1991, dictates that health care institutions must take steps to educate all adult patients on their right to accept or refuse medical care. The written information concerning advance directives must be provided to an adult individual by healthcare facilities.

The requirements of the PSDA are as follows:

- Patients are given written notice on admission. Patient rights include the rights to:
  - *Facilitate their own health care decisions.*
  - *Accept or refuse medical treatment.*
  - *Make an advance health care directive.*
- Facilities must inquire as to the whether the patient already has an advance health care directive, and make note of this in their medical records.
- Facilities must provide education to their staff and affiliates about advance health care directives.

- Health care providers are not allowed to discriminately admit or treat patients based on whether or not they have an advance health care directive.

If an individual at the time of admission or is otherwise unable to express whether or not he/she has already executed an advance directive, information about advance directives may be given to the individual's family members.

ADVANCE DIRECTIVES: A BRIEF OVERVIEW
Living Will
A written document which includes the medical treatment the person would want and not want to receive.
Durable Power of Attorney
Gives the power (authority) to another person for making medical decisions for the patient in the event of the patient unable to take the decision himself. The name of the document used for such purpose is known as, **Protective Medical Decisions Document (PMDD).**

Examples of what can be incorporated within the advance directive can be:

1. **Do Not Resuscitate (DNR)**
   This document indicates medical professionals not to perform CPR on the patient.
2. **Do Not Intubate (DNI)**
   This document indicates medical professionals not to perform intubation on the patient.

FALSE IMPRISONMENT
Restraint a person without proper authorization and consent. All patients have their rights and respecting their rights is crucial.

PHYSICAL RESTRAINTS
Restraints are procedures that restrict a patient's movement. Restraints may assist a person from getting injured or injuring others. Restraints are used as the last alternative.

Types of Physical Restraints
- Belts restraints, vests restraints, jackets restraints, and mitts restraints for the patient's hands

Restraints are only performed with a doctor's order. Restraints are also be used to prevent harmful movement of the patient. While on the contrary, it may also be used to control the movement of the resident. Restraints should not cause injury or should not be used to discipline the residents. Health care providers should first try other methods to control a patient and ensure safety.

When restraints are used, they must:

- Limit only the movements that may cause harm to the patient or caregiver.
- Be removed as soon as the patient and the caregiver are safe.

Patients who are on restraints need special care to ensure:

- They can have a proper bladder and bowel movement.
- They are given proper hygiene (care).
- They are given the right amount of nutrition they need.
- They are positioned as comfortable as possible.
- They do not harm themselves.

CHEMICAL RESTRAINT

Is a form of restraint in which medications are used to restrict the patient's movements or freedom to move.

Respondeat Superior: Employers are liable for the actions of an employee within the course and scope of their employment.

Res ipsa Loquitor: Latin for "the thing speaks for itself".

Abandonment: Occurs when a healthcare personnel leaves the patient without providing the care that was needed.

Scope of Practice

Defines the procedures, actions, and processes that are permitted to perform under the licensed profession. Each state has its scope of practice for the licensed individual.

Good Samaritan Act(s)

Good Samaritan laws are laws or acts that protect those individual/s who choose to serve and tend to help others who are injured or ill. Good Samaritan laws vary from jurisdiction to jurisdiction.

Uniform Anatomical Gift Act

The Uniform Anatomical Gift Act (UAGA or the Act) was passed in the US in 1968 and has since been revised in 1987 and in 2006. "Anatomical gift" means a donation of all or part of a human body (organs, tissues, and other human body parts) to take effect after the donor's death for the purpose of transplantation, therapy, research, or education.

Americans with Disabilities Act (ADA)

The Americans with Disabilities Act of 1990 (ADA) is a federal civil rights law that prohibits discrimination against individuals with disabilities in everyday activities, including medical services. The ADA is a wide-ranging civil rights law that prohibits discrimination based on disability. It affords similar protections against discrimination to Americans with disabilities as the Civil Rights Act of 1964, which made discrimination based on race, religion, sex, national origin, and other characteristics illegal.

5 Titles of the ADA

Title I—Employment
Title II—Public entities
Title III—Public accommodations
Title IV—Telecommunications
Title V—Miscellaneous provisions

The ADA requires access to medical care services and the facilities where the services are provided. Private hospitals or medical offices are covered by Title III of the ADA as places of public accommodation. Public hospitals and clinics and medical offices operated by state and local governments are covered by Title II of the ADA as programs of the public entities. Both Title II and Title III of the ADA and Section 504 require that medical care providers provide individuals with disabilities:

1. full and equal access to their health care services and facilities; and
2. reasonable modifications to policies, practices, and procedures when necessary to make health care services fully available to individuals with disabilities, unless the modifications would fundamentally alter the nature of the services (i.e. alter the essential nature of the services).

Accessible examination room has features that make it possible for patients with mobility disabilities, including those who use wheelchairs, to receive appropriate medical care. These features allow the patient to enter the examination room, move around in the room, and utilize the accessible equipment provided. The features that make this possible are:

1. an accessible route to and through the room;
2. an entry door with adequate clear width, maneuvering clearance, and accessible hardware;

3. appropriate models and placement of accessible examination equipment (See Part 4 for detailed discussion of accessible examination equipment.); and

4. adequate clear floor space inside the room for side transfers and use of lift equipment.

New and altered examination rooms must meet requirements of the ADA Standards for Accessible Design. Accessible examination rooms may need additional floor space to accommodate transfers and for certain equipment, such as a floor lift. The number of examination rooms with accessible equipment needed by the medical care provider depends on the size of the practice, the patient population, and other factors. One such exam room may be sufficient in a small doctor's practice, while more will likely be necessary in a large clinic.

Entry Doors

Under the ADA Standards for Accessible Design, an accessible doorway must have a minimum clear opening width of 32 inches when the door is opened to 90 degrees. Maneuvering clearances on either side of the door that comply with the ADA Standards must be provided. In addition, the door hardware must not require tight twisting, pinching, or grasping in order to use it. Keep in mind that the hallway outside of the door and the space inside the door should be kept free of boxes, chairs, or equipment, so that they do not interfere with the maneuvering clearance or accessible route.

Clear Floor and Turning Space Inside Examination Rooms

In order for accessible equipment to be usable by an individual who uses a wheelchair or other mobility device, that individual must be able to approach the exam table and any other elements of the room to which patients have access. The exam table must have sufficient clear floor space next to it so that an individual using a wheelchair can approach the side of the table for transfer onto it. The minimum amount of space required is 30 inches by 48 inches. Clear floor space is needed along at least one side of an adjustable height examination table. Because some individuals can only transfer from the right or left side, providing clear floor space on both sides of the table allows one accessible table to serve both right and left side transfers. Another way to allow transfers to either side of exam tables, particularly when more than one accessible examination room is available, is to provide a reverse furniture layout in another accessible examination room.

The room should also have enough turning space for an individual using a wheelchair to make an 180-degree turn, using a clear space of 60 inches in diameter or a 60-inch by 60-inch T-shaped space. Movable chairs and other objects, such as waste baskets, should be moved aside if necessary to provide sufficient clear floor space for maneuvering and turning. When a portable patient lift or stretcher is to be used, additional clear floor space will be needed to maneuver the lift or stretcher. Ceiling-mounted lifts, on the other hand, do not require the additional maneuvering clear floor space because these lifts are mounted overhead.

Features of an Accessible Examination Room

1 A clear floor space, 30" X 48" minimum, adjacent to the exam table and adjoining accessible route make it possible to do a side transfer.

2 Adjustable height accessible exam table lowers for transfers.

3 Providing space between table and wall allows staff to assist with patient transfers and positioning. When additional space is provided, transfers may be made from both sides.

4 Amount of floor space needed beside and at the end of exam table will vary depending on the method of patient transfer and lift equipment size.

5 Accessible route connects to other accessible public and common use spaces.

6 Accessible entry door has 32" minimum clear opening width with the door open at 90 degrees.

7 Maneuvering clearances are needed at the door to the room.

An accessible exam table or chair should have at least have the following:

1. Ability to lower to the height of the wheelchair seat, 17-19 inches from the floor; and

2. Elements to stabilize and support a person during transfer and while on the table, such as rails, straps, stabilization cushions, wedges, or rolled up towels.

Typical Transfer Techniques: Staff Assistance and Patient Lifts

Some individuals will need additional assistance to get on and off an exam table, even if it lowers to 17-19 inches from the floor. The kind of assistance needed will depend on the patient's disability. The provider should ask the patient if he or she needs assistance, and if so, what is the best way to help and what extra equipment, if any, is needed.

Some individuals will need only a steady hand from a staff person in order to transfer safely to the exam table. Other individuals will need simple tools such as a transfer board (a product made of a smooth rigid material which acts as a supporting bridge between a wheelchair and another surface, along which the individual slides) or sheet. Individuals using a transfer board may need assistance from a staff person Patients who can complete an independent transfer may prefer to do so for reasons of safety and simplicity.

Using Patient Lifts

Medical providers may need a lift in order to transfer some patients safely onto an exam table. Patient lifts may move along the floor or be mounted on an overhead track attached to the ceiling or to a free-standing frame. A staff person operates the lift. To use the lift, a sling is positioned under the individual while sitting in the wheelchair. Then the sling is attached to the lift so the staff person can move the individual to the examination surface. Once over the surface, the individual is lowered onto the table, stabilized, and then the sling is detached from the lift. The sling may remain under the patient during the exam or may be removed, depending on the exam. A variety of slings are available to provide different kinds of support. Using lifts provides better security for the patient than being lifted by medical staff because there is less likelihood that the individual will be dropped or hurt in the process. Patient lifts also protect health care providers from injuries caused by lifting patients.

Scales

A patient's weight is essential medical information used for diagnostics and treatment. Too often, individuals who use wheelchairs are not weighed at the doctor's office or hospital, even though patients without disabilities are routinely weighed, because the provider does not have a scale that can accommodate a wheelchair. Medical providers should have an accessible scale with a platform large enough to fit a wheelchair, and with a high weight capacity for weighing an individual while seated in his or her wheelchair. Other options may include a scale integrated into a patient lift, hospital bed, or exam table.
Accessible Scale
1   Sloped surface provides access to scale platform -- no abrupt level changes at floor or platform.
2   Edge protection at drop off.

3   Large platform to accommodate various wheelchair sizes.
4   Provide maneuvering space to pull onto and off the scale.

Staff Training

A critical, but often overlooked component to ensuring success is adequate and ongoing training of medical practitioners and staff. Purchasing accessible medical equipment will not provide access if no one knows how to operate it. Staff must also know which examination and procedure rooms are accessible and where portable, accessible medical equipment is stored. Whenever new equipment to provide accessible care is received, staff should be immediately trained on its proper use and maintenance. New staff should receive training as soon as they come on the job and all staff should undergo periodic refresher training during each year. Finally, training staff to properly assist with transfers and lifts, and to use positioning aids correctly will minimize the chance of injury for both patients and staff. Staff should be instructed to ask patients with disabilities if they need help before providing assistance and, if they do, how best they can help. People with mobility disabilities are not all the same - they use mobility devices of different types, sizes and weight, transfer in different ways, and have varying levels of physical ability. Make sure that staff know, especially if they are unsure, that it is not only permissible, but encouraged, to ask questions. Understanding what assistance, if any, is needed and how to provide it, will go a long way toward providing safe and accessible health care for people with mobility disabilities.

NEW: The Americans with Disabilities Act (ADA) Amendments Act of 2008 was signed into law on September 25, 2008 and becomes effective January 1, 2009.

References:
a.   *Washington State Legislature, Revised Code of Washington (RCW), Title 68, Chapter 68.64, Section 68.64.010*
b.   *Centers for Disease Control and Prevention:* http://www.cdc.gov/tb/education
c.   *Civil Rights Act of 1964 Archived 14 November 2009 at WebCite*
d.   *Americans with Disabilities Act, Access To Medical Care For Individuals With Mobility Disabilities, July 2010*
e.   *CFR Title 42; Chapter IV; Subchapter G; Part 483; Subpart B*
f.   *The Joint Commission. The Comprehensive Accreditation Manual for Hospitals: Human Resources.*

CHAPTER 3
END OF CHAPTER REVIEW QUESTIONS

Question Set 1: Essay Questions
50 points (5 points each)

1. Explain in brief about different types of consents?

2. Explain the features of an accessible examination room according to ADA.

3. What is the standard of care?

4. How to protect patient confidentiality?

5. What are the basic elements of negligence?

6. Explain different types of damages?

7. Summarize your findings in a case involving medical negligence.

8. Summarize your findings in a case involving medical malpractice.

9. Explain in brief Scope of Practice, Good Samaritan Act(s) and Uniform Anatomical Gift Act?

10. Explain the difference between assault and battery?

SECTION 1

CHAPTER 4: INTRODUCTION TO HUMAN ANATOMY & PHYSIOLOGY

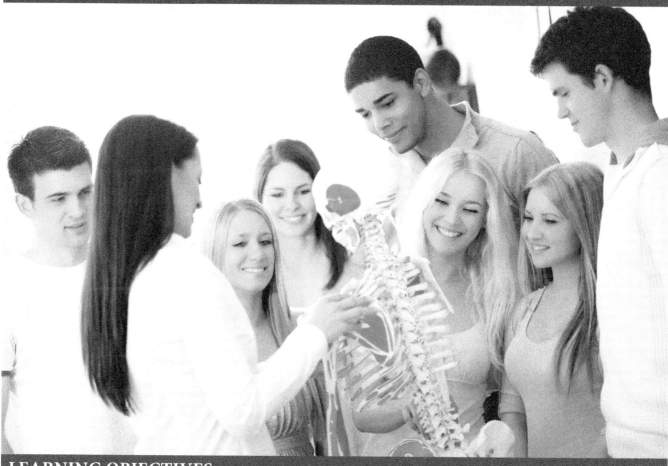

LEARNING OBJECTIVES

At the end of this chapter the student will be able to describe in brief:

- Muscular System Overview
- Skeleton System Overview
- Nervous System Overview
- Heart Overview
- Vascular System Overview
- Integumentary System Overview
- Urinary System Overview
- Digestive System Overview
- Endocrine System Overview
- Pulmonary System Overview

INTRODUCTION TO HUMAN ANATOMY & PHYSIOLOGY

HUMAN ANATOMY: MUSCULAR SYSTEM

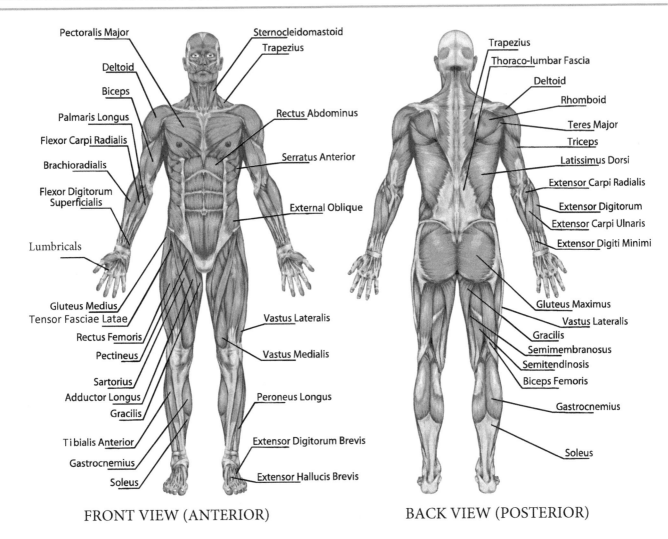

FRONT VIEW (ANTERIOR)   BACK VIEW (POSTERIOR)

FIGURE 4. 1 HUMAN BODY MUSCLES

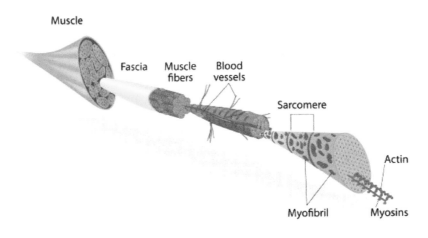

FIGURE 4. 1a MUSCLE ANATOMY

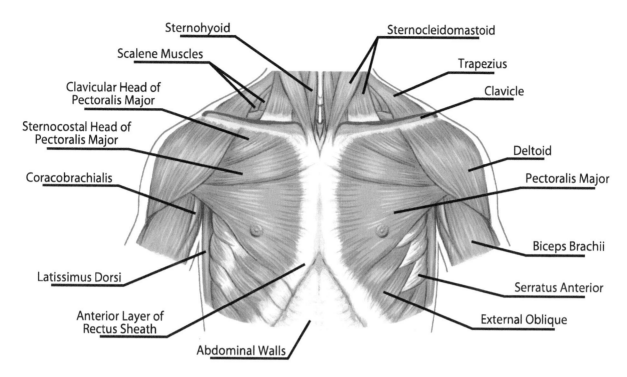

FIGURE 4.2 UPPER BODY MUSCLES FRONT VIEW (ANTERIOR)

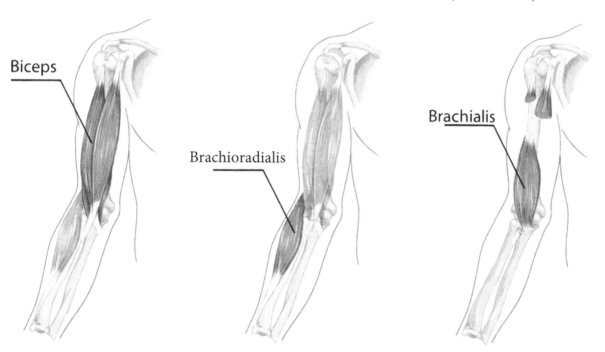

FIGURE 4.3 UPPER ARM MUSCLES FRONT VIEW (ANTERIOR)

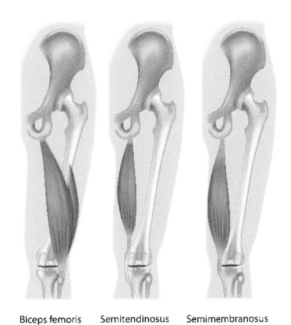

Biceps femoris   Semitendinosus   Semimembranosus

FIGURE 4.4 UPPER LEG MUSCLES BACK VIEW (POSTERIOR)

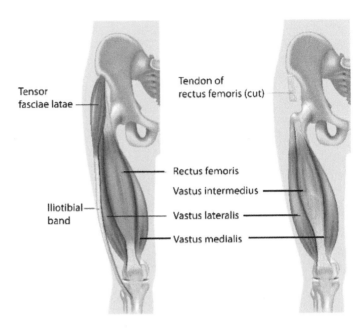

Tensor fasciae latae

Tendon of rectus femoris (cut)

Rectus femoris

Vastus intermedius

Iliotibial band

Vastus lateralis

Vastus medialis

FIGURE 4.5 UPPER LEG MUSCLES FRONT VIEW (ANTERIOR)

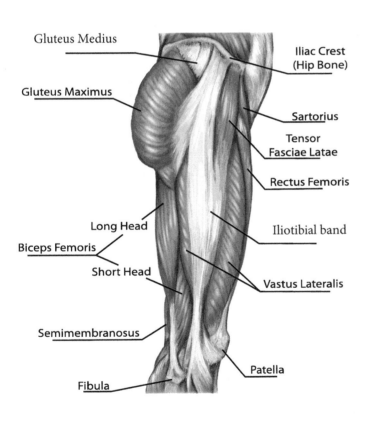

Gluteus Medius

Iliac Crest (Hip Bone)

Gluteus Maximus

Sartorius

Tensor Fasciae Latae

Rectus Femoris

Long Head

Biceps Femoris

Iliotibial band

Short Head

Semimembranosus

Vastus Lateralis

Fibula

Patella

FIGURE 4.6 UPPER LEG MUSCLES SIDE VIEW (LATERAL)

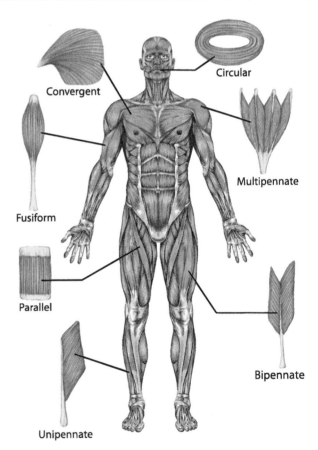

Convergent

Circular

Fusiform

Multipennate

Parallel

Unipennate

Bipennate

FIGURE 4.7 HUMAN BODY MUSCLES ACCORDING TO

THEIR SHAPES

MUSCLES AND THEIR ACTIONS

MUSCLES OF THE BACK	
Muscle	**Action**
Erector Spinae	Extension of the vertebral column
Iliocostalis	Extends and laterally flexes the trunk and neck
Multifidus	Extends and laterally flexes trunk to the same side
Semispinalis	Extends the trunk and laterally flexes the trunk
Spinalis	Extends and laterally flexes trunk and neck
Splenius	Extends and laterally flexes neck and head, head rotation to the same side

MUSCLES OF THE UPPER LIMB	
Muscle	**Action**
Anconeus	Forearm extension
Biceps Brachii	Forearm flexion, arm flexion (long head), supination
Brachialis	Forearm flexion
Brachioradialis	Forearm flexion and brings forearm into mid-prone position
Coracobrachialis	Arm flexion and adduction
Deltoid	Anterior portion: arm flexion and medial rotation; Middle portion: arm abduction; Posterior portion: arm extension and lateral rotation
Infraspinatus	Lateral rotation of the arm
Latissimus Dorsi	Arm extension and medial rotation
Levator Scapulae	Elevates the scapula
Palmaris Longus	Wrist flexion
Pectoralis Major	Adduction and medial rotation of humerus; draws scapula anteriorly and inferiorly
Pectoralis Minor	Moves the scapula forward, and downward.
Pronator Quadratus	Forearm pronation
Pronator Teres	Forearm pronation
Rhomboideus Major	Retracts and rotates the scapula inferiorly
Rhomboideus Minor	Retracts and rotates the scapula inferiorly

Serratus Anterior	Moves the scapula forward and upward; abduction and rotation of scapula
Serratus Posterior Inferior	Depresses down lower ribs
Serratus Posterior Superior	Elevates the upper ribs
Subscapularis	Medial rotation of arm and adduction of arm; assists extension of the arm
Supinator	Forearm supination
Supraspinatus	Arm abduction
Teres Major	Arm adduction, and medial rotation of the arm
Teres Minor	Lateral rotation of the arm
Trapezius	Scapula elevation, retraction and rotation
Triceps Brachii	Extends (extension) the forearm; long head extends and adducts arm

MUSCLES OF THE HEAD AND NECK

Muscle	Action
Masseter	Mandible elevation
Rectus Capitis Anterior	Head flexion
Rectus Capitis Lateralis	Head lateral flexion
Sternocleidomastoid	Bilateral muscle contraction: neck flexion and head extension. Unilateral muscle contraction: rotates head and neck to the opposite side and flexes to the same side.
Temporalis	Mandible elevation and retraction

MUSCLES OF THE THORACIC REGION

MUSCLE	ACTION
Diaphragm	Pushes the abdominal viscera inferiorly (inspiration)
External Intercostal	Stabilizes intercostal spaces during respiration. Assists in inspiration by elevating ribs
Internal Intercostal	Stabilizes intercostal spaces during inspiration. Assists in forced inspiration by elevating ribs

MUSCLES OF THE ABDOMINAL REGION

MUSCLE	ACTION
External Abdominal Oblique	Forward flexion and lateral flexion of the trunk

Internal Abdominal Oblique	Forward flexion and lateral flexion of the trunk
Psoas Major	Hip joint flexion
Pyramidalis	Pulls the linea alba inferiorly
Quadratus Lumborum	Lateral flexion of the trunk
Rectus Abdominis	Flexion of the trunk
Transversus Abdominis	Abdomen compression

MUSCLES OF THE LOWER LIMB

Muscle	Action
Adductor Brevis	Femur adduction and flexion
Adductor Longus	Femur adduction and flexion
Adductor Magnus	Femur adduction
Biceps Femoris	Extension of the thigh, flexion of the leg
Fibularis (Peroneus) Tertius	Eversion of the foot
Gastrocnemius	Flexion of the leg; plantar flexion of the foot
Gemellus, Inferior	Lateral rotation of the femur
Gemellus, Superior	Lateral rotation of the femur
Gluteus Maximus	Extension of the thigh; lateral rotation of the femur
Gluteus Medius	Abduction of the femur; medial rotation of the thigh
Gluteus Minimus	Abduction of the femur; medial rotation of the thigh
Gracilis	Adduction of the thigh, flexion and medial rotation of the thigh, flexion of the leg
Iliacus	Flexion of the thigh
Iliopsoas	Flexion of the thigh; flexion and laterally flexes the lumbar vertebral column
Obturator Externus	Lateral rotation of the thigh
Obturator Internus	Lateral rotation and abduction of the thigh when flexed
Pectineus	Adduction, flexion, and medial rotation of the thigh
Piriformis	Lateral rotation and abduction of the thigh
Plantaris	Flexion of the leg; plantar flexion of the foot
Popliteus	Lateral rotation of the femur on tibia (if tibia is fixed); Medial rotation of the tibia on femur (if femur is fixed)

Psoas Major	Flexion of the thigh; flexion & laterally flexes the lumbar vertebral column
Quadratus Femoris	Lateral rotation of the thigh
Quadriceps	Extension of the knee; rectus femoris contraction causes flexion at the thigh
Rectus Femoris	Extension of the leg, flexion of the thigh
Sartorius	Flexion, abduction and lateral rotation of the thigh; flexion of the leg
Semimembranosus	Extension of the thigh, flexion of the leg
Semitendinosus	Extension of the thigh, flexion of the leg
Soleus	Plantar flexion of the foot
Tensor Fasciae Latae	Flexion, abduction, and medial rotation of the thigh
Tibialis Anterior	Dorsiflexion and inversion the foot
Tibialis Posterior	Plantarflexion of the foot; inversion of the foot
Vastus Intermedius	Leg extension
Vastus Lateralis	Leg extension
Vastus Medialis	Leg extension

Some important terms and their meanings:

Bone:	The dense, semirigid, porous, calcified connective tissue forming the major portion of the skeleton.
Ligament:	Band of tough, flexible, fibrous connective tissue that connects a bone to another bone.
Tendon:	Tough band of fibrous connective tissue that connects muscle to bone.
Cartilage:	Flexible connective tissue that covers the ends of bones at a joint.
Membrane:	Layer of tissue covering a surface.
Joint Fluid:	Viscid lubricating fluid secreted by the synovial membrane, it lubricates and cushions the joint.
Bursae:	A bursa is a small sac that is filled with fluid. This sac acts like a cushion between two structures such as the bone and muscles, skin, or tendon(s).
Strain:	Occurs in a muscle.
Sprain:	Occurs in a ligament.
Muscle fibres	Type 1: slow contraction (endurance activity), **Type 2a: fast contraction (strength activity)**, Type 2b: very fast contraction (power activity).

ANATOMICAL MOVEMENTS

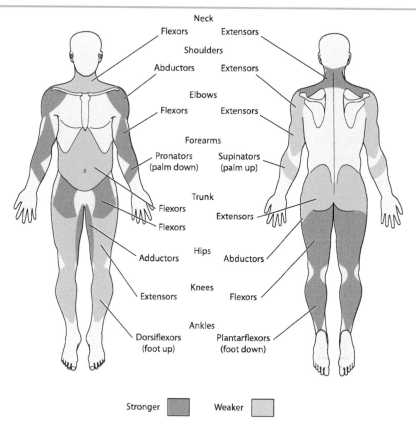

FIGURE 4.8 ANATOMICAL MOVEMENTS

MOVEMENT TERMINOLOGIES	
TERMS	MEANING
Flexion	Bones coming together or when the joint angle decreases.
Extension	When joint angle increases.
Abduction	Movement away from the midline of the body.
Adduction	Movement towards the midline of the body.
Internal rotation	Inward rotation, towards the midline of the body.
External rotation	Outward rotation, away from the midline of the body.
Circumduction	Combination of all the movements.
Pronation	Elbow at mid flexed position and palm facing downwards.
Supination	Elbow at mid flexed position and palm facing upwards.
Dorsi-flexion	Ankle joint flexes towards the leg (shin bone) or toes pointing towards the leg.
Plantar-flexion	Opposite of dorsiflexion.
Inversion	Turning of the ankle joint inward.
Eversion	Turning of the ankle joint outward.

Table 4.1

HUMAN ANATOMY: SKELETON SYSTEM

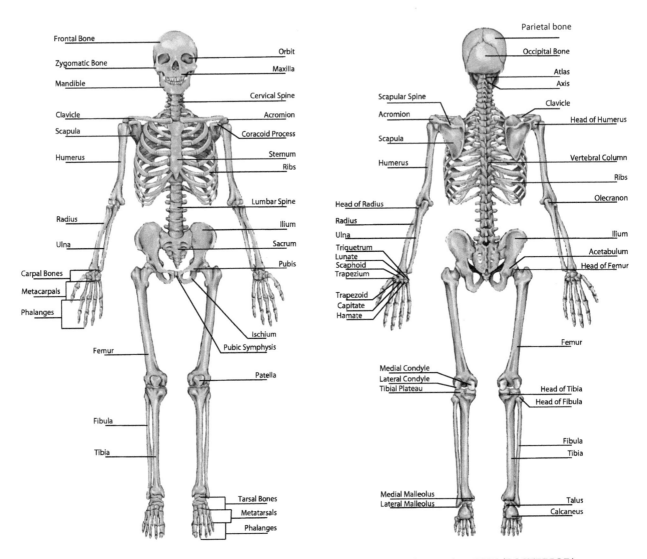

FIGURE 4.9 SKELETON SYSTEM FRONT VIEW (ANTERIOR) & BACK VIEW (POSTERIOR)

SKELETON SYSTEM IS DIVIDED INTO TWO SECTIONS

AXIAL SKELETON

A. SKULL
B. SPINAL COLUMN
C. SACRUM
D. RIBS
E. STERNUM

APPENDICULAR SKELETON

A. SHOULDER GIRDLE:
- CLAVICLE
- SCAPULA

B. PELVIC GIRDLE:
- PELVIS

C. ARMS:
- HUMERUS
- ULNA
- RADIUS

- CARPALS
- METACARPALS
- PHALANGES

D. LEGS:
- FEMUR
- PATELLA
- TIBIA
- FIBULA
- TARSALS
- METATARSALS
- PHALANGES

HUMAN ANATOMY: NERVOUS SYSTEM

Nervous system is made up of two parts:

a)   Central Nervous System (CNS) -brain and spinal cord

b)   Peripheral Nervous System (PNS) -motor neurons and sensory neurons

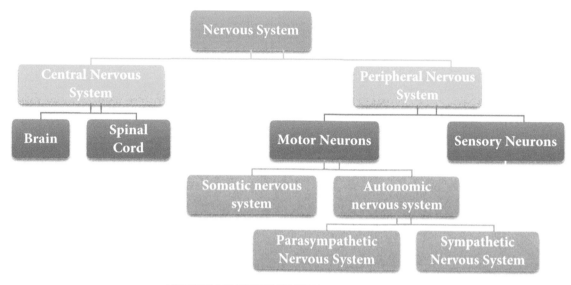

FIGURE 4.10 NERVOUS SYSTEM DIVISIONS

THE CENTRAL NERVOUS SYSTEM (CNS)

Is a part of the nervous system. It consists of two main components:

1. The spinal cord
    *   Carry and transfer signals between the brain and the rest of the body.
2. The brain
    *   Brain is located in the skull. The brain continues as the spinal cord in the vertebral canal through the foramen magnum of the skull bone.

THE PERIPHERAL NERVOUS SYSTEM (PNS)

Subdivided into the:

1) Motor
    A. Is further divided into somatic and autonomic
        a. Somatic: Controls voluntary movement to muscles.
        b. Autonomic: Controls involuntary movement to muscles (smooth muscles, cardiac muscles, glands and adipose tissues). It is divided into
            i.   Sympathetic nervous system(fight and flight).
            ii. Parasympathetic nervous system (rest and digest).
    B. Motor neurons travels from the CNS to the muscles and glands.
2) Sensory
    a. Sensory neurons travel from stimulus receptors (site of stimulus) to the CNS to inform about the stimuli received. Common sensations that can act as a stimuli are: vision, auditory (hearing), somatic sensation (touch), gustatory (taste), olfaction (smell) and vestibular (balance-/movement).

HUMAN ANATOMY: HEART (CARDIOVASCULAR)

The pathway of blood flow through the heart

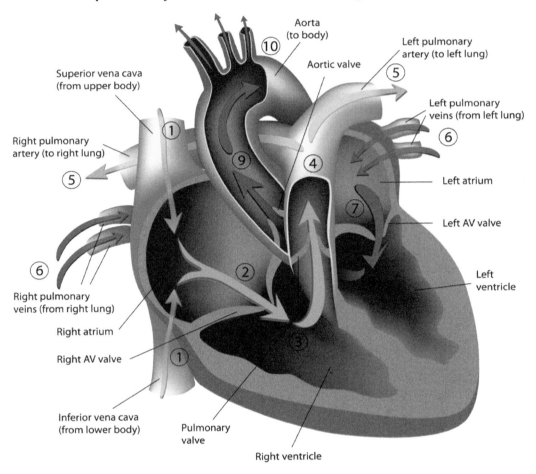

FIGURE 4.11 ANATOMY OF HEART

	RIGHT	LEFT
UPPER CHAMBERS	**ATRIUM** Receives deoxygenated blood from superior and inferior vena cava.	**ATRIUM** Receives oxygenated blood from both (right and left) lungs via the pulmonary vein.
LOWER CHAMBERS	**VENTRICLE** Receives the deoxygenated blood from right atrium via the tricuspid valve and pumps it out of the heart via the pulmonary artery to the right and the left lung.	**VENTRICLE** Receives oxygenated blood from left atrium via the bicuspid valve and pumps it out of the heart to the rest of the body via the aorta.

Table 4.2 HEART: INTERNAL BLOOD FLOW

HUMAN ANATOMY: BLOOD VESSELS (CARDIOVASCULAR)

Vessels of the circulatory system are the aorta, arteries, arterioles, capillaries, venules, veins, and vena cava.

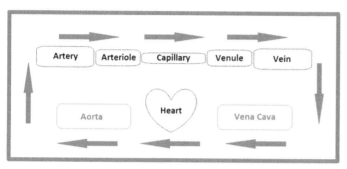

FIGURE 4.12
Direction of blood flow from the heart and back into the heart

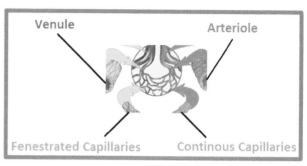

FIGURE 4.13
Venule, Capillaries, and Arteries

ARTERIAL SYSTEM

Arterial system is comprised of the aorta, arteries, and arterioles. Walls of the aorta and arteries are formed by three layers.

FUNCTIONS:

- Carries oxygenated blood (oxygen-rich blood) from the heart to the rest of the body.

STRUCTURE:

- **Layers of the arteries are as follows:**
    1. Outer tunica adventitia
    2. Middle tunica media, which is formed by smooth muscles.
    3. Inner tunica intima, which is made up of endothelium.

The diameter of the arterial branches decrease (becomes narrow) and the walls become thinner while reaching the organ. The largest artery (aorta) has the largest diameter and is gradually decreased into the terminal arterioles. Arterioles are further continued as capillaries. Capillaries are the sites of nutrient and waste exchange between the blood and body cells.

VASODILATION:

Vasodilation refers to the **widening (increase in diameter)** of the blood vessels.
Dilation (increase in diameter) of the blood vessels causes the flow of blood to increase due to a decrease in vascular resistance. Hence, vasodilation **(increase in diameter)** of blood vessels (artery) causes a decrease in blood pressure.

VASOCONSTRICTION:

Vasoconstriction refers to the **narrowing (decrease in diameter)** of the blood vessels.
Constriction (decrease in diameter) of the blood vessels causes the flow of blood to decrease due to increase in vascular resistance. Hence, vasoconstriction (decrease in diameter) of blood vessels (artery) causes an increase in blood pressure.

VENOUS SYSTEM

Capillaries further continue as venule, veins and vena cava (superior and inferior venae cavae).

FUNCTIONS:

- Carries deoxygenated blood from the rest of the body to the heart.

STRUCTURE:

- Layers of the veins are as follows:
  1. Outer tunica adventitia
  2. Middle tunica media
  3. Inner tunica intima

CAPILLARY TYPES:

1. **Continuous Capillaries**
2. **Fenestrated Capillaries**

FUNCTIONS:

- The main function of the capillaries is to give oxygen to the tissues from the artery and collect carbon dioxide from the tissues back into the vein.

STRUCTURE:

- **Layer**

Consists of a single *layer* of endothelial cell.

	Artery	Vein	Capillaries
Lumen	Narrow	Wide	Very Narrow
Function	Carry Oxygen	Carry Carbon dioxide	Diffuses Oxygen and Collected Carbon Dioxide
Pressure	High Pressure	Low Pressure	Gradually Falls
Permeability	No	No	Yes

Table 4.3 DIFFERENCE BETWEEN ARTERY, VEIN, AND CAPILLARIES

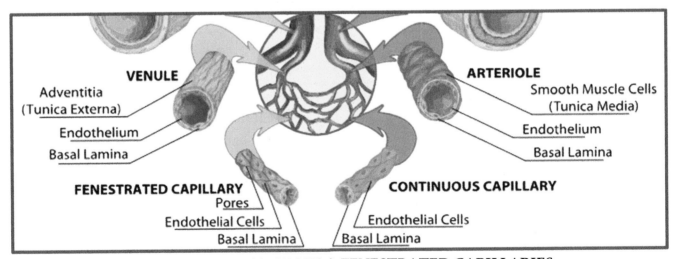

FIGURE 4.14 CONTINUOUS & FENESTRATED CAPILLARIES

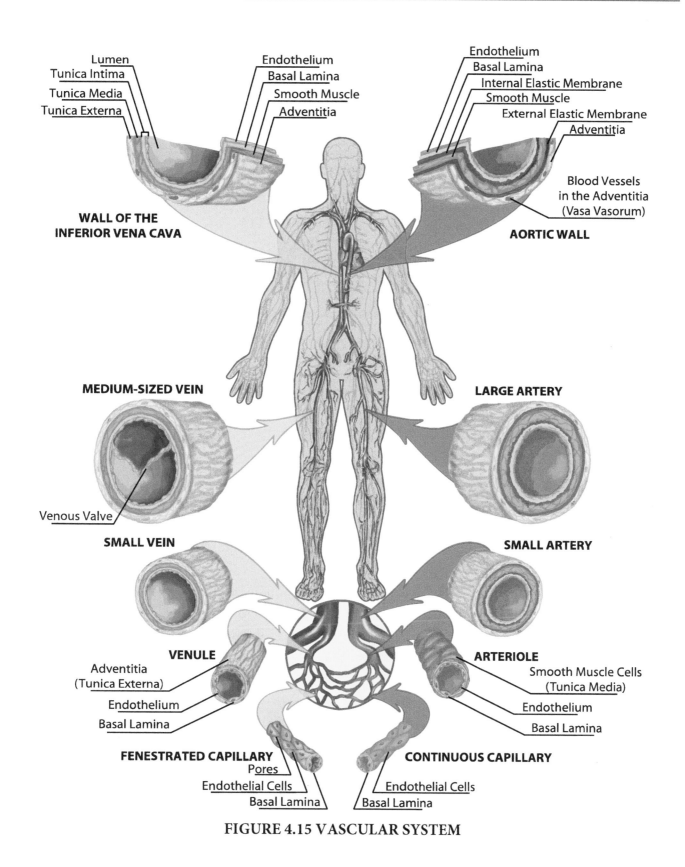

FIGURE 4.15 VASCULAR SYSTEM

HUMAN ANATOMY: INTEGUMENTARY SYSTEM

The Integumentary system is an organ that includes skin, its derivatives (sweat and oil glands), nails, and hair.

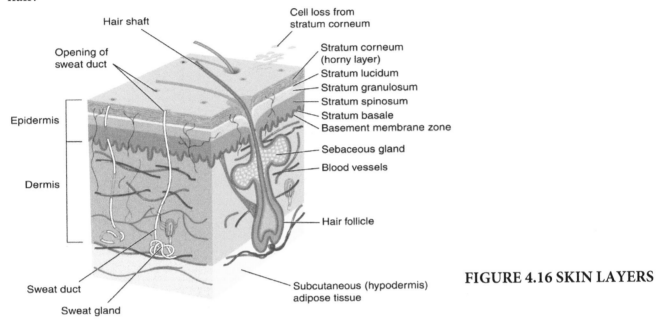

FIGURE 4.16 SKIN LAYERS

SKIN LAYERS

INNERMOST LAYER: HYPODERMIS/SUBCUTANEOUS TISSUE

The hypodermis is the innermost layer of the skin. It is composed of adipose tissue. The hypodermis consists of fat tissue below the dermis that serves the function of insulating the body from extreme temperatures, conserves energy and provides shock absorption. Cells of the hypodermis layer stores nutrients and energy. The hypodermis layer is slightly thicker in females than males.

MIDDLE LAYER: DERMIS

The dermis is the middle layer of the skin located between the hypodermis and the epidermis. This layer on average is about 2-4 mm thick.

THE DERMIS CONSISTS OF THE FOLLOWING LAYERS:

OUTER PAPILLARY LAYER: Consists of loose connective tissue that supports and nourishes the epidermis.

- Contain capillaries and innervated (nerves) skin surface.
- Has dermal papillae projecting between epidermal ridges.
- Contains the free sensory nerve endings and structures called meissners corpuscles. If these corpuscles are stimulated, they register the sensation of touch. According to some theories, the number of these corpuscles are age related and drops leading to decrease in the sensation of touch as age advances.

DEEP RETICULAR LAYER: Consists of interwoven meshwork of dense irregular connective tissue containing both collagen and elastic fibers.

- Elastic fibers: This fiber give the skin ability to return to its original form after a stretch force is applied.
- Collagen fibers: Collagen fibers extends into the subcutaneous layer below. The collagen gives the skin strength. The presence of glycosaminoglycans, a moisture binding molecule, it further enables the collagen fibers to retain water. This retaining of water provides moisture to the uppermost layer of the skin.
- Nerves, Blood and lymph vessels.

Glands of the dermis:

Two types:

1. Sweat glands
2. Sebaceous glands

The sweat gland secretes sweat which is composed of water, salt, and other chemicals along with some waste products. As sweat evaporates off the skin, it helps cool the body.
The sweat glands also known as sudoriferous glands produces sweat in response to heat and stress.

Two Types of Sweat Glands

1. Apocrine Sweat Gland: secrete odorous sweat
2. Eccrine Sweat Gland: secrete odorless sweat

The sebaceous glands secrete oil and wax-like secretion called sebum. Sebum keeps the skin moist and soft and acts as a barrier against foreign substances (germs).

The hair follicles present in this layer helps in regulating body temperature, providing protection from injury, and increase sensation. The blood vessels found in this layer provide nutrients required for the skin and assist in regulating body temperature. Hot climate causes the blood vessels to go into vasodilation allowing more blood to circulate near the surface of the skin, so that the heat can escape. Cold climate causes the blood vessels to go into vasoconstriction, which results in retaining the temperature of the body.

OUTERMOST LAYER: EPIDERMIS

The epidermis is the outermost layer of the skin. Consists of five horizontal layers.

1ST Layer: **Stratum Basale**

2ND Layer: **Stratum Spinosum**

3RD Layer: **Stratum Granulosum**

4TH Layer: **Stratum Lucidum**

5TH Layer: **Stratum Corneum**

Melanocytes are found in stratum basale layer of the epidermis and are responsible for the producing a skin pigment called **melanin**. This pigment helps in protection of the skin against ultraviolet radiation (UV rays).

HUMAN ANATOMY: URINARY SYSTEM

KIDNEYS

A pair of organs found in the abdominal cavity. Located against the back muscles on either side of the spine.

URETERS

Two tubes that run from the kidney to the bladder. Urine is conveyed through the ureters by peristalsis and gravity.

URINARY BLADDER

The bladder is a hollow sac situated towards the front of the lower part of the abdomen. The bladder stores urine.

URETHRA

Urine is conveyed from the bladder through the urethra. On an average, the female urethra is about 10cms long and male urethra is about 20cms long. The opening at the end of the urethra is called the urinary meatus.

THE NEPHRON

The nephron is the basic working unit of the kidney. Blood enters the nephron and passes through the structures of the nephron to be filtered. Most of the water and many substances that are needed by the body are returned to the circulation. Various factors affect the production of urine. It includes; age, illness, amount and type of fluids (ingested), the amount of salt intake, and medications.

FUNCTION

- Removes metabolic wastes from the circulatory system.
- Plays a part in red blood cell formation.
- Assists in the regulation of blood pressure.
- Maintains the balance of body fluids in the body.

EXCRETION OF URINE

Urination (also called 'voiding' or 'micturition') is the process of emptying the bladder. As the bladder fills with urine, nerve impulses carry the message to the central nervous system (CNS) that the bladder is full. The central nervous system then sends a message back to the bladder via the motor nerves causing the bladder to contract and the sphincter to relax. This is a 'reflex' that gives rise to the urge to urinate.

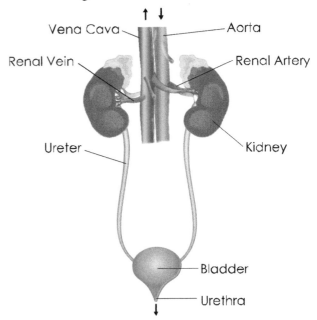

FIGURE 4.16 PARTS OF URINARY SYSTEM

HUMAN ANATOMY: DIGESTIVE SYSTEM

MOUTH

The process of digestion begins in the mouth where food is chewed until it reaches a consistency whereby it can be swallowed. The following accessory structures aid this early stage of digestion:

- **Tongue**: a muscle that is covered by taste buds. It assists the process of chewing and maneuvering food to a position where it can be swallowed easily.
- **Salivary glands**: begin the process of chemical digestion through the secretion of the enzyme, salivary amylase. This enzyme begins the process of breaking down carbohydrates. Saliva also moistens the food which helps it to be swallowed more easily.
- **Teeth**: breaks food down mechanically into smaller particles that may be ingested more easily.
- **Pharynx**: allows the passage of both food and air.
- **Esophagus**: a tube that leads to the stomach.

ESOPHAGUS

The esophagus is the tube connecting the mouth to the stomach. It lies in front of the vertebral column and behind the trachea and heart.

STOMACH

Food remains in the stomach for between 3 to 4 hours. During this time it is further broken down by the muscular churning action of the stomach. Powerful gastric juices are also secreted by the cells of the stomach, which contribute to chemical digestion. The food ends up in a semi-liquid form that is called "**chyme**".

INTESTINES

Digested material is moved through the intestine via a process of wavelike muscular contractions called peristalsis. The process of digestion is completed in the small intestine. At this stage the nutrients that the body needs are absorbed through the walls of the small intestine.

The waste material then moves into the large intestine where water is reabsorbed, thereby changing it into a more solid form, ready to be excreted through the rectum.

LIVER

Large gland that is divided into **4 lobes**. It carries out many vital metabolic functions such as:

- Manufactures bile that break down fats.
- Helps maintain normal blood glucose levels.
- Produces the blood proteins; prothrombin and fibrinogen which have a role in blood clotting.

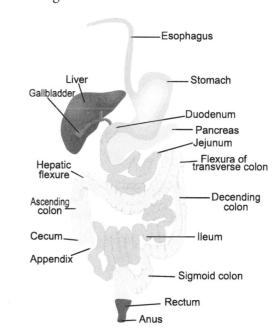

FIGURE 4.17 PARTS OF DIGESTIVE SYSTEM

- Stores iron derived from food or the byproduct of the breakdown of worn out red blood cells.
- Stores vitamins A, D, E, & K that have been extracted from ingested food.

GALLBLADDER

The gallbladder concentrates and stores bile that is produced in the liver. It then releases the bile when it is needed for digestion after a fatty meal.

PANCREAS

The pancreas is an endocrine and exocrine gland. It produces pancreatic juices, containing enzymes that play a vital role in the chemical digestion of food. The pancreas also produces the hormones; insulin and glucagon directly into the bloodstream.

Function of digestive system

The Digestive System performs the following vital activities:

- **Ingestion**: to take in and absorb food.
- **Digestion** which may take two forms:
  1. **Mechanical breakdown** of food by chewing and the action of muscles within the digestive tract.
  2. **Chemical breakdown** of food by enzymes produced at various stages of the digestive tract.

Absorption is where substances pass through the gastrointestinal tract into the bloodstream. 90 % of the absorption of all nutrients take place in the small intestine.

Elimination is the process by which undigested food leaves the body. This elimination is known as defecation.

Swallowing

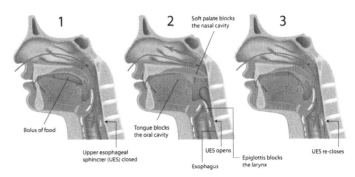

Fig 4.17a STAGES OF SWALLOWING

HUMAN ANATOMY: ENDOCRINE SYSTEM

The endocrine system is composed of glands and hormones. Hormones are secreted by endocrine glands directly into the bloodstream. The body contains many different types of hormones that are designed to regulate the body's activities. Each hormone is specialized to target particular types of cells, like a lock and key. The hormone will only work if it comes into contact with the target cells.

HORMONES

Hormones are chemical substances secreted by endocrine glands directly into the blood. Hormones are classified as proteins and steroids. Hormones are aimed at the 'receptors' of target organs. These receptors are located on the outer surface of the cells of those organs.

GLANDS

Glands are located throughout the body.

The **pituitary gland** is the master gland and is located in the brain behind the eyes at the base of the frontal lobe. It is divided into two parts - the anterior and the posterior pituitary. Each part secretes specific hormones that affect the action of other glands in the body.

The **hypothalamus** is located above the pituitary. It releases hormones that either stimulate or inhibit the release of hormones by the anterior pituitary.

The **thyroid gland** is located in the neck near the 'Adams Apple'. It produces a hormone that regulates growth and general metabolism.

The **thymus** is located in the chest above the xiphoid process and gets smaller after puberty, but plays a part in the body's immune system.

The **parathyroid** is located within the thyroid capsule. It produces a hormone that regulates the level of phosphorus and calcium in the blood along with one of the hormones of the thyroid gland.

The **pancreas** produces insulin and glucagon, which help regulate blood glucose levels. **Insulin acts to lower** blood sugar level, and **glucagon acts to raise** blood sugar level.

The **adrenal glands** lie on top of the kidneys and secrete hormones that help the body grow and adapt to stress.

The **ovaries** in the female secrete estrogen and progesterone. The rise and fall of these hormones determine the menstrual cycle and are important in causing the release of the ovum (egg) and in the maintenance of pregnancy. They are also responsible for the development of secondary sex characteristics.

The **testes** in the male produce testosterone, which causes the production of sperm. Testosterone is also responsible for the development of secondary sex characteristics.

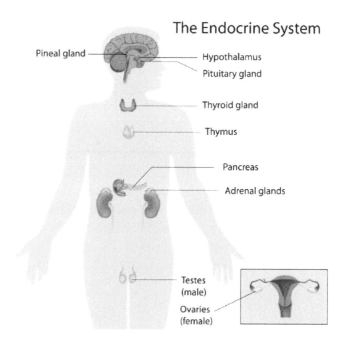

FIGURE 4.18 ENDOCRINE GLANDS

HUMAN ANATOMY: PULMONARY SYSTEM

The respiratory system is composed of various structures and organs that ensure that the body is able to maintain its internal environment through the exchange of air between the lungs and the atmosphere. In order to survive, the body needs a constant supply of oxygen, which it obtains from the air. The body also needs to dispose of carbon dioxide, made as a waste product from the process of cell metabolism. The inhalation of oxygen and the exhalation of carbon dioxide, occurs through the process of respiration or breathing.

STRUCTURE

The respiratory system is comprised of the:

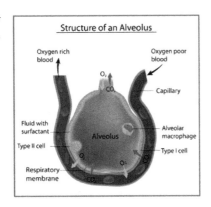

- nose
- nasopharynx
- mouth
- sinuses
- larynx
- trachea
- bronchi
- lungs
- alveoli

The respiratory system consists the upper and the lower respiratory tracts.

- **The upper respiratory tract** consists of the respiratory organs located outside the chest cavity (nose, nasal pharynx, larynx and upper trachea).
- **The lower respiratory tract** consists of organs located in the chest cavity: the lower trachea, bronchi, bronchioles, alveoli and the lungs. The lower parts of the bronchi, the bronchioles and alveoli are all located in the lungs. The alveoli are the point at which gas exchange takes place. Pleura is a membrane that covers the lungs. The muscles that form the chest cavity are also part of the lower respiratory tract. The respiratory center in the brain, which is located in the medulla oblongata, regulates breathing.

FUNCTION

The function of the respiratory system (pulmonary system) is to supply oxygen and to collect carbon dioxide from cells.

RESPIRATION

Respiration involves the passage of air in and out of the lungs. Air enters the body via the nasal passages, where it is warmed, moistened and filtered. Air then passes down through the pharynx and into the larynx and trachea. The air continues into the right and left bronchi and then into the lungs. In the lungs the bronchi then branch into smaller bronchioles, that each have air sacs called alveoli, attached to them. The exchange of oxygen and carbon dioxide takes place at this level, between the alveoli and the blood capillaries. Through this process oxygen enters the bloodstream and can be transported around the body.

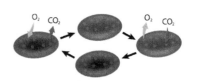

FIGURE 4.19a Gas Exchange at alveolar level

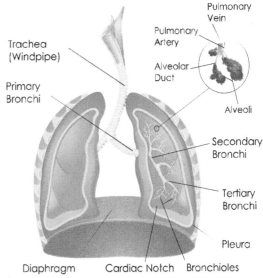

FIGURE 4.19b Pulmonary System

References; http://www.niams.nih.gov/health_info/bursitis/bursitis_ff.asp

CHAPTER 4

END OF CHAPTER REVIEW QUESTIONS

Question Set 1: Fill in the Missing Answer
58 points (1 point each)

MUSCLE NAME	THEIR ACTIONS
1. Erector Spinae	
2. Iliocostalis	
3. Multifidus	
4. Brachialis	
5. Brachioradialis	
6. Coracobrachialis	
7. Deltoid	
8. Infraspinatus	
9. Latissimus Dorsi	
10. Levator Scapulae	
11. Subscapularis	
12. Supinator	
13. Supraspinatus	
14. Teres Major	
15. Teres Minor	
16. Trapezius	
17. Triceps Brachii	
18. Masseter	
19. Rectus Capitis Anterior	
20. Rectus Capitis Lateralis	
21. Sternocleidomastoid	
22. Temporalis	
23. Diaphragm	
24. External Intercostal	
25. Internal Intercostal	
26. External Abdominal Oblique	
27. Internal Abdominal Oblique	
28. Psoas Major	
29. Quadratus Femoris	
30. Quadriceps	
31. Rectus Femoris	
32. Sartorius	
33. Semimembranosus	
34. Semitendinosus	
35. Soleus	
36. Tensor Fasciae Latae	
37. Tibialis Anterior	
38. Tibialis Posterior	

39. Vastus Intermedius	
40. Vastus Lateralis	
41. Vastus Medialis	
42. Pectoralis Major	
43. Pectoralis Minor	
44. Pronator Quadratus	
45. Pronator Teres	
46. Rhomboideus Major	
47. Rhomboideus Minor	
48. Serratus Anterior	
49. Pectoralis Major	
50. Pectoralis Minor	
51. Pronator Quadratus	
52. Adductor Brevis	
53. Adductor Longus	
54. Adductor Magnus	
55. Gastrocnemius	
56. Gluteus Maximus	
57. Gluteus Medius	
58. Gluteus Minimus	

Question set 2: Fill in the Answers in column "A"   13 points (1 point each)

Column A	Column B
1.	Bones coming together or when the joint angle decreases.
2.	When joint angle increases.
3.	Movement away from the midline of the body.
4.	Movement towards the midline of the body.
5.	Inward rotation towards the midline of the body.
6.	Outward rotation away from the midline of the body.
7.	Combination of all the movements.
8.	Elbow at mid flexed position and palm facing downwards.
9.	Elbow at mid flexed position and palm facing upwards.
10.	Ankle joint flexes towards the leg (shin bone) or toes pointing towards the leg.
11.	Opposite of dorsiflexion.
12.	Ankle joint turns inward.
13.	Ankle joint turns outward.

Question set 3: Multiple Choice   7 points (1 point each)

1) Bones in the leg includes all the following except:
   a. Femur
   b. Humerus
   c. Tibia
   d. Fibula

2) Bones in the arm includes all the following except:
   a. Ulna
   b. Radius
   c. Carpals
   d. Patella

3) Which of the following event occurs in the right ventricle
   a. Receives deoxygenated blood from superior and inferior vena cava.
   b. Receives oxygenated blood from both (right and left) lungs via the pulmonary vein.
   c. Receives the deoxygenated blood from right atrium via the tricuspid valve and pumps it out of the heart via the pulmonary artery to the right and the left lung.
   d. Receives oxygenated blood from left atrium via the bicuspid valve and pumps it out of the heart to the rest of the body via the aorta.

4) Which of the following structure carries oxygenated blood (oxygen-rich blood) from the heart to the rest of the body.
   a. artery
   b. vein
   c. nerve
   d. capillary

5) The main function of the _____ is to give oxygen to the tissues from the artery and collect carbon dioxide from the tissues back into the vein.
   a. arteries
   b. veins
   c. nerves
   d. capillaries

6) The function of the urinary bladder is to _____ urine.
   a. Produce
   b. Store
   c. Eliminate
   d. Process

7) Which of the following is not a function of the urinary system?
   a. Removes metabolic wastes from the circulatory system.
   b. Plays a part in red blood cell formation.
   c. Assists in the regulation of blood pressure.
   d. Chemical breakdown of food by enzymes produced at various stages.

Question set 4: True or False (T/F) CIRCLE ANSWERS   20 points (1 point each)

1. A ligament connects a bone to a muscle.
   Answer: TRUE OR FALSE

2. Tendon is a flexible connective tissue that covers the ends of bones at a joint.
   Answer: TRUE OR FALSE

3. The thyroid gland is the master gland and is located in the brain behind the eyes at the base of the frontal lobe. It is divided into two parts - the anterior and the posterior pituitary.
   Answer: TRUE OR FALSE

4. The pituitary gland lies in the neck near the 'Adams Apple'. It produces a hormone that regulates growth and general metabolism.
   Answer: TRUE OR FALSE

5. The pancreas produces insulin and glucagon, which help regulate blood glucose levels. Insulin acts to lower blood sugar level and glucagon acts to raise blood sugar level.
   Answer: TRUE OR FALSE

6. The adrenal glands lie on top of the kidneys and secrete hormones that help the body grow and adapt to stress.
Answer: TRUE OR FALSE

7. The ovaries in the male secrete estrogen and progesterone.
Answer: TRUE OR FALSE

8. The testes in the male produce testosterone, which causes the production of sperm. Testosterone is also responsible for the development of secondary sex characteristics.
Answer: TRUE OR FALSE

9. The urinary bladder concentrates and stores bile that is produced in the liver. It then releases the bile when it is needed for digestion after a fatty meal.
Answer: TRUE OR FALSE

10. The large intestine is a large gland that is divided into four lobes. It carries out many vital metabolic functions such as: Manufactures bile that breaks down fats. Helps maintain normal blood glucose levels.
Answer: TRUE OR FALSE

11. The neuron is the basic working unit of the kidney. Blood enters the nephron under pressure and passes through the structures of the nephron to be filtered.
Answer: TRUE OR FALSE

12. The dermis is middle layer of the skin located between the hypodermis and the epidermis. This layer on average is about 2-4 mm thick.
Answer: TRUE OR FALSE

13. Elastic fibers contains elastin that gives the skin its ability to return back to its original shape after application of stretching force.
Answer: TRUE OR FALSE

14. The ureter is the tube connecting the mouth to the stomach. It lies in front of the vertebral column and behind the trachea (breathing tube) and heart.
Answer: TRUE OR FALSE

15. Vasodilation refers to the narrowing of blood vessels.
Answer: TRUE OR FALSE

16. Urination also called defecation is the process of emptying the bladder.
Answer: TRUE OR FALSE

17. Esophagus – breaks food down mechanically into smaller particles that may be ingested more easily.
Answer: TRUE OR FALSE

18. Food remains in the esophagus for between 3 to 4 hours. During this time it is further broken down by the muscular churning action of the stomach. Powerful gastric juices are also secreted by the cells of the stomach, which contribute to chemical digestion. The food ends up in a semi-liquid form that is called chyme.
Answer: TRUE OR FALSE

19. Kidney stores vitamins A, D, E, & K that have been extracted from food ingested.
Answer: TRUE OR FALSE

20. The upper respiratory tract contains the respiratory organs located outside the chest cavity: the nose and the nasal cavities, pharynx, larynx and upper trachea.
Answer: TRUE OR FALSE

SECTION 1

CHAPTER 5: Medical Conditions, Diseases & Disorders

Learning Objectives: At the end of this chapter the student will be able to briefly describe the following

- Osteoarthritis
- Osteoporosis
- Osteomyelitis
- Myofascial pain syndrome
- Tendinitis
- Bursitis
- Muscle strain
- Scoliosis
- Kyphosis
- Torticollis
- Medial epicondylitis (GF)
- Carpal tunnel syndrome
- Spondylolysis/listhesis
- Slipped disc
- Whiplash Injury
- Sacroiliitis
- Types of Fractures
  - Open fracture
  - Closed fracture
- Hemophilia
- Adult Attention Deficit Hyperactivity Disorder (ADHD)
- Anaphylaxis
- Amyotrophic Lateral Sclerosis
- Alzheimer's Disease
- Ankylosing Spondylitis
- Gout
- Rheumatoid Arthritis (RA)
- Systemic Lupus Erythematosus
- Aseptic Necrosis
- Asthma
- Balance Disorder
- Vertigo
- Meniere's Disease
- Facial Nerve (Bells palsy)
- Bipolar Disorder

- Urinary Incontinence
- Shoulder Bursitis
- Coronary Artery Bypass Graft
- Cancer
- Tarsal Tunnel Syndrome
- Cataracts
- Chronic Fatigue Syndrome (CFS)
- Congestive Heart Failure (CHF)
- Gallstones
- Claudication
- Crohn's Disease
- Complex Regional Pain Syndrome (CRPS)
- Compartment Syndrome
- Contact Dermatitis
- Deep Vein Thrombosis (DVT)
- Diabetes
- Guillain-Barre Syndrome
- Hyperglycemia
- Multiple Sclerosis
- Neuropathic Pain
- Peripheral Neuropathy
- Orthostatic Hypotension
- Osgood-Schlatter Disease
- Paget's Disease
- Osteochondritis Dissecans
- Osteopenia
- Overactive Bladder
- Parkinson's Disease
- Peripheral Vascular Disease
- Plantar Fasciitis
- Pneumothorax
- Pneumonia
- Psoriatic Arthritis
- Radiculopathy

- Raynaud's Phenomenon
- Sciatica
- Tuberculosis (TB)
- Tennis Elbow
- Transient Ischemic Attack (TIA)
- Trigeminal Neuralgia
- Urinary Retention
- Varicose Veins
- Vasculitis
- Paralysis
- Classifying Paralysis
  - Monoplegia
  - Hemiplegia
  - Paraplegia
  - Quadriplegia/Tetraplegia
- Diabetic Neuropathy
- Fibromyalgia
- HIV

MEDICAL CONDITIONS, DISEASES & DISORDERS (BRIEF DESCRIPTION)

OSTEOARTHRITIS

EXPLAIN — Breakdown of cartilage (a smooth, cushioning substance) on the end of bones where they meet to form a joint, making the normally smooth surface rough or uneven, due to the development of spurs at the edge of the bones in a joint.

CAUSES — Excess weight or obesity, joint injury, repetitive kneeling or squatting and repetitive heavy lifting.

SYMPTOMS
1. Joint tenderness and joint stiffness.
2. Decrease in joint range of motion.
3. A grating sound known as crepitus found within the joint.

OSTEOPOROSIS

EXPLAIN — A condition that occurs as a result of lower bone mass and this further causes bone deterioration which in turn leads to bone fragility and eventually an increased risk of fracture(s).

CAUSES — Bones start to lose more calcium than is deposited and gradually lose strength.

SYMPTOMS — Bone fracture (wrist, hip or spine): the curvature of the spine (dowager's hump) or loss of height.

OSTEOMYELITIS

EXPLAIN — A condition that occurs as a result of an infection in the bone due to invasion of bacteria, fungus, etc.

CAUSES — Bone trauma, for example, gunshot wound.

SYMPTOMS — Shivering, chills, bone pain, soreness, swelling, and redness.

MYOFASCIAL PAIN SYNDROME

EXPLAIN — A condition characterized by myofascial trigger points that are located within the taut bands of skeletal muscle fibers. Trigger points are painful.

CAUSES
- An injury to the muscles, ligaments or tendons.
- Stress and anxiety.

SYMPTOMS
- Pain that lasts long.
- Muscle is sensitive or tender to touch.
- Pressure on a trigger point can cause pain.
- Affected area suffers decreased range of motion.
- Affected muscle undergo a feeling of weakness.

TENDINITIS

EXPLAIN — Inflammation or irritation of a tendon.

CAUSES — Overuse and/or injury.

SYMPTOMS — Pain and tenderness.

BURSITIS

EXPLAIN	Inflammation or irritation of a bursa.
CAUSES	Overuse and/or injury.
SYMPTOMS	• Localized pain and swelling (examples are **Tennis Elbow** and **Golfer's Elbow**)

MUSCLE STRAIN

EXPLAIN	A strain is caused by twisting, pulling or stretching a muscle or tendon. Strains can be acute or chronic.
CAUSES	Twisting, pulling or stretching these tissues can cause a strain.
SYMPTOMS	Pain, muscle spasms, swelling, limited motion and trouble moving the muscle. Symptoms varies with severity of strain.

SCOLIOSIS

EXPLAIN	A condition that leads to a sideward bending (curve) of the spine. The bending (curves) can be an **S or C-shaped.**
CAUSES	Idiopathic (Unknown), Causes of curves are classified as either nonstructural or structural.
SYMPTOMS	• Uneven shoulders • One shoulder blade appears prominent (protruding) than the other • Tilted waist or uneven waist • One hip higher than the other • Prominent ribs • The curve is more pronounced when the child bends forward. The curve usually is s or c shaped.

KYPHOSIS

EXPLAIN	Kyphosis is a curvature of the spine that develops into a bowing (rounding) of the back, which leads to a 'hunchback' or slouching posture. **(Forward Bending).**
CAUSES	Week muscles, bad posture, injury, degenerative changes, spondylolisthesis, fracture.
SYMPTOMS	Pain, difficulty breathing, tenderness, stiffness in spine, fatigue.

TORTICOLLIS

EXPLAIN	Torticollis also known as wryneck, is a deformity of the neck in which the sternocleidomastoid neck muscles are spastic or shortened. Two types acquired or congenital.
CAUSES	Acquired (injury or infection), Congenital (present at birth).
SYMPTOMS	The stiffness of the neck muscle on one side (unilateral), twitching or contraction of the muscles, neck pain, and head pain. It causes the head to tilt to one side and the chin to turn (rotate) on the opposite side.

MEDIAL EPICONDYLITIS (GOLFERS ELBOW)

EXPLAIN	A tendinosis that results in painful elbow condition occurring on the medial aspect (inner side) of the elbow.
CAUSES	Inflammation and injury to the tendons.
SYMPTOMS	Localized elbow pain on the inner aspect (medial epicondyle) of the elbow.

CARPAL TUNNEL SYNDROME

EXPLAIN A condition in which the median nerve (which runs from the arm into the hand) is compressed as it passes through the carpal tunnel at the wrist.

CAUSES Workplace factors, inflammatory conditions, anatomic factors.

SYMPTOMS
- Tingling, burning, itching and numbness in the fingers (thumb and the index and middle fingers) and palm of the hand.
- Pain in the wrist or hand, which may radiate up the arm or down to your fingers, and can be severe.
- Sense of weakness in the hands and a loss of grip strength, which can makes it difficult to form a fist, grasp small objects or some other activities.
- Symptoms may be worse at night when people may sleep with their wrists flexed.

SPONDYLOLYSIS/LISTHESIS

EXPLAIN Spondylolisthesis is a forward displacement of the proximal vertebra above over the distal vertebra. Spondylolysis is a defect in the pars inter-articularis.

CAUSES Congenital, stress, genetic, dysplastic.

GRADES
Spondylolisthesis Grades:
1. **Grade I** — 1 percent to 25 percent slip
2. **Grade II** — 26 percent to 50 percent slip
3. **Grade III** — 51 percent to 75 percent slip
4. **Grade IV** — 76 percent to 100 percent slip

SLIPPED DISC

EXPLAIN A disc herniation is a displaced fragment of the center part or nucleus of the disc that is pushed through a tear in the outer layer or annulus fibrosus of the disc. The stages of disc herniation are stage 1: degeneration, stage 2: prolapse (bulging disc herniation), stage 3: extrusion, stage 4: sequestration.

SYMPTOMS Tingling, aching or burning sensations in the affected area, radiating pain.

WHIPLASH INJURY

EXPLAIN Acceleration or deceleration injury to the cervical region.

CAUSES Car accidents, trauma.

SYMPTOMS Neck pain, inflammation, radiating pain and numbness if the nerve is involved.

SACROILIITIS

EXPLAIN The sacroiliac joint (SIJ) is a deep joint in the buttock between the tailbone (sacrum) and the pelvic wing bone (ilium). Sacroiliitis is the inflammation of one or both of your sacroiliac joints

CAUSES Injury, pregnancy, arthritis, infection.

SYMPTOMS Pain is felt in the buttocks region or in the lower back area, and this pain may even extend down to one or both legs.

FRACTURE: a complete or partial break in the bone.

TYPES OF FRACTURES:

- Open fracture (compound): the bone tissue protrudes through the skin.
- Closed fracture (simple): the bone tissue does not protrude through the skin (intact skin).

OTHER TERMINOLOGIES AND CLASSIFICATION OF FRACTURES:

- Complete: a type of fracture in which the bone breaks into two or more pieces. The break is complete across the bone.
- Comminuted: a type of fracture in which the bone breaks into several pieces or into small fragments.
- Greenstick: a type of fracture in which the bone bends and breaks without separating into separate parts or pieces. Usually seen in children.
- Spiral: a type of fracture that occurs as a result of torsion force (twisting).
- Transverse: a type of fracture that occurs across a bone.
- Impacted (buckle): one broken part or fragment of the bone tissue is driven into another part or fragment.
- Pott's fracture: a fracture at the distal end of the fibula (lateral malleoli/medial malleoli).
- Colle's fracture: a fracture of the distal end of the radius that causes posterior displacement of the distal fragment resulting in a silver fork deformity.
- Smith fracture: a fracture of the distal end of the radius that causes anterior displacement of the distal fragment.
- Barton's fracture: a fracture of the distal end of the radius and dislocation of the radioulnar joint.
- Chauffeur's fracture: a fracture of the distal radial styloid process of the radius bone of the forearm.
- Galeazzi's fracture: a fracture of the radius in the distal third along with subluxation or dislocation of the distal radioulnar joint.
- Monteggia's fractures: a fracture of the ulna at the proximal third along with subluxation or dislocation of the proximal radioulnar joint.
- Stress (hairline) fracture: a partial fracture resulting from repeated stress.

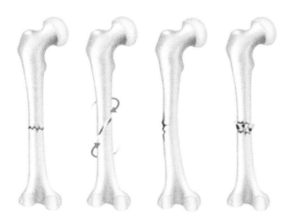

Transverse   Spiral   Greenstick Comminuted

Fig 5.1: Fracture Illustrations (4 types)

COMPLICATIONS:

The major complication of a fracture would be an injury to the nearby or surrounding organs, structures and/or tissues.

BRIEF DESCRIPTIONS

HEMOPHILIA

Human blood consists of various proteins that are known as clotting factors; these clotting factors help to stop bleeding. Hemophilia is considered an inherited bleeding disorder in which the blood does not clot appropriately due to lack or low levels of certain clotting factors. This can lead to spontaneous bleeding as well as bleeding following injuries or surgery.

ADULT ATTENTION DEFICIT HYPERACTIVITY DISORDER (ADHD)

Considered a behavioral condition characterized by distractibility, impulsivity, and/or hyperactivity. ADHD affects about 2% - 6% of the population. There are three kinds of ADHD: inattentive type, hyperactive/impulsive type, and the combined type.

ANAPHYLAXIS

Is a life threatening allergic reaction affecting numerous body systems at one time. This can be fatal and is considered the most severe allergic reaction and is potentially life threatening. Anaphylaxis is rare.

AMYOTROPHIC LATERAL SCLEROSIS

A rapidly progressive, invariably fatal neurological disease that attacks the nerve cells responsible for controlling voluntary muscles. Amyotrophic lateral sclerosis (ALS) is sometimes called Lou Gehrig's disease. The muscles gradually weaken, waste away (atrophy) and twitch. Eventually, the ability of the brain to start and control voluntary movement is lost. Muscles under voluntary control are affected, and patients lose their strength and the ability to move their arms, legs, and body.

ALZHEIMER'S DISEASE

Alzheimer's disease (AD) is an age-related, non-reversible brain disorder that develops over a period of years. Initially, people experience memory loss and confusion, which may be mistaken for the kind of memory changes that are sometimes associated with normal aging. However, the symptoms of AD gradually lead to behavior and personality changes, a decline in cognitive abilities such as decision-making and language skills, and problems recognizing family and friends. AD ultimately leads to a severe loss of mental function. These losses are related to the worsening breakdown of the connections between certain neurons in the brain and their eventual death. AD is one of a group of disorders called dementias that are characterized by cognitive and behavioral problems. It is the most common cause of dementia among people age 65 and older.

ANKYLOSING SPONDYLITIS

A form of chronic inflammation that involves the spine and the sacroiliac joints. Chronic inflammation causes pain and stiffness in and around the spine, including the neck and back. After prolong period of time, chronic inflammation of the spine (spondylitis) can lead to a complete fusion of the vertebrae; this is referred to as ankylosis. The fusion of vertebrae causes loss of mobility of the spine. Ankylosing spondylitis is considered a type of arthritis condition that tend to cause chronic inflammation of the spine.

GOUT

Gout is considered a type of arthritis. Gout causes joint inflammation, asymmetrical in nature (usually in one joint). Severe gout can affect many joints at once. This is known as polyarticular gout. Gout is a painful condition that occurs when the bodily waste product uric acid is deposited as needle-like crystals in the joints and/or soft tissues. In the joints, these uric acid crystals cause inflammatory arthritis, which in turn leads to intermittent swelling, redness, heat, pain, and stiffness in the joints.

RHEUMATOID ARTHRITIS (RA)

Rheumatoid arthritis (RA) is an inflammatory disease that causes pain, swelling, stiffness, and loss of function in the joints. It occurs when the immune system, which normally defends the body from invading organisms, turns its attack against the membrane lining the joints. The course of rheumatoid arthritis can range from mild to severe. In most cases it is chronic, meaning it lasts a long time. For many people, periods of relatively mild disease activity are punctuated by flares, or times of heightened disease activity. In others, symptoms are constant.

Features of Rheumatoid Arthritis

- Tender, warm and swollen joints.
- Symmetrical pattern of affected joints.

- Joint inflammation often affecting the wrist and finger joints.
- Joint inflammation sometimes affecting other joints, including the neck, shoulders, elbows, hips, knees, ankles, and feet.
- Fatigue, occasional fevers or loss of energy.
- Pain and stiffness lasting for more than 30 minutes in the morning or after a duration of long rest.
- Symptoms lasts for many years.
- Variability of symptoms among people with the disease.

SYSTEMIC LUPUS ERYTHEMATOSUS

Systemic lupus erythematosus (SLE) is the form of the disease that most people are referring to when they say "lupus". The word "systemic" means the disease can affect many parts of the body. The symptoms of SLE may be mild or severe. Few common symptoms of lupus; painful or swollen joints and muscle pain, unexplained fever, red rashes, most commonly on the face, chest pain upon deep breathing, unusual loss of hair, pale or purple fingers or toes from cold or stress (raynaud's phenomenon), sensitivity to the sun, swelling (edema) in legs or around eyes, mouth ulcers, swollen glands, extreme fatigue.

ASEPTIC NECROSIS

Osteonecrosis is a disease resulting from the temporary or permanent loss of blood supply to the bones. Without blood, the bone tissue dies, and ultimately the bone may collapse. If the process involves the bones near a joint, it often leads to the collapse of the joint surface. Osteonecrosis is also known as avascular necrosis, aseptic necrosis, and ischemic necrosis.

ASTHMA

Asthma is a complex chronic airway inflammation disorder characterized by the hyper-responsiveness of the airway and periods of bronchospasm. This causes reversible airway obstruction. Asthma causes periods of recurring wheezing, coughing, tightness in the chest region, dyspnea (shortness of breath).

BALANCE DISORDER

A type of disorder in which an individual may feel dizzy or not able to balance independently. The individual may be at stand still like either in a lying or standing position, but may feel that he or she is spinning or moving. There are certain factors that may cause such balance disorders for example ear infection, certain drugs and also several health related conditions.

VERTIGO

Vertigo is an abnormal sense of rotation, rocking, or spinning experienced by an individual while in standstill position (lying or standing position).

MENIERE'S DISEASE

Episodes of vertigo, hearing loss, tinnitus, and a feeling of fullness in the ear. It may be associated with a change in fluid volume within parts of the labyrinth.

FACIAL NERVE (Bell's Palsy)

The facial nerve is a nerve that controls the muscles on the side of the face. Bell's palsy is a form of temporary facial paralysis of the facial nerves. It is the most common cause of facial paralysis. Generally, Bell's palsy affects only one of the paired facial nerves and one side of the face, however, in rare cases, it can affect both sides. Symptoms of Bell's palsy usually begin suddenly and reach their peak within 48 hours. Symptoms vary from person to person and can range in severity from mild weakness to total paralysis. These symptoms include twitching, weakness, or paralysis, drooping eyelid or corner of the mouth, drooling, dry eye or mouth, impairment of taste, and excessive tearing in the eye. Bell's palsy often causes significant facial distortion.

BIPOLAR DISORDER

A person may experience symptoms which cause a shift in mood, energy, and several functions. It can involve a mood swing that ranges from depression characteristics to manic characteristics.

URINARY INCONTINENCE

Urinary incontinence is the inability of an individual to hold urine. There are several causes associated with this, some of the causes are overactive or weak bladder muscles, prostate conditions or damage to the nerve controlling the bladder. There are 4 types of urinary incontinence: Functional incontinence, Urge incontinence, Stress incontinence, and Overflow incontinence. Remember: FUSO

SHOULDER BURSITIS

A bursa is a small, fluid-filled sac that acts as a cushion between a bone and other moving parts: muscles, tendons, or skin. Bursae are found throughout the body. Bursitis occurs when a bursa becomes inflamed (redness and increased fluid in the bursa). Shoulder Bursitis is caused due to injury or inflammation of a bursa around the shoulder joint.

CORONARY ARTERY BYPASS GRAFT (CABG)

Artery supplying oxygen to the heart muscles are known as coronary arteries. A plaque (buildup) can be formed within the arteries blocking the flow of blood to the heart musculature. CABG also known as Coronary artery bypass graft is a surgery performed to re-establish the blood supply to the heart musculature.

CANCER

A condition that starts, when a cell growth is out of control. The growth seen is abnormal and causes invasion into other tissues. There are several types of cancers.

TARSAL TUNNEL SYNDROME

Compression of the posterior tibial nerve while its passage through the tarsal tunnel leads to a tarsal tunnel syndrome. The tarsal tunnel is located posteriorly to the medial malleolus and beneath the retinaculum of the flexor muscles of the foot. This may cause numbness, burning and tingling sensation.

CATARACTS

A condition characterized by clouding of the lens of the eye. Most commonly as a result of aging process. It can occur in one eye of both eyes. There are various symptoms (blurred vision, cloudy vision, poor night vision, etc.) associated with cataract.

CHRONIC FATIGUE SYNDROME (CFS)

Chronic fatigue syndrome (CFS), is a debilitating and complex disorder characterized by extreme fatigue that does not subside with bed rest, unlike regular fatigue that usually subsides with rest.

CONGESTIVE HEART FAILURE (CHF)

A condition in which the heart is unable to meet the oxygen and nutrient requirements of the organs and tissues. There are several causes associated with it.

GALLSTONES

Stones formed within the gallbladder are known as gallstones. The most common type of gallstones are composed of cholesterol or pigments. The pain associated with the gall stones are referred to as biliary colic.

CLAUDICATION

A condition in which an individual experiences pain and cramping in the leg. This is usually due to insufficient blood supply to the muscles. It is known as intermittent claudication since the symptoms are felt while performing an activity and subsides at rest. In severe stages the pain can also be felt while the individual is resting.

CROHN'S DISEASE

A chronic inflammatory disease of the gastrointestinal tract, commonly affecting the small intestine and the start of the large intestine. Some common symptoms are diarrhea, abdominal cramping, abdominal pain and weight loss.

COMPLEX REGIONAL PAIN SYNDROME (CRPS)

Complex regional pain syndrome (CRPS) is a chronic pain condition most often affecting one of the limbs (arms, legs, hands, or feet), usually after an injury or trauma to that limb. CRPS is believed to be caused by damage to, or malfunction of, the peripheral and central nervous system. CRPS is characterized by prolonged or excessive pain and mild or dramatic changes in skin color, temperature, and/or swelling in the affected area.

COMPARTMENT SYNDROME

An injury may lead to internal bleeding, if the bleeding is excessive it may cause an increase in the pressure within the muscle compartment. The increase in pressure may compress the underlying nerve leading to an injury or damage. Symptoms; extreme pain, cramping, numbness and tightness.

CONTACT DERMATITIS

Contact dermatitis is a red, itchy rash or irritation due to contact with an allergen or irritant substance that produces a skin response. There are two types of contact dermatitis.

- Irritant contact dermatitis
- Allergic contact dermatitis

DEEP VEIN THROMBOSIS (DVT)

Thrombosis is a formation of a clot within the vein; this may cause a decrease in blood flow which may lead to blockage of the blood vessel. Thrombo-Embolism, on the other hand, is a process in which the thrombus dislodges from its original site and floats freely in the form of an embolus throughout the circulatory system. The free floating mass embolus can lodge itself in a blood vessel that results in the blockage of that particular blood vessel. Embolus blocks the blood supply to a particular organ which is called embolism. If the emboli lodges in the heart it can cause heart attack, in the brain can cause stroke and in lungs can cause pulmonary embolism.

There are two types of thrombosis formed in the vein:

- Deep vein thrombosis
- Superficial vein thrombosis

DIABETES

A disease characterized by an increase in body's blood glucose level. The two main types of diabetes are type 1 and type 2.

- **Type 1 diabetes:** Insulin Dependent (pancreas produce no to little insulin)
- **Type 2 diabetes:** Insulin Resistant (body unable to use insulin)

GUILLAIN-BARRE SYNDROME

Guillain-Barre syndrome is a disorder in which the body's immune system attacks the parts of the peripheral nervous system. The first symptoms of this disorder include varying degrees of weakness or tingling sensation in the legs. In many instances, the weakness and abnormal sensations spread to the arms and upper body. These symptoms can increase in intensity until the muscles cannot be used at all and the person is almost totally paralyzed. In these cases, the disorder is life-threatening and is considered a medical emergency. The patient is often put on a ventilator to assist with breathing. Most individuals, however, have a good recovery from even the most severe cases of Guillain-Barre syndrome (GBS), although some continue to have some degree of weakness. Guillain-Barre syndrome is rare.

HYPERGLYCEMIA

A condition characterized by high levels of blood glucose. Common, signs and symptoms of hyperglycemia, include:

- Increased levels of blood glucose.
- Increased levels of sugar in the urine.
- Increase in frequency of urination.
- Increased thirst.

MULTIPLE SCLEROSIS

Multiple sclerosis (MS) is a disease of demyelination of the neurons (brain and spinal cord nerve cells) resulting in disrupt communication between the brain and other parts of the body. Most people experience their first symptoms of MS between the ages of 20 and 40; the initial symptom of MS is often blurred or double vision, red-green color distortion, or even blindness in one eye. Most MS patients experience muscle weakness in their extremities and difficulty with coordination and balance. These symptoms may be severe enough to impair walking or even standing. In the worst cases, MS can produce partial or complete paralysis. Most people with MS also exhibit paresthesia's, transitory abnormal sensory feelings such as numbness, prickling, or "pins and needles" sensations. Some may also experience pain. Speech impediments, tremors, and dizziness are other frequent complaints. Occasionally, people with MS have hearing loss. Approximately half of all people with MS experience cognitive impairments such as difficulties with concentration, attention, memory, and poor judgment, but such symptoms are usually mild and are frequently overlooked. Depression is another common feature of MS.

NEUROPATHIC PAIN

Pain arising as a result of damage or dysfunction or injury to the nerve fibers. This may cause numbness, tingling, lack of sensation or pain.

PERIPHERAL NEUROPATHY

Is a condition of peripheral nervous system. The function of the peripheral nervous system (PNS) is to transmit information from the brain and spinal cord to every other part of the body. In peripheral neuropathy, the patient has impaired function and symptoms depending on the type of nerves (motor, sensory, or autonomic) that are damaged. Some people may experience temporary numbness, tingling, and pricking sensations, sensitivity to touch, or muscle weakness. Others may suffer more extreme symptoms, including burning pain (especially at night), muscle wasting, paralysis, or organ or gland dysfunction.

ORTHOSTATIC HYPOTENSION

Orthostatic hypotension is a sudden fall in blood pressure that occurs when a person stands. It is due to a lesion of the baroreflex loop, which senses a change in blood pressure and adjusts heart rate and activates sympathetic nerve system fibers to cause the blood vessels to narrow and correct blood pressure. It may also be caused by hypovolemia (a decreased amount of blood in the body), resulting from the excessive use of diuretics, vasodilators, or other types of drugs, dehydration, or prolonged bed rest. Symptoms, which occur after sudden standing, include dizziness, lightheadedness, blurred vision, and syncope (temporary loss of consciousness).

OSGOOD-SCHLATTER DISEASE

A condition that affects the upper portion of the shin bone (at the insertion of patellar tendon). Symptoms may include knee pain, swelling, and tenderness.

PAGET'S DISEASE

Paget's disease of bone is a chronic condition of bone characterized by excessive bone resorption followed by an increase in bone formation. Overactive osteoclastic activity followed by compensatory osteoblastic activity lead to a formation of bone that is large, weak and less compact. These bones are more prone to fracture.

OSTEOCHONDRITIS DISSECANS

A condition whereby a small segment of bone begins to fragment along with the articular cartilage due to lack of blood supply. Most common joints affected are the knee, ankle and elbow joints.
There are two main types:
- Adult form
- Juvenile form

OSTEOPENIA

A condition characterized by a lower bone mineral density leading to characterized bone weakening and increased the risk of bone fractures.

OVERACTIVE BLADDER

A condition characterized by involuntary contraction of the bladder that is sudden in nature that leads to urinary incontinence. Individual may feel a need to urinate more frequently, and urine may leak after an urge for urination.

PARKINSON'S DISEASE

Parkinson's disease is a neurodegenerative disorder which leads to progressive deterioration of motor functions. Parkinson's disease (PD) belongs to a group of conditions called motor system disorders, which are the result of the loss of dopamine-producing brain cells. The four primary symptoms of PD are a tremor, or trembling in hands, arms, legs, jaw, and face; rigidity, or stiffness of the limbs and trunk; bradykinesia, or slowness of movement; and postural instability, or impaired balance and coordination. Other symptoms may include depression and other emotional changes; difficulty in swallowing, chewing and speaking; urinary problems or constipation; skin problems; and sleep disruptions.

PERIPHERAL VASCULAR DISEASE

A disease characterized by the formation of plaque build-up that leads to narrowing or occlusion of the arteries. This narrowing or occlusion of the arteries limits the flow of blood to the organs. A plaque build-up within the arteries is known as atherosclerosis.

PLANTAR FASCIITIS

Plantar fascia is a ligament that connects the heel to the front of the foot, thereby supporting the arches of the foot. Inflammation of the plantar fascia is called as plantar fasciitis. This may result in heel pain and tightness of the plantar fascia.

PNEUMOTHORAX

Pneumothorax is the collection of air in the pleural cavity (thoracic cavity) as more and more air accumulates within the pleural cavity it causes the lung(s) to collapse.

PNEUMONIA

Infection of one or both lungs that eventually, leads to inflammation of the airspaces. Common signs of pneumonia can include cough, fever, and trouble breathing. Pneumonia may be caused by viruses, bacteria, or fungi. Certain people are more likely to become ill with pneumonia: adults 65 years of age or older, children younger than 5 years of age, individuals who have underlying medical conditions (like asthma, diabetes or heart disease), individuals who smoke cigarettes.

PSORIATIC ARTHRITIS

Psoriatic arthritis is a form of arthritis (joint inflammation) that can occur in individuals who have the skin disease known as psoriasis. Psoriasis is a common condition characterized by scaly red and white skin patches (chronic, autoimmune skin disease that speeds up the growth cycle of skin cells). Psoriatic arthritis can affect any joint in the body, including the spine.

RADICULOPATHY

Pain, numbness, tingling or weakness caused due to a compression of the nerve in the spine is termed as radiculopathy. Most commonly seen in the cervical spine and lower lumbar spine due to the compression of a nerve in a particular area.

RAYNAUD'S PHENOMENON

A disorder characterized by brief episodes of vasospasm (narrowing of the blood vessels). Vasospasm of the arteries reduces blood flow to the fingers and toes as a result of exposure to temperature change (cold or hot) or emotional events. As a result of vasospasm, skin discoloration is seen in which the skin color turns white due to lack of blood supply, then turns blue due to prolonged lack of blood supply and finally turns red after regaining its blood flow.

SCIATICA

Sciatica is characterized by pain, numbness, weakness, or tingling sensation along the course of the sciatic nerve. The cause of sciatica may include injury or compression of the nerve. Symptoms start in the lower back and extends down towards the leg and further down into the calf, foot, or even toes.

TUBERCULOSIS (TB)

TB is an airborne infectious disease that is contagious in nature. It can spread from one person to another. A bacteria known as Mycobacterium tuberculosis causes TB. This disease usually affects the lungs, but can spread to different parts of the body.

TENNIS ELBOW

Tennis elbow is also known as lateral epicondylitis causes soreness or pain on the lateral aspect of the elbow. This occurs as a result of strain due to overuse of the tendon.

TRANSIENT ISCHEMIC ATTACK (TIA)

A type of stroke which is temporary in nature due to stoppage of blood flow to the brain for a short period of time. This may cause numbness, weakness, confusion, slurred speech, vision problems, dizziness, loss of balance or coordination.

TRIGEMINAL NEURALGIA

Trigeminal neuralgia (TN), also called tic douloureux, is a chronic pain condition that causes extreme, sporadic, sudden burning or shock-like face pain. The pain seldom lasts more than a few seconds or a minute or two per episode. The intensity of pain can be physically and mentally incapacitating. TN pain is typically felt on one side of the jaw or cheek. Episodes can last for days, weeks, or months at a time and then disappear for months or years. In the days before an episode begins, some patients may experience a tingling or numbness sensation or a somewhat constant and aching pain. The attacks often worsen over time, with fewer and shorter pain-free periods before they recur. The intense flashes of pain can be triggered by vibration or contact with the cheek (such as when shaving, washing the face or applying makeup), brushing teeth, eating, drinking, talking, or being exposed to the wind.

URINARY RETENTION

Urinary retention is the inability to empty the bladder completely. Urinary retention can be acute or chronic. Acute urinary retention occurs suddenly and lasts for only a short time. Chronic urinary retention can be a long-lasting medical condition. Causes may include nerve problems, medications, weak bladder muscles or obstruction of the urethra.

VARICOSE VEINS

Veins have one-way valves that help the blood to flow in one direction only. If the valves are weak or damaged, blood can back up and pool within the veins causing the veins to swell; this can eventually lead to varicose veins. Varicose veins usually occur in the legs. Varicose veins cause mild to moderate pain, skin ulcers, and blood clots.

VASCULITIS

Vasculitis is the inflammation of blood vessels. "Inflammation" refers to the body's response to injury, including injury to the blood vessels. Inflammation may involve pain, redness, warmth, swelling, and loss of function in the affected tissues. In vasculitis, inflammation can lead to serious problems. **Complications** depend on which blood vessels, organs, or other body systems are affected. If a blood vessel is inflamed, it can narrow or close off. This limits or prevents blood flow through the vessel. Rarely, the blood vessel will stretch and weaken, causing it to bulge. This bulge is known as an **aneurysm**.

PARALYSIS

Loss of muscular function is known as paralysis. Sensory function loss may accompany the motor function loss. Few causes of such a loss of muscular activity is due to the problems associated with the nerves and or spinal cord.

CLASSIFYING PARALYSIS

There are also a number of medical terms used to describe different types of paralysis:-

- Monoplegia – one limb is paralyzed.
- Hemiplegia – the arm and leg on one side of the body is paralyzed.
- Paraplegia – both legs and sometimes the pelvis and some section of the lower body is paralyzed.
- Quadriplegia/Tetraplegia – both the arms and legs are paralyzed.

DIABETIC NEUROPATHY

Diabetic neuropathy is a peripheral nerve disorder caused by diabetes or poor blood sugar control. Diabetic neuropathy can be classified as peripheral, autonomic, proximal, or focal. Each affects different parts of the body in various ways. People with diabetes can, over time, develop nerve damage throughout the body. Some people

with nerve damage have no symptoms. Others may have symptoms such as pain, tingling, or numbness, loss of feeling in the hands, arms, feet, and legs. The loss of sensation in the feet may also increase the possibility of foot injuries that is unnoticed and eventually develops into an ulcer(s) or lesion(s) which then becomes infected. In some cases, diabetic neuropathy can be associated with weakness in the foot muscles and walking difficulties.

FIBROMYALGIA

Fibromyalgia syndrome is a chronic disorder characterized by widespread pain, diffuse tenderness, fatigue, sleep disturbances, psychological distress and it can also interfere with an individual's ability to carry out daily activities.

HIV

HIV stands for human immunodeficiency virus that causes AIDS. This leads to acquired immunodeficiency syndrome or AIDS. HIV attacks the immune system by destroying CD4 positive (CD4+) T cells that help in fighting off infection. The destruction of these cells leaves people infected with HIV vulnerable to other infections, diseases, and other complications. AIDS is the final stage of HIV infection.

References

1. Reference: National Institute of Neurological Disorders and Stroke, Amyotrophic Lateral Sclerosis (ALS)
2. Reference: National Institute of Neurological Disorders and Stroke, Alzheimer's Disease.
3. Reference: National Institute of Arthritis and Musculoskeletal and Skin Diseases (NIAMS), NIH Publication No. 10–7609
4. Reference: National Institute of Arthritis and Musculoskeletal and Skin Diseases (NIAMS), NIH Publication No. 12–5027
5. Reference: National Institute of Arthritis and Musculoskeletal and Skin Diseases (NIAMS), NIH Publication No. 14-4179
6. Reference: National Institute of Arthritis and Musculoskeletal and Skin Diseases (NIAMS), NIH Publication No. 13–4178
7. Reference: National Institute of Arthritis and Musculoskeletal and Skin Diseases (NIAMS), NIH Publication No. 09–4857
8. Reference: National Institute on Deafness and Other Communication Disorders, NIH Pub. No. 14-4374
9. Reference: National Institute of Neurological Disorders and Stroke, Bell's Palsy.
10. Reference: National Institute of Arthritis and Musculoskeletal and Skin Diseases (NIAMS), NIH Publication No. 13-6240
11. Reference: National Institute of Neurological Disorders and Stroke, NIH Publication No. 13-4173, No. 12-4898

12. *Reference: National Institute of Neurological Disorders and Stroke, Guillain-Barre Syndrome.*
13. *Reference: National Institute of Neurological Disorders and Stroke, Multiple Sclerosis.*
14. *Reference: National Institute of Neurological Disorders and Stroke, Peripheral Neuropathy.*
15. *Reference: National Institute of Neurological Disorders and Stroke, Orthostatic Hypotension.*
16. *Reference: National Institute of Neurological Disorders and Stroke, Parkinson's disease.*
17. *Reference: National Institute of Arthritis and Musculoskeletal and Skin Diseases (NIAMS), NIH Publication No. 14–AR-8001, No. 13–4862*
18. *Reference: Centers for Disease Control and Prevention* www.cdc.gov
19. *www.aids.gov*

Disclaimer: Information provided in this chapter is. Information provided here is for informational and educational purposes only, not intended to serve as medical advice and is not to be used for diagnosis or treatment of any condition or symptom.

CHAPTER 5
END OF CHAPTER REVIEW QUESTIONS

Question Set 1: Match the following (Types of Fractures)   10 points 1 point each

Answer	Column 1	Column 2
	1. Smith	a type of fracture in which the bone breaks into two or more pieces. The break is complete across the bone.
	2. Colle's	a type of fracture in which the bone breaks into several pieces or into small fragments.
	3. Transverse	a type of fracture in which the bone bends and breaks without separating into separate parts or pieces. Usually seen in children.
	4. Comminuted	a type of fracture that occurs as a result of torsion force (twisting).
	5. Barton's	a type of fracture that occurs across a bone (right angles to the long axis of the bone).
	6. Spiral	one broken part or fragment of the bone tissue is driven into another part or fragment.
	7. Complete	a fracture at the distal end of the fibula (lateral malleoli/medial malleoli).
	8. Greenstick	a fracture of the distal end of the radius that causes posterior displacement of the distal fragment resulting in a silver fork deformity.
	9. Impacted	a fracture of the distal end of the radius that causes anterior displacement of the distal fragment.
	10. Pott's	a fracture of the distal end of the radius and dislocation of the radioulnar joint.

Question Set 2: Essay Questions   54 points 3 points each

Explain in brief about the following conditions and disorders:

a. Osteoarthritis

b. Rheumatoid arthritis

c. Osteoporosis

d. Osteomyelitis

e. Myofascial pain syndrome

f. Tendinitis

g. Bursitis

h. Muscle strain

i. Scoliosis

j. Kyphosis

k. Torticollis

l. Medial epicondylitis

m. Carpal tunnel syndrome

n. Spondylolysis/listhesis

o. Slipped disc

p. Whiplash

q. Sacroiliitis

r. Classify paralysis

Question Set 3: Fill in the Blanks   20 points 1 point each

1. A _____ is a displaced fragment of the center part or nucleus of the disc that is pushed through a tear in the outer layer or annulus fibrosus of the disc.

2. _____ considered a behavioral condition characterized by distractibility, impulsivity, and/or hyperactivity.

3. _____ is sometimes called Lou Gehrig's disease.

4. _____ is a form of chronic inflammation that involves the spine and the sacroiliac joints. Chronic inflammation causes pain and stiffness in and around the spine, including the neck and back.

5. _____ is an inflammatory disease that causes pain, swelling, stiffness, and loss of function in the joints.

6. _____ is the form of the disease that most people are referring to when they say "lupus".

7. _____is a complex chronic airway inflammation disorder characterized by the hyper-responsiveness of the airway and periods of bronchospasm.

8. _____ is a form of temporary facial paralysis of the facial nerves.

9. There are 4 types of urinary incontinence: Functional incontinence, Urge incontinence, Stress incontinence, and _____ incontinence.

10. Compression of _____ while its passage through the tarsal tunnel leads to a tarsal tunnel syndrome.

11. The pain associated with the gall stones are referred to as _____.

12. _____ is a condition in which an individual experiences pain and cramping in the leg. This is usually due to insufficient blood supply to the muscles.

13. _____ is a chronic inflammatory disease of the gastro-intestinal tract, commonly affecting the small intestine and the start of the large intestine.

14. _____ is a red, itchy rash or irritation due to contact with an allergen or irritant substance that produces a skin response. There are two types of contact dermatitis.

15. _____ is a formation of clot within the vein, this may cause a decrease in blood flow which may lead to blockage of the blood vessel. _____ on the other hand is a process in which the thrombus dislodges from its original site and floats freely in the form of an embolus throughout

the circulatory system. The free floating mass embolus can lodge itself in a blood vessel that results in the blockage of that particular blood vessel. _____ blocks the blood supply to a particular organ which is called _____.

16. _____is a condition characterized by high levels of blood glucose.

17. _____ is a disease of demyelination of the neurons (brain and spinal cord nerve cells) resulting in disrupt communication between the brain and other parts of the body.

18. _____ is a condition characterized by a lower bone mineral density leading to characterized bone weakening and increased risk of bone fractures.

19. Parkinson's disease is a neurodegenerative disorder which leads to progressive deterioration of _____ functions.

20. _____ is a type of stroke which is temporary in nature due to stoppage of blood flow to the brain for a short period of time. This may cause numbness, weakness, confusion, slurred speech, vision problems, dizziness, loss of balance or coordination.

Question Set 4: True or False   26 points 1 point each

1. Osteoarthritis is the breakdown of cartilage on the end of bones where they meet to form a joint.
   Answer: True or False

2. Osteoporosis is a condition that occurs as a result of lower bone mass and this further causes bone deterioration which in turn leads to bone fragility and eventually an increased risk of fracture(s).
   Answer: True or False

3. Rheumatoid arthritis is an infection in the bone caused by bacteria, sometimes other organisms such as a fungus may be the cause.
   Answer: True or False

4. Tendinitis are characterized by myofascial trigger points that are located within the taut bands of skeletal muscle fibers.
   Answer: True or False

5. Bursitis inflammation of a tendon.
   Answer: True or False

6. Kyphosis is a sideward curve of the backbone or spine.
   Answer: True or False

7. 'Hunchback' or slouching posture results from Sacroiliitis.
   Answer: True or False

8. Medial epicondylitis (golfers elbow) is a painful elbow condition occurring on the medial aspect (inner side) of the elbow.
   Answer: True or False

9. Torticollis is also known as wryneck.
   Answer: True or False

10. Carpal tunnel syndrome is a condition in which the ulnar nerve (which runs from the arm into the hand) is compressed as it passes through the carpal tunnel at the wrist.
    Answer: True or False

11. Spondylolisthesis is a backward displacement of the proximal vertebra above over the distal vertebra.
Answer: True or False

12. Chauffeur's fracture is a fracture of the distal radial styloid process of the radius bone.
Answer: True or False

13. Galeazzi's fracture is a fracture of the radius in the proximal third along with subluxation or dislocation of the distal radioulnar joint.
Answer: True or False

14. Monteggia's fractures is a fracture of the ulna at the distal third along with subluxation or dislocation of the proximal radioulnar joint.
Answer: True or False

15. Hemophilia is considered an inherited bleeding disorder in which the blood does not clot appropriately due to lack or low levels of certain clotting factors.
Answer: True or False

16. Anaphylaxis is a life-threatening allergic reaction affecting numerous body systems at one time.
Answer: True or False

17. Osteonecrosis is a disease resulting from the temporary or permanent loss of blood supply to the bones.
Answer: True or False

18. Vertigo is an abnormal sense of rotation, rocking, or spinning experienced by an individual while in standstill position (lying or standing position).
Answer: True or False

19. Gout causes joint inflammation, symmetrical in nature (usually in one joint). Severe gout can affect many joints at once.
Answer: True or False

20. Alzheimer's disease (AD) is an age-related, reversible brain disorder that develops over a period of years.
Answer: True or False

21. Asthma is a complex chronic airway inflammation disorder characterized by the hyper-responsiveness of the airway and periods of bronchospasm.
Answer: True or False

22. Artery supplying oxygen to the heart muscles is known as superior and inferior vena cava.
Answer: True or False

23. Contact dermatitis is a red, itchy rash or irritation due to contact with an allergen or irritant substance that produces a skin response.
Answer: True or False

24. Cataract is a condition characterized by clouding of the lens of the eye.
Answer: True or False

25. Neuropathic pain arises as a result of damage or dysfunction or injury to the nerve fibers.
Answer: True or False

26. Osgood-Schlatter disease of bone is a chronic condition of bone characterized by excessive bone resorption followed by an increase in bone formation.
Answer: True or False

SECTION 2
CHAPTER 6: PHYSICAL ASSESSMENT AND EXAMINATION

Learning Objectives: At the end of this chapter the student will be able to describe the following

(1) Physical assessment techniques
(2) Medical Documentation:
    a. SOAP Notes
(3) Vital Signs
    a. Temperature
        i.   Heat production in human body
        ii. Heat distribution in human body
        iii. Stages of fever
        iv. Assessment of body temperature
        v.   Assessment sites
        vi. Oral temperature
        vii. Axillary temperature
        viii. Rectal
        ix. Tympanic
        x.   Forehead
        xi. Types of thermometer
        xii. Electronic
        xiii. Tympanic membrane
        xiv. Temporal artery
        xv. Chemical
        xvi. Disposable chemical single use
        xvii. Temperature sensitive strip
(4) Pulse
    a. Mechanism of pulse
    b. Major factors affecting pulse rate
    c. Application of pressure
    d. Pulse sites
    e. Assessment of pulse
        i.   Rate
        ii. Rhythm
        iii. Volume
(5) Respiration
    a. Mechanism of respiration
    b. Phases of respiration
    c. Types of respiration
    d. Assessment of respiration
        i.   Respiratory Rate
        ii. Respiratory Rhythm and Depth
    e. Respiratory abnormalities
    f. Factors affecting respiratory rate
    g. Cyanosis
    h. Breath Sounds

        i.   Normal
        ii. Abnormal
(6) Blood Pressure
    a. Mechanism of blood pressure
    b. Pulse pressure
    c. Mean arterial pulse pressure
    d. Factors affecting blood pressure
    e. Blood pressure recording equipment
        i.   Sphygmomanometer
        ii. Mercury
        iii. Aneroid
        iv. Digital
        v.   Cuff sizes
        vi. Stethoscope
        vii. Type of chest piece
    f. Korotkoff sounds of blood pressure
    g. Automated oscillometric blood pressure device
(7) Pulse oximetry
    a. Factors affecting pulse oximetry
(8) Measuring height and weight
(9) Body mass index
(10) Measuring head circumference in pediatrics
(11) Pulmonary function test
    a. Lung volumes
    b. Lung capacities
    c. Spirometry
    d. Pulmonary function test objectives
        i.   Pulmonary function test (steps)
        ii. Pulmonary function test: Points to consider before the test
        iii. Pulmonary function test: Points to consider during the test
        iv. Pulmonary function test: Points to consider post test
(12) Autoclaving and sterilization procedures
    a. Risk associated with autoclave
    b. Phases of autoclave
        i.   Phase 1: Loading
        ii. Phase 2: Operating
        iii. Phase 3: Unloading
    c. Spill clean up

PHYSICAL ASSESSMENT & EXAMINATION

Physical Assessment Techniques

Inspection is a method of visual assessment of the patient.
- ✓ Visual examination is performed while assessing the respiratory rate of a patient.

Palpation is a method of using one's hand to examine the patient's body.
- ✓ Pulse is assessed by touching a patient.
  - • Two types: Light & Deep Palpation

Percussion is a method of tapping on a surface of the human body to determine the underlying structure.
- ✓ Two Types:
  - • Direct percussion
  - • Indirect percussion

Auscultation is a method of listening to the internal sounds of the body, mostly using a stethoscope.
- ✓ Two Types:
  - • Direct auscultation: The ear is directly placed on the patient's skin.
  - • Indirect auscultation: Listening with a device placed over the patient's skin.

MEDICAL DOCUMENTATION (SOAP NOTES)

S = Subjective
O = Objective
A = Assessment
P = Plan

Subjective component:-

Includes the Chief Complaint abbreviated as CC of the patient. A statement quoted by the patient for the reason of his or her visit to the facility. In this stage, the physician will take a History of Present Illness.

A review of body systems is performed which includes all pertinent and negative symptoms. Pertinent medical history, surgical history, family history, and social history, along with current medications and allergies, are also recorded.

Objective component:-

The objective component includes: Findings from physical examinations-
I. Vital signs.
II. Measurements (such as height and weight).
III. Laboratory results
IV. Diagnostic test results

Assessment component:-

Summary of the patient's main symptoms and diagnosis, including the differential diagnosis. It may also include patient's current progress and overall progress towards the patient's goal from the physician's point of view.

Plan component:-

Plan of what the physician will perform, this may include:
- ✓ Recommended lab work
- ✓ Radiological work up
- ✓ Referrals given
- ✓ Recommended treatment
- ✓ Procedures performed
- ✓ Recommended medications prescribed
- ✓ Discharge notes
- ✓ Treatment progression
- ✓ Treatment outcome
- ✓ Long vs short term goal

VITAL SIGNS

The word "vital" means important or crucial. Assessment, Measurement and Monitoring (AMM) of vital signs are essential for health care technician(s), and assistant(s) working with a variety of population. Vital signs are performed by health-care professional in both settings (inpatient and outpatient settings).

The vital signs are as follows:
- • **Temperature,**
- • **Heart/Pulse Rate,**
- • **Respiratory Rate And**
- • **Blood Pressure**

Other examinations include:
- • **Pain Assessment**
- • **Level of Consciousness**

Relevant information obtained by assessing, measuring and monitoring the vital signs play a crucial role as an **indicator** for the patient's health status.

Recording: Good record keeping is essential for effective monitoring and interpretation of vital signs about a patient's health status.

The term assessment is typically used to indicate a broader process involving

- **Inspection**
- **Palpation**
- **Auscultation**
- **Percussion**

All health care assistants and technicians that assess, measure and monitor infants, children, adult and geriatric populations must be well trained to become competent in the accurate assessment, recording and monitoring of the vital signs (Temperature, Pulse rate, Respirations and Blood Pressure). Hint: TPR, BP.

Health care assistants and technicians should be aware of normal physiological parameters for temperature, pulse, respiratory rate and blood pressure for various age groups. Health care assistants and technicians should be mindful of the fact that practitioners take appropriate action in response to changes in vital signs, hence performing them properly are crucial. A systematic procedure is used when assessing, measuring and recording vital signs. Visual observation, palpation (touch), listening and communication, are utilized by the healthcare assistants or technicians when assessing and measuring vital signs.

The aim should be to **correctly** and **appropriately** assess and measure vital signs. Vital signs vary during the course of illness and should be closely observed by the healthcare assistants or technicians. Significant changes should be reported immediately as this may indicate a change in the patient's health status.

A change in vital signs may be an indicator of health issues that may occur as a result of systemic disorders or conditions.

Health care assistants and technicians should follow specific guidelines when measuring vital signs:

1. Correct order of assessment (TPR,BP)
   a. Temperature
   b. Pulse Rate
   c. Respiration Rate
   d. Blood Pressure
2. Equipment used should be in working condition.
3. Factors affecting vital signs must be identified and rectified.
4. Gain consent before performing vital signs.

5. Health care assistants and technicians should familiarize themselves with normal ranges of vital signs in different age groups.

TEMPERATURE

Temperature is recorded in Celsius or Fahrenheit. Celsius, also known as centigrade, is a scale and unit of measurement for temperature. Celsius was named after the astronomer Anders Celsius. The degree **Celsius** (°C) can refer to a specific temperature on the Celsius scale.

Fahrenheit (°F) was named after the physicist Daniel Gabriel Fahrenheit; it is a temperature based scale. The Fahrenheit scale is used for climatic, industrial and medical purposes.

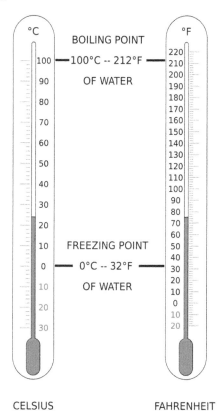

Figure 5.0 Thermometer in Celsius and Fahrenheit

Conversion Formula

°F to °C
Deduct 32, then multiply by 5, and divide by 9
Formula: (°F - 32) x 5/9 = °C

°C to °F
Multiply by 9, then divide by 5, and add 32
Formula: °C x 9/5 + 32 = °F

CELSIUS	FAHRENHEIT
34.0° C	93.2° F
35.0° C	95.0° F
36.0° C	96.8° F
36.5° C	97.7° F
37.0° C	98.6° F
37.5°C	99.5° F
38.0° C	100.4° F
38.5° C	101.3° F
39.0° C	102.2° F
40.0° C	104.0° F
41.0° C	105.5° F
42.0° C	107.6° F
43.0° C	109.4° F
44.0° C	111.2° F

Figure 5.0a Celsius/Fahrenheit equivalent temperature.

ORAL	RECTAL	AXILLARY
98.6°F	99.5°F	97.7°F
37.0°C	37.5°C	36.5°C

Figure 5.0b Temperature in different areas

The body keeps its core temperature constant at about 37°C by physiological adjustments controlled by the hypothalamus located in the brain. Hypothalamus (thermostat) is the temperature control center in the human body. The temperature control center usually allows the body temperature to vary by only about 1°F to 2°F Fahrenheit.

The thermostatic set point of the thermoregulatory center is set which causes the core temperature of the human body to regulate within the normal range.

- When body temperature begins to increase above the thermostatic set point, heat dissipating mechanisms are initiated within the human body.
- When the temperature decreases below the thermostatic set point, there is increased heat production within the human body.

HEAT PRODUCTION IN HUMAN BODY

Increase in body temperature may result due to the following factors:-

1. **Muscular activity**: Muscle contraction leads to an increase in tissue metabolism which in turn increases heat production, this may occur as a result of:-
   a. Shivering
   b. Muscular exercises
   c. Vigorous activity
2. **Ingestion of food**: Body metabolism increase during the process of digestion, resulting in increased body temperature.
3. **Time of day**: Body temperature is also affected by time of the day and sometimes also varies due to climatic conditions. During sleep, body temperature tends to be lower due to decreased muscle contractions.
4. **Emotion**: Release of epinephrine due to stimulation of the sympathetic nervous system increases the metabolic activities of body tissues causing an increase in body temperature. Be sure to observe this factor in young children who cry when their temperature is being recorded. If a child is ill and cries during the procedure, the recorded temperature may falsely get elevated due to crying (emotional status change).
5. **Hormones**: Basal metabolic rate increases due to increased production of thyroxin by the thyroid gland thereby causing an increase in body temperature.
6. **Infection or Fever**: Causes an increase in body temperature.
7. **Age**: Infants and young children normally have a higher body temperature than adults.
8. **Pregnancy**: During pregnancy, the cell metabolism of the body increases resulting in increased body temperature.
9. **Menstruation**: During ovulation, a female body increases in body temperature.
10. **Normal body temperature**: Some individuals normally have a high temperature, to find this the healthcare assistant or technician should compare the individual's current temperature with the past medical records of temperature.

Decrease in body temperature may result due to the following factors:-

1. **Illness for long duration**: Prolong inactivity and decrease muscle contraction.
2. **Fasting**: Decrease in nutrients.
3. **Sleep**: Decrease muscle contraction during sleep.
4. **Nervous system**: Neurological conditions and drugs acting on the nervous system.
5. **Climatic Condition**: Cold weather.

6. **Age**: Elderly individuals have low temperature due to lack of physical activity, loss of subcutaneous fat, loss of thermoregulatory control and other associated factors.

7. **Normal body temperature**: Some individuals normally have a high temperature, to find this the healthcare assistant or technician should compare the individual's current temperature with the past medical records of temperature.

HEAT DISTRIBUTED THROUGHOUT THE BODY

Temperature changes slightly due to the environmental and metabolic factors. Some factors as discussed may increase core temperature by up to three degrees, while some factors may decrease core temperature by a degree. If temperature crosses these ranges, it may lead to life-threatening conditions.

HEAT LOSS FROM HUMAN BODY

Waste product elimination: urine and feces cause loss of heat from the body.

Expiration: expelling carbon dioxide from lungs causes loss of heat.

Perspiration: evaporation of moisture from the surface of the skin causes a cooling effect.

Body Temperature Range

The main purpose of measuring the temperature of human body is to establish the patient's baseline temperature and to detect any abnormally high or low body temperature. The average body temperature is 98.6° F (37° C). Body temperature is typically recorded using the Fahrenheit system of temperature measurement.

Alterations in Body Temperature

1. **Hypothermia**: body temperature less than 95° F (35° C).

2. **Normal temperature**: body temperature is 36.5–37.5 °C (97.7 – 99.5 °F).

3. **Hyperthermia**: body temperature is greater than 37.5–38.3 °C (99.5–100.9 °F).

4. **Pyrexia**: body temperature greater than 100.4° F (38° C) indicates a fever.

5. **Hyperpyrexia**: body temperature reading greater than 104.0-106.7° F (40.0 - 41.5° C) is a serious condition, and a temperature greater than 109.4° F (43° C) is fatal.

6. **Fever**: Fever, or pyrexia, denotes that a patient's temperature has increased to greater than 100.4° F (38° C). Individual having fever is said to be in a **state of FEBRILE**, whereas an individual who is not in a state of fever is called **AFEBRILE**.

STAGES OF FEVER

A fever can be divided into the following three stages:

1. **Chill Phase (onset stage)**: The onset of fever is when the temperature first begins to rise. The increase in temperature may be slow or sudden; the patient may often experience chills (feeling of coldness) and increase in pulse rate and respiratory rate.

2. **Course of Fever**:
   Pattern in course of fever:-
   - Continuous
   - Remittent (Fever fluctuates)
   - Intermittent

   During the course of fever stage, the pulse and respiratory rate increases and the patient's skin feel warm and flushed. The patient may also experience one or more of the following: flushed appearance, increased thirst, loss of appetite, headache, aching muscles, drowsiness, restlessness, and malaise. The word "**Malaise**" refers to a vague feeling of generalized body discomfort, weakness, and fatigue.

3. **Termination or decline stage**:
   - Crisis: a sudden fall in temperature.
   - Lysis: a slow and gradual fall in temperature.

   The patient during this stage perspires and sometimes may become dehydrated.

ASSESSMENT OF BODY TEMPERATURE

Assessment Sites

There are five sites for measuring body temperature:
1. Oral
2. Axilla
3. Rectum
4. Ear (tympanic)
5. Forehead

The site chosen for measuring a patient's temperature depends on the:
1. Patient's age
2. Condition
3. State of consciousness
4. Type of thermometer

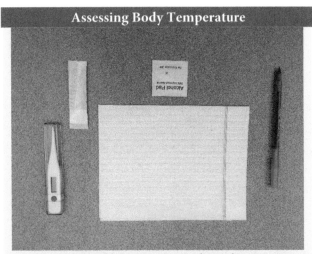

Assemble equipment and supplies

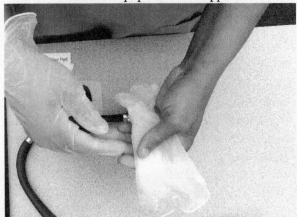

Wear gloves

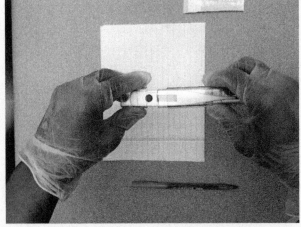

Remove the thermometer from its cover

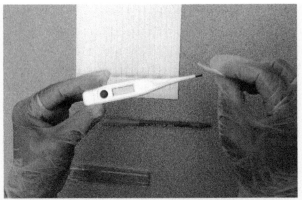

Disinfect the thermometer probe

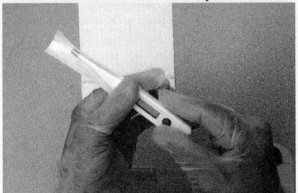

Put on probe cover

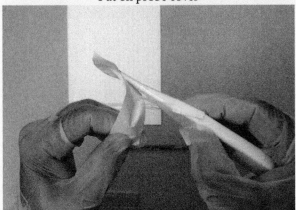

Peel of covering from probe cover

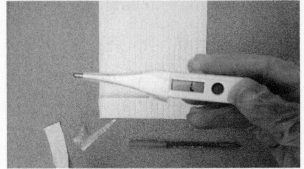

Press start button to start the thermometer

Oral Temperature

The oral method is the most common and reliable route of measuring body temperature. The thermometer should be placed under the tongue, posteriorly into the sublingual pocket on either side (right or left) to get the most accurate reading. Placing the thermometer in this location brings the thermometer in close vicinity of the sublingual artery. While the thermometer is in place, instruct the patient to keep his or her mouth closed during the procedure to avoid exposure of thermometer with the atmospheric air. Healthcare assistant or technician should be careful in placement of thermometer as placing the thermometer probe anteriorly may yield lower temperature. Few factors that can affect the true recording of temperature from this site includes drinking hot liquid, consuming food and smoking prior to the procedure being performed.

Axillary Temperature

The axillary route is recommended for patients in whom oral route is contraindicated or not accessible for some reason. Temperature is recorded from the axilla by placing the thermometer probe in the center of the armpit and adducting the arm close to the chest wall. The literature suggests that this is an unreliable site for estimating core body temperature because there are no main blood vessels around this area (Sund-Levander and Grodzinsky, 2009). The temperature at this site can be affected due to sweating and improper thermometer placement. Axillary temperature is recommended for infants. The axillary site should be used for patients with conditions of the oral cavity (injury, surgery or inflammation), or open-mouth-breathing patients. **This site measures an approximate of 1° F lower than the oral site.**

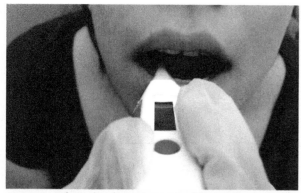
Place the thermometer sublingually

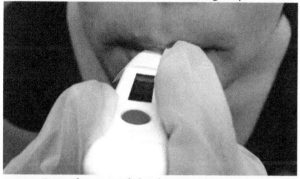
Purse-lip around the thermometer probe

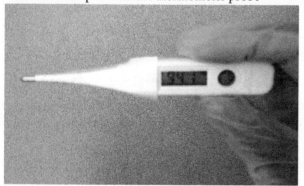
Remove thermometer from mouth and read temperature

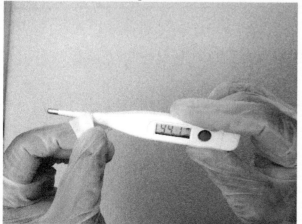
Remove and discard probe cover

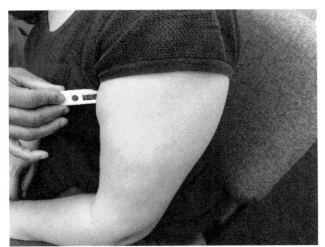

Figure 5.1 Assessing Axillary Temperature

Rectal Temperature

The rectal temperature is considered to be the most accurate measurement of core temperature. The procedure is a bit lengthier than that of other sites. It is also not favored by many patients and is one of the most unfavorable routes of measuring temperature. Some factors may not allow the probe to touch the wall of the rectum (for e.g presence of feces) leading to inaccurate results. The rectal site is the most accurate due to the presence of blood vessels and closed cavity surrounding the probe at insertion.

Contraindicated: if the patient has diarrhea, rectal disease, or has recently had rectal surgery, or a heart condition as insertion of the probe may cause stimulation of vagus nerve.

Indicated: infants or young children, patients who are unconscious and irrational, a patient who have difficulty in breathing with mouth closed, and when greater accuracy in body temperature is desired. **This site measures an approximate of 1° F higher than the oral site.**

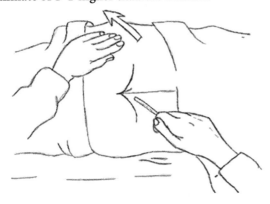

Figure 5.1a Assessing Rectal Temperature

Tympanic Temperature

The ear is the site considered when using a tympanic membrane thermometer. Ear provides a closed cavity that is easily accessible with the tympanic thermometer. This method is quick, easy to perform and minimally non-invasive. It can record fluctuations in core body temperature since the site is close to the hypothalamus, unlike rectal temperature which cannot record fluctuations in core body temperature due to its location. Factors like the presence of ear wax can lead to erroneous results from this site, make sure to inspect the ear for earwax.

Indications: children younger than 6 years, uncooperative patients or patients in whom oral and axillary site are not accessible.

Contraindications: ear infection, ear inflammation, and ear injury.

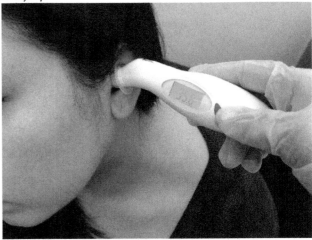

Figure 5.2 Assessing Tympanic Temperature

Forehead Temperature

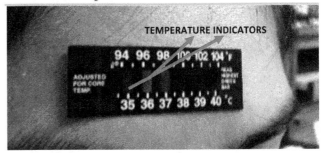

Figure 5.2a Forehead Thermometer Strip

The temperature from this site is taken by placing a special thermometer over the forehead in close vicinity of the temporal artery, due to the constant flow of blood in the temporal artery the site provides accurate results.

Indications: can be used for any population.

This site measures an approximate of 1°F higher than oral body temperature and 2°F higher than axillary temperature.

Types of Thermometers

The four types of thermometers available for measuring body temperature are:

1. Electronic Thermometer
2. Tympanic Membrane Thermometer
3. Temporal Artery Thermometer
4. Chemical Thermometer

Traditional thermometers are no longer used due to its hazardous effects since mercury in the thermometer is not safe for the environment and human body.

Electronic Thermometer

Most commonly used thermometer in an inpatient and outpatient settings by healthcare assistants and technicians. It is portable and can measure temperature from sites like oral, axillary and rectal. The thermometer consists of a LCD (liquid-crystal display) screen which displays the temperature from the chosen site. Sensors present in the probe of the thermometer records the temperature. Different color probe covers are:

- BLUE COLOR: **Oral or Axillary Probe Cover**
- RED COLOR: **Rectal Probe Cover**

A disposable plastic probe cover is placed over the probe to prevent the transmission of microorganisms from one patient to another. To record the temperature, the probe of the thermometer is inserted or placed into the site (oral, axillary, rectal, or tympanic) and left in place until an audible sound is heard, on which the thermometer is removed, and the temperature is seen on the LCD (liquid-crystal display) screen. The next step is to record the temperature. Moreover, discard the probe cover into a waste container.

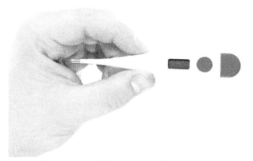

Figure 5.3 Electronic Thermometer

Tympanic Membrane Thermometer

The aural site is used for the tympanic thermometer. It is a choice of thermometer used in children over 2 years of age and adults. It is minimally invasive, painless with quick results. The thermometer consists two of main parts: a handle and a probe. The probe is placed into the external ear canal; the activation button is then clicked and left till the thermometer displays the temperature; a probe cover is used on the probe to prevent cross-contamination amongst patients prior to placing the thermometer into the site. Once the temperature is displayed the probe cover is discarded into the waste container and the temperature is recorded.

Temporal Artery Thermometer

Temporal artery thermometer consists of a handle and a probe unit; the probe unit should be clean and inspected prior to its placement on the forehead. Apply probe cover onto the probe unit or wipe with a disinfectant wipe. Hold the probe gently against the forehead of the patient and press the "ON" switch button and keep the "ON" button pressed. While doing so move the thermometer across the forehead, this movement is required for the thermometer to record the highest temperature (peak temperature) emitted from the temporal artery. If required the probe unit is placed behind the earlobes (just below the mastoid process). Wait for the thermometer to display the recorded temperature (peak temperature), discard the probe cover. Finally, document the recorded temperature.

The second location behind the ear is taken into consideration when the forehead is sweating or displaying false temperature due to evaporation of perspired moisture from the surface of the forehead.

Chemical Thermometers

Chemical thermometers contain chemicals that are heat sensitive and include:-

- A disposable chemical single-use thermometer.
- A temperature-sensitive strip.

Disposable Chemical Single-Use Thermometers

One end of the thermometer is the sensor, while the other end of the thermometer is the dotted matrix. The temperature change in the sensor brings change in the dotted matrix by increased filling of the empty dots on the matrix by color, and the number of dots filled on the dotted matrix indicates the temperature change of the individual. Each dot filled on the thermometer indicates a temperature change. The thermometer is placed under the tongue or in the axilla for the temperature to be recorded in the dotted matrix, the manufacturer generally instructs the length of time the thermometer should be placed at the site. Care should be taken to avoid touching the dotted matrix end of the thermometer. Once the procedure is completed, the thermometer should be discarded.

Temperature-Sensitive Strips

The strip is placed over the forehead, and the color change in the test strip of the thermometer indicates the temperature being recorded, the thermometer is held in place till the color no longer changes. These changes display the temperature on the thermometer. Recorded temperature is less accurate from other methods.

Care should be taken in storage of these thermometers:-

- Place in cool areas.
- Avoid direct sunlight exposure or hot climate.

Competency Checklist: Oral Temperature

1. Assemble equipment and supplies
2. Wash hands / Wear gloves (follow standard precautions)
3. Greet the patient
4. Identify yourself (name & designation)
5. Identify patient (full name & date of birth)
6. Explain procedure & inquire about activity, diet & medication
7. Ask the patient about recent activities
8. Remove thermometer from case
9. Inspect & disinfect the thermometer
10. Apply thermometer probe cover
11. Switch thermometer on
12. Check display window for "ready" signal
13. Insert sublingually
14. Wait for the thermometer to beep
15. Withdraw thermometer/read the results
16. Remove probe cover and discard in biohazard waste
17. Disinfect the thermometer
18. Remove gloves and discard
19. Wash hands
20. Record results in patient's chart accurately

PULSE

Mechanism of the Pulse

The left side of the heart has two chambers, the left atrium, and the left ventricle. The left atrium is a thin walled and low-pressure chamber. It receives oxygenated blood from the lungs through pulmonary veins (right and left). This is an exception in the human body, where a vein carries oxygenated (oxygen-rich) blood. Blood from left atrium enters the left ventricle through the mitral valve (bicuspid valve). The wall of the left ventricle is very thick. The left ventricle pumps the oxygenated blood to different parts of the body through the aorta to the arterial system; this causes a pulsating wave like effect called "BEAT" through the artery. This "BEAT" is the heart rate which is determined by assessing pulse rate. Pulse is the rhythmic expansion and contraction of an artery caused by the impact of blood pumped by the heart.

Key factors Affecting Pulse Rate

- Muscular Activity
- Emotional Status
- Hormonal Changes
- Fever
- Age
- Pregnancy
- Medications
- Body Size
- Body Position
- Weather (Temperature)
- Vagal Stimulation
- Dehydration
- Body Temperature

Application of pressure

Gentle pressure should be applied with 2–3 fingers depending on the site to be assessed.

- If the pressure applied is more than what is required, it may lead to cut off, the closing of the blood supply with minimum or no pulse.
- If the pressure is applied less than what is required, it may result in difficulty in detecting the pulse.

PULSE SITES

The pulse can be felt when an examiner places their evaluating middle and index finger over a superficial artery and hold it firmly against a firm body tissue (bone).

Radial

Radial pulse (radial artery) is the most easily accessible and commonly used pulse site. The radial pulse can be located by placing the index and middle fingers at the base of the thumb over the wrist (approximately).

Press the index and middle fingers down in the grove between the middle tendons and the bone (RADIUS). A pulse should be felt.

Count the number of beats for 60 seconds this will give the heart rate.

Another method is to count the number of beats for 30 seconds and then multiply the number of beats by 2. This will give the heart rate for a minute, beats per minute (bpm). If an individual has 42 beats in 30 seconds, the heart rate would be as follows:

Pulse Rate = # of heart beats in 30 seconds X 2

$$= 42 \times 2$$

$$= 84 \text{bpm (Beats per minute)}$$

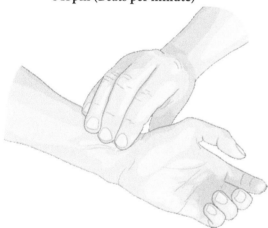

Figure 5.4 Radial Pulse Location

Apical

To locate the apical pulse, the chest piece of the stethoscope is placed gently and firmly over the apex of the heart, located at the fifth intercostal space (between the ribs) on the left side of the chest on the midclavicular line. The sound heard will be "lubb and dubb", this should be counted as one beat only.

The beats should be counted for over a period of 60 seconds; this site is used for small children usually below age 3 and infants due to their faster heart rate. Other indications may include patients suffering from cardiac conditions.

Brachial

The brachial pulse (brachial artery) can be located in the antecubital space, which is the space located at the inner aspect of the elbow. This site is most commonly used to obtain blood pressure.

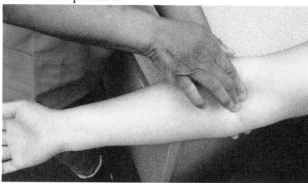

Figure 5.5 Brachial Pulse Location

Ulnar

The ulnar pulse can be located by placing the index and the middle finger at the base of the little finger over the wrist, the reason for checking this pulse is to find out the circulation status of the hand.

Temporal

The temporal pulse is located in temple area of the forehead.

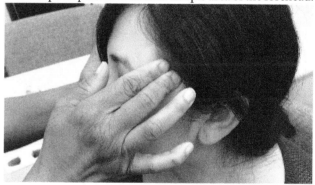

Figure 5.6 Temporal Pulse Location

Carotid

The carotid pulse is located between the larynx and sternocleidomastoid on the anterior side of the neck, slightly to one side of the midline (trachea).

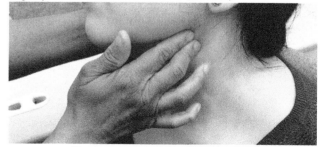

Figure 5.7 Carotid Pulse Location

Femoral

The femoral pulse is in the mid-groin region and should be firmly compressed to assess the pulse.

Popliteal

The popliteal pulse can be located on the posterior aspect of the knee and can be felt easily if the knee is slightly flexed.

Posterior Tibial

The posterior tibial pulse is located on the posterior aspect of the ankle joint.

Dorsalis Pedis

The dorsalis pedis pulse is located on the superior surface of the foot, usually found between the first and second metatarsal bones.

Assessment of Pulse

Assessment of pulse includes three main components:
1. **Pulse Rate**
2. **Pulse Rhythm**
3. **Pulse Volume**

PULSE RATE

Normal Pulse Rate: 60 -100 beats per minute.
Bradycardia: less than 60 beats per minute.
Tachycardia: more than 100 beats per minute.
Pulse rate is higher in infants and lower in elderly.

PULSE RHYTHM

Pulse rhythm is the spacing of the beats.
Regular: equal spacing of beats or even beats.
Irregular: uneven spacing of beats or uneven beats.

PULSE VOLUME

Pulse volume is the amount of blood present in the arteries and the strength of the contractions in the heart with the current elasticity of blood vessels.
Regular and Strong Pulse: Normal blood volume
Full and Bounding Pulse: Increase blood volume
Weak and Thready Pulse: Decrease blood volume

COMPETENCY CHECKLIST: PULSE RATE

1. Assemble equipment and supplies (timer/stopwatch).
2. Wash hands (follow standard precautions).
3. Greet the patient.
4. Identify yourself (name & designation).

5. Identify patient (full name & date of birth).
6. Explain procedure & inquire about activity, diet & medication.
7. Position patient comfortably.
8. Locate the pulse using proper finger placement.
9. Palpate & describe the quality of pulse.
10. Count beats per minute.
11. Record results in a patient chart.
12. Wash hands.

RESPIRATION

Mechanism of Respiration

Respiration is the process by which oxygen is inhaled in, and carbon dioxide is exhaled out.

PHASES OF RESPIRATION

Respiration occurs in two phases:
1. **Inspiration:** during which air (oxygen) enters the lungs.
2. **Expiration:** during which air (carbon dioxide) leaves the lungs.

During normal breathing, inspiration is an active phase and expiration is a passive phase. Inspiration phase causes expansion of thoracic cage.

Expansion of thoracic cage takes place in the following diameters:

Anteroposterior Diameter of Thoracic Cage
• Increases by elevation of ribs
Transverse Diameter of Thoracic Cage
• Increases by elevation of ribs
Vertical Diameters of Thoracic Cage
• Increases by descent of diaphragm

One complete respiration consists of one inhalation and one exhalation.

TYPES OF RESPIRATION

Respiration is classified into two types:
1. External respiration that involves the exchange of respiratory gasses, i.e. oxygen and carbon dioxide **between lungs and the blood.**
2. Internal respiration, which involves the exchange of gasses **between blood and the tissues.**

Assessment of Respiration

The patient should not be informed about the assessment of respiration as this may change the breathing pattern. It is best to assess the respiratory rate right after the pulse rate is assessed.

Respiratory Rate

1. **Eupnea (Normal):** 12-20 respirations per minute.
2. **Bradypnea:** less than 12 respirations per minute.
3. **Tachypnea:** more than 20 respirations per minute.
4. **Apnea:** no breathing.

Respiratory Rhythm & Depth

    a. Rhythm
        i. Regular
        ii. Irregular
    b. Depth
        i. Normal
        ii. Deep
        iii. Shallow

Respiratory Abnormalities

1. **Eupnea:** Rate: 12-20, rhythm: even and regular, depth: normal.
2. **Hyperpnea:** Increase in pulmonary ventilation due to increase in rate and force of respiration (occurs mainly due to insufficient oxygen supply and increase in carbon dioxide in blood):-
    a. normal after exercise and
    b. abnormal in fever and conditions affecting heart & lungs.
3. **Hypopnea:** Decrease in rate and depth of breathing (shallow and slow).
4. **Hyperventilation:** Abnormally fast and increased depth of breathing, may lead to dizziness, discomfort and chest pain. A large amount of air moves in and out of lungs.
5. **Hypoventilation:** Decrease in pulmonary ventilation caused by a decrease in rate or force of breathing. Thus, the amount of air moving in and out of lungs is reduced.
6. **Asphyxia:** Combination of hypoxia and hypercapnea, due to obstruction of the air passage.
7. **Dyspnea:** Difficulty in breathing.
8. **Cheyne-Stokes breathing:** A periodic breathing characterized by rhythmic hyperpnea and apnea.
9. **Biot breathing:** is another form of periodic breathing characterized by a period of apnea and

hyperpnea. After an apneic period, hyperpnea occurs abruptly.

10. **Orthopnea:** difficulty breathing in a specific position (supine or sitting).

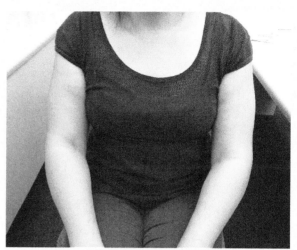

Inhalation (Inspiration)
Check for rise in shoulder or chest

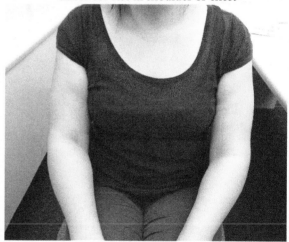

Exhalation (Expiration)
Check for drop in shoulder or chest

Figure 5.8

Factors Affecting Respiratory Rate

a. Muscular Activity
b. Emotional Status
c. Fever
d. Age
e. Pregnancy
f. Medications
g. Body Size
h. Body Position

Skin Color of the Patient

Cyanosis is a condition which leads to bluish discoloration of the skin and mucous membrane. During the assessment of respiratory rate the patient's skin color should be observed. If the oxygen supply to the tissues (hypoxia) reduces it results in a condition known as cyanosis (bluish discoloration of the skin and mucous membrane).

Cyanosis is first observed in the:

- Fingertips (Nail Beds)
- Lips
- Cheeks
- Ear Lobes
- Nose

Breath Sounds

A. Normal breath sounds are classified as:
1. Tracheal
2. Bronchial
3. Bronchovesicular
4. Vesicular Sounds

B. Abnormal breath sounds are referred to as adventitious sounds and signify the presence of a respiratory disorder.
1. Crackles (Rales)
2. Wheezes (Rhonchi)
3. Stridor
4. Pleural Rubs
5. Voice Sounds
6. Egophony
7. Bronchophony
8. Whispered Pectoriloquy

COMPETENCY CHECKLIST: RESPIRATION

1. Assemble equipment and supplies.
2. Wash hands (follow standard precautions).
3. Greet the patient.
4. Identify yourself (name & designation).
5. Identify patient (full name & date of birth).
6. Ask the patient about recent activities influencing respiratory rate.
7. Position patient comfortably.
8. Observe the rise and fall of the chest (inspiration and expiration) this counts as one breath.
9. Assess & verbally describe the quality of respiration.
10. The respirations should be counted for a full minute in order to have an accurate recording.
11. Record results in a patient chart.

BLOOD PRESSURE

Mechanism of Blood Pressure

Blood pressure is the measurement of the force which the blood exerts on the walls of the arteries; this force is produced by the "systolic phase" of the cardiac cycle during which the left ventricle contracts to eject the blood out of the heart through the aorta. This exertion pressure towards the wall of the arteries is known as **systolic pressure**. The other phase of the blood pressure measurement is the relaxation phase in which the ventricles relaxes, this is called "**diastolic phase**". The measurement of pressure in this phase is called as "diastolic pressure". Blood pressure is important since it is this pressure which helps in propelling the blood in a forward direction so that each and every organ, cell and tissue receive oxygenated blood.

Cardiac Cycle	Blood Pressure	Readings
Systolic Phase	Systolic Pressure	120mmhg
Diastolic Phase	Diastolic Pressure	80mmhg

Table 5.0 Blood Pressure Reading

When recording blood pressure the readings are to be recorded as follows:-
- **Systolic Reading (Numerator)**
- **Diastolic Reading (Denominator)**

If the blood pressure is recorded as **120/80 mmHg**. The numerator "**120**" is the "**systolic pressure**", the pressure recorded during the contraction phase of the heart. The denominator "**80**" is the "**diastolic pressure**" recorded during the relaxation phase of the heart. The unit of measuring blood pressure is **millimeters of mercury (mmHg)**.

Blood Pressure Category	Systolic mm Hg (upper #)
Normal	less than 120
Pre-hypertension	120 – 139
High Blood Pressure (Hypertension) Stage 1	140 – 159
High Blood Pressure (Hypertension) Stage 2	160 or higher
Hypertensive Crisis (Emergency care needed)	Higher than 180

Blood Pressure Category	Diastolic mm Hg (lower #)
Normal	less than 80
Pre-hypertension	80 – 89
High Blood Pressure (Hypertension) Stage 1	90 – 99
High Blood Pressure (Hypertension) Stage 2	100 or higher
Hypertensive Crisis (Emergency care needed)	Higher than 110

Blood pressure chart

High blood pressure (HBP) is a condition that can cause heart conditions, nervous system conditions, renal conditions and others. It can damage various organs (parts) of the body.

Pulse Pressure

Pulse pressure is the difference between the systolic pressure and diastolic pressure.

Normal pulse pressure: 40 mmHg (120 – 80 = 40). A pulse pressure between 30 and 40 mmHg is considered to be within normal range. Recent studies have shown that pulse pressure may help in predicting coronary heart disease.

Mean arterial blood pressure (MAP)

Mean arterial blood pressure is the average pressure existing in the arteries. The formula to calculate mean arterial blood pressure.

= diastolic pressure + 1/3 of pulse pressure

Example: If an individual has a diastolic blood pressure of 90 mmHg and pulse pressure of 45 mmHg

Answer: **90 + 45/3 = 105 mmHg** (MAP)

Factors Affecting Blood Pressure

1. Overweight or obese.
2. Lack of physical activity.
3. Too much salt in the diet.
4. Too much alcohol consumption.
5. Stress
6. Family history of high blood pressure.
7. Chronic kidney disease.
8. Adrenal and thyroid disorders.
9. Age: blood pressure increases with age.
10. Gender: before menopause, female blood pressure is lower than male. After menopause, women usually have an equal or sometimes higher blood pressure than male of the same age.
11. Diurnal variations: changes in blood pressure is seen.
12. Digestion: increase in blood pressure due to increase in metabolism.
13. Sleep: decrease in blood pressure.
14. During the day: blood pressure is usually low in the morning than during the day (due to activities which leads to increase in the blood pressure).
15. Emotional status: Some emotions like anxiety, fear and anger will increase the blood pressure, while some emotions will decrease blood pressure.
16. Exercise: Muscle contractions during exercise increases cardiac output which causes an increase in blood pressure.
17. Prescribed & Over-the-Counter Medications: Some medications may increase, whereas other medications may decrease the blood pressure.

Blood Pressure Recording Equipment

The equipment used are stethoscope and a sphygmomanometer. There are 3 types of sphygmomanometers:

- Aneroid
- Mercury
- Digital

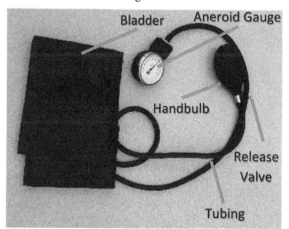

Figure 5.9 Aneroid Blood Pressure Unit

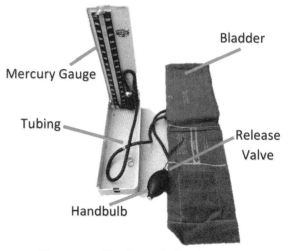

Figure 5.10 Traditional Blood Pressure Unit

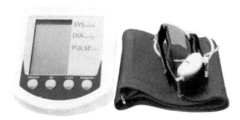

Figure 5.11 Digital Blood Pressure Unit

Sphygmomanometer

1. **Bladder:** The bladder is also known as a cuff. The bladder is a part wrapped around the arm and inflated with air when taking the patient's blood pressure.
2. **Handbulb:** The handbulb is a part used to inflate the bladder. To inflate the bladder the handbulb should be firmly pressed; this leads to the entry of air into the bladder resulting in inflation of the bladder.
3. **Rubber tubes:** Two tubes
   Tube 1: Connected to the handbulb on one end and bladder on the other hand.
   Tube 2: Connected to the gauge on one end and bladder on the other hand.
4. **Release valve:** Is a part that functions as a "lock and key" for inflating and deflating the bladder air. If the valve is locked, squeezing the bulb will inflate the air into the bladder and unlocking the valve will lead to deflating the bladder.
5. **Gauge:** The gauge measures the air pressure in the bladder. There are two types of gauges (mercury gauge and aneroid gauge).
   A. **Mercury.** The mercury gauge has a column of mercury in a glass tube.
   B. **Aneroid.** The aneroid manometer gauge is circular in shape with a dial.

Cuff Sizes

Cuff sizes are available in a variety of sizes.
To measure blood pressure, the cuff should encircle at least 80% of the arm circumference and should be wide enough to cover 2/3rd of the distance from the axilla to the antecubital space.
1) **CUFF SIZE SMALL**
   - Reading falsely high
2) **CUFF SIZE LARGE**
   - Reading falsely low

The cuff should be applied over the brachial artery to allow for complete compression of the brachial artery. If the arm is bigger in circumference, the patient's blood pressure can be measured using the forearm on the radial artery, but this may lead to a false increase in the systolic recording.

Stethoscope

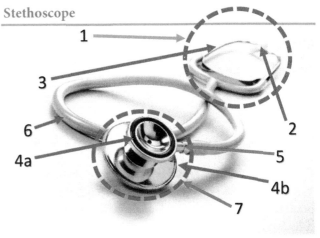

Figure 5.12 Stethoscope

The acoustic stethoscope is commonly used for measuring blood pressure measurement.
Part of a stethoscope are:
1. **Headset:** is the proximal metallic part of the stethoscope. The two rubber tubing's fit on this part. It also consists of the two ear tips.
2. **Eartip:** is the part which fits into the ear for hearing the sound picked up by the chest piece.
3. **Eartube:** is the part that extends from the eartip to the start (proximal end) of the rubber tubing.
4. **Bell (4a) & Diaphragm (4b):** the bell is used to hear **low-frequency sounds** by means of a **light contact** with the skin and the diaphragm is used to hear **high frequency sounds** by means of a **firm contact** with the skin.
5. **Stem:** extends from the distal end of the tubing to the chestpiece.
6. **Tubing:** is a hollow tube, can be made of up plastic or rubber.
7. **Chestpiece:** a part of the stethoscope, placed on the anatomical location.

Types of Chest Piece

There are two types of chest pieces:
Type 1. With a diaphragm and a bell
Type 2. Diaphragm only
The chest piece must be rotated (**turn on**) to ensure that it is in a proper position for the sound to be audible through the diaphragm or the bell.
- The **diaphragm** of the chest piece is used to hear **high-pitched sounds.**

- The **bell** of the chest piece is used for hearing **low-pitched sounds.**

Korotkoff Sounds of Blood Pressure

Korotkoff sounds are used to determine systolic and diastolic blood pressure readings.

1) **1st sound** heard when the cuff is deflated at 2-3 mmHg/sec and is recorded as **systolic pressure**.

2) **2nd sound** is the last sound heard, this is recorded as **diastolic pressure**.

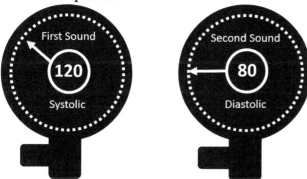

Figure 5.12a 1st and 2nd Heart Sound

Practice is required to familiarize with both the sounds and should be practiced more frequently during training sessions.

Automated Oscillometric Blood Pressure Device

The device automatically records the blood pressure by inflating and deflating on its own, the recording of the pressure is done via sensors present in the device. The device has a screen on which the results are displayed which can then be recorded in the patient's record or blood pressure log or flow sheet.

Advantages of using an automated oscillometric blood pressure device:-

1. Automatic recording
2. Automatic inflation
3. No skills required for listening sounds
4. Time saving
5. Eliminates use of stethoscope

Disadvantages of using an automated oscillometric blood pressure device:-

1. May not be accurate at times.
2. Automated oscillometric devices are expensive.

BLOOD PRESSURE COMPETENCY CHECK

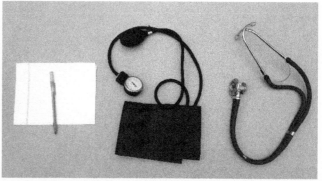

Assemble Equipment and Supplies

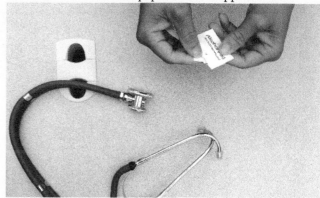

Use an alcohol pad

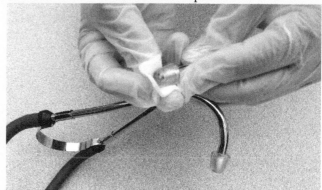

Disinfect ear piece of stethoscope

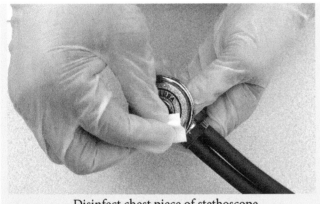

Disinfect chest piece of stethoscope

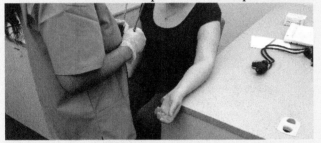

Have patient sit in a comfortable position

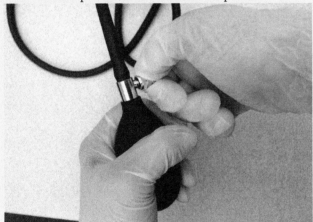

Locking the blood pressure cuff

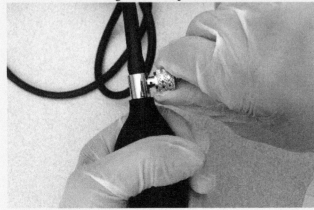

Unlocking the blood pressure cuff

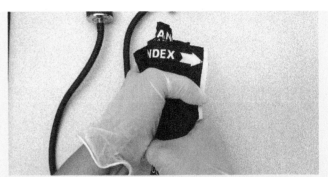

Squeeze out all the air from the cuff

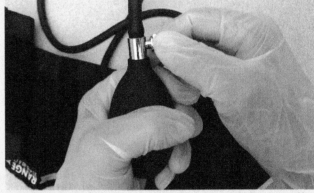

Double check and close the knob, before inflating cuff

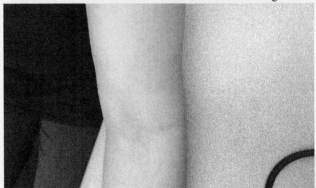

Select site of cuff placement

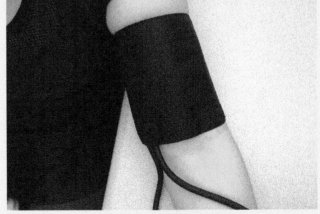

Place cuff on the site

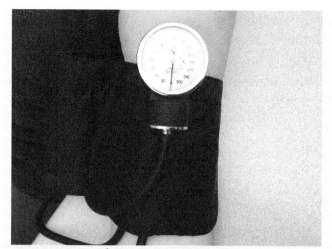

Place meter appropriately

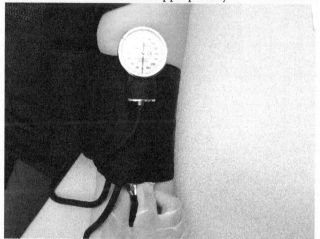

Place the diaphragm of the stethoscope on the brachial
artery.
Listen to the systolic and diastolic blood pressure
Finally, record systolic and diastolic blood pressure

Blood Pressure Recording Unit Digital Blood Pressure Unit

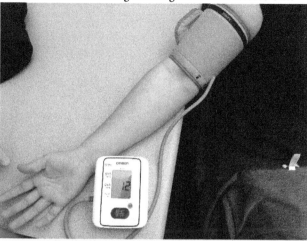

Using a digital blood pressure machine place cuff on site

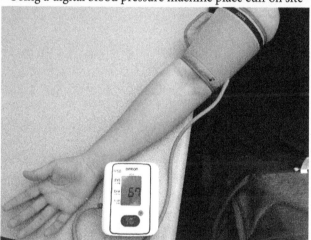

Press start and wait

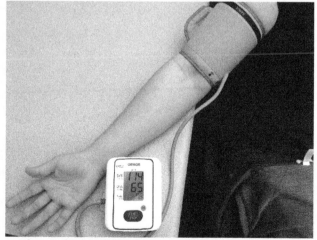

The machine will display systolic(Upper number) and
diastolic(Lower number) blood pressure.

COMPETENCY CHECKLIST: BLOOD PRESSURE

1. Assemble equipment and supplies.
2. Disinfect earpieces and head of the stethoscope.
3. Wash hands (follow standard precautions).
4. Greet the patient.
5. Identify yourself (name & designation).
6. Identify patient (full name & date of birth).
7. Explain procedure & inquire about activity, diet & medication.
8. Position patient comfortably.
9. Squeeze all air from bladder cuff of the sphygmomanometer.
10. Close valve of the sphygmomanometer.
11. Expose patient's arm and apply cuff at the appropriate location.
12. Palpate/Locate brachial artery by using index & middle finger.
13. Tap the head of the stethoscope for audible sound.
14. Position stethoscope on the brachial artery.
15. Inflate cuff as directed.
16. Open valve slowly as directed to deflate the cuff.
17. Note first sound heard in the earpieces of the stethoscope (systolic pressure).
18. Note last sound heard in the earpieces of the stethoscope (diastolic pressure).
19. Release remaining air.
20. Remove stethoscope and cuff from patient's arm (fully deflate the cuff).
21. Clean equipment/ return to storage.
22. Record results.

PULSE OXIMETRY

A pulse oximeter is a device that monitors the level of oxygen saturation (percentage of hemoglobin that is oxygen-saturated) of a patient's arterial blood. Pulse oximetry is a painless and non-invasive method for monitoring a patient's O_2 saturation.

The probe of the pulse oximetry should be secured onto the capillary bed (fingertip).

The interpretation of results are as follows:-

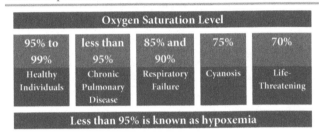

Oxygen Saturation Level				
95% to 99% Healthy Individuals	less than 95% Chronic Pulmonary Disease	85% and 90% Respiratory Failure	75% Cyanosis	70% Life-Threatening
Less than 95% is known as hypoxemia				

Factors Affecting Pulse Oximetry:-

1. Incorrect positioning of the probe
2. Fingernail polish or artificial nails
3. Poor peripheral blood flow
4. Ambient (surrounding) light
5. Patient movement

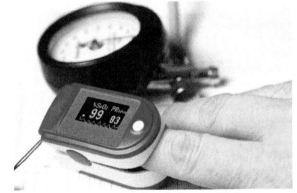

Figure 5.13 Pulse Oximetry Unit

MEASURING HEIGHT AND WEIGHT

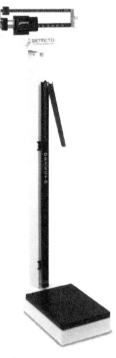

Purpose:

a. To determine if the patient is underweight or overweight.

b. For dosage of certain medication.

c. To check for increase or decrease in edema as some conditions may cause edema leading to increase in total body weight.

d. In addition to height and weight, the head circumference is also measured in infants to check the growth.

• Growth pattern not within the normal range may indicate deficiencies.

e. Height can also indicate a postural problem. If the height readings are lower than the reading taken in the past, it may indicate conditions such as kyphosis or other postural problems (temporary or permanent).

f. Height and weight readings are also used to calculate the body mass index (BMI).

Equipment used to measure weight and height are:

- **Weighing Scale**
- **Stadiometer:** Portable or Wall Mounted

MEASURING HEIGHT

A. Measuring Height: Standing Position

a. Use a height measuring device (Stadiometer).

b. Ask the patient to stand on the platform of the device with erect posture and look straight. **Four Points of Contact on the scale: Head, Shoulder blades, Buttock and Heel.**

c. Instruct to remove footwear or hair accessories that can interfere with the measurement.

d. Measure the height by reading the scale appropriately (From the Foot to Crown of the Head).

e. Double check your work.

B. Measuring Height: Supine Position

a. Position individual on side-lying or back (supine).

b. Remove patient's shoes.

c. Use appropriate measuring device or make two points with a pencil (one point just above the head and one point just below the foot), using a measuring tape measure the distance between these two points. Care should be taken to ensure that the patient is in the supine position with arms by the side and legs straight.

d. Measure the height by reading measurement appropriately.

e. Once done, reposition the patient back to the normal position.

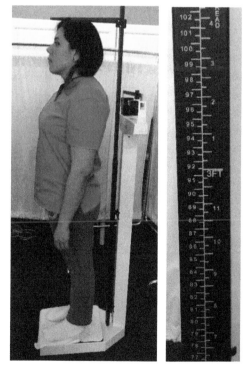

Figure 5.14 Measuring Height (Standing Position)

MEASURING WEIGHT

1. Identify your patient.
2. Introduce yourself.
3. Explain the procedure and gain consent.

4. Balance the scale to zero.
5. Weigh individual: STANDING VS SUPINE

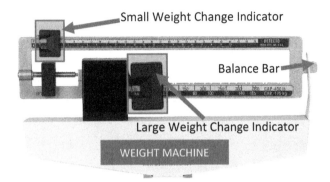

Small Weight Change Indicator

Balance Bar

Large Weight Change Indicator

WEIGHT MACHINE

Figure 5.15 Weight Scale (Weigh the individual by moving the large weight indicator and small weight indicator until the bar balances).

A. Individual, who is able to stand to be weighed:

a. Place a disposable towel on the scale platform.
b. Have the patient stand on the scale platform without any footwear or any object that can add extra weight. Make sure to check that this additional weight object is not of medical necessity, if it is, leave it and record the patient's weight with the object, finally subtract the objects weight from the readings you obtained while the patient was on the scale. Provide assistance if the patient needs it for getting onto the scale platform.
c. Read weight measurement.
d. Make sure to provide appropriate assistance as required for the patient to get off the weighing scale platform.
e. Record the patient's name, time of recording and weight.

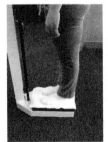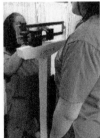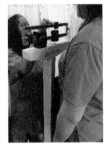

Figure 5.16 Weight Recording

B. Individual, who is weighed by wheelchair or bed scale:

a. Make sure to sanitize the equipment before its use (wheelchair/bed scale).

b. Assist individual on wheelchair scale or bed scale appropriately.
c. Read weight measurement.
   • If using the wheelchair scale, subtract the weight of the unoccupied wheelchair from the recording obtained.
   • If using a bed or chair scale just record the reading as seen on the equipment display.
   • If using a chair scale or bed scale, have the patient positioned appropriately on the scale for accurate recording.
d. Assist resident off wheelchair/bed scale as appropriate.
e. Return scale balance to zero.
f. Record the patient's name, time of recording and weight.

BODY MASS INDEX

Body Mass Index (BMI) is a number calculated from a person's weight and height. BMI is a fairly reliable indicator of body fatness for most people. BMI does not measure body fat directly, but research has shown that BMI correlates to direct measures of body fat, such as underwater weighing and dual energy x-ray absorptiometry (DXA).[1,2] BMI can be considered an alternative to direct measures of body fat. Additionally, BMI is an inexpensive and easy-to-perform method of screening for weight categories that may lead to health problems. BMI is used as a screening tool to identify possible weight problems for adults. However, BMI is not a diagnostic tool. For example, a person may have a high BMI. However, to determine if excess weight is a health risk, a healthcare provider would need to perform further assessments. These assessments might include skinfold thickness measurements, evaluations of diet, physical activity, family history, and other appropriate health screenings.

Calculation of BMI:
BMI is calculated the same way for both adults and children. The calculation is based on the following formulas:

Kilograms and meters (or centimeters)
Formula: weight (kg) / [height (m)]^2

With the metric system, the formula for BMI is weight in kilograms divided by height in meters squared. Since height is commonly measured in centimeters, divide height in centimeters by 100 to obtain height in meters.

Example: Weight = 68 kg, Height = 165 cm (1.65 m)
Calculation: $68 \div (1.65)^2 = 24.98$

Pounds and inches
Formula: weight (lb) / [height (in)]² x 703

Calculate BMI by dividing weight in pounds (lbs) by height in inches (in) squared and multiplying by a conversion factor of 703.

Example: Weight = 150 lbs, Height = 5'5" (65")
Calculation: [150 ÷ (65)²] x 703 = 24.96

Measurement Units	Formula and Calculation
Kilograms and meters (or centimeters)	Formula: weight (kg) / [height (m)]² With the metric system, the formula for BMI is weight in kilograms divided by height in meters squared. Since height is commonly measured in centimeters, divide height in centimeters by 100 to obtain height in meters. Example: Weight = 68 kg, Height = 165 cm (1.65 m) Calculation: 68 ÷ (1.65)² = 24.98
Pounds and inches	Formula: weight (lb) / [height (in)]² x 703 Calculate BMI by dividing weight in pounds (lbs) by height in inches (in) squared and multiplying by a conversion factor of 703. Example: Weight = 150 lbs, Height = 5'5" (65") Calculation: [150 ÷ (65)²] x 703 = 24.96

The standard weight status categories associated with BMI ranges, for adults, are shown in the following table.

BMI	Weight Status
Below 18.5	Underweight
18.5 – 24.9	Normal
25.0 – 29.9	Overweight
30.0 and Above	Obese

The correlation between the BMI number and body fatness is fairly strong; however, the correlation varies by sex, race, and age. These variations include the following examples:

- At the same BMI, women tend to have more body fat than men.
- At the same BMI, older people, on an average, tend to have more body fat than younger adults.

- Highly trained athletes may have a high BMI because of increased muscularity rather than increased body fat.

It is also important to remember that BMI is only one factor related to risk for the disease. For assessing someone's likelihood of developing overweight or obesity-related diseases, the National Heart, Lung, and Blood Institute guidelines recommend looking at two other predictors:

- The individual's waist circumference (because abdominal fat is a predictor of risk for obesity-related diseases).
- Other risk factors the individual has for diseases and conditions associated with obesity (for example, high blood pressure or physical inactivity).

References

1. Mei Z, Grummer-Strawn LM, Pietrobelli A, Goulding A, Goran MI, Dietz WH. Validity of body mass index compared with other body-composition screening indexes for the assessment of body fatness in children and adolescents. American Journal of Clinical Nutrition 2002;7597–985.
2. Garrow JS and Webster J. Quetelet's index (W/H2) as a measure of fatness. International Journal of Obesity 1985;9:147–153.
3. Prentice AM and Jebb SA. Beyond Body Mass Index. Obesity Reviews. 2001 August; 2(3): 141–7.
4. Gallagher D, et al. How useful is BMI for comparison of body fatness across age, sex and ethnic groups? American Journal of Epidemiology 1996;143:228–239.
5. World Health Organization. Physical status: The use and interpretation of anthropometry. Geneva, Switzerland: World Health Organization 1995. WHO Technical Report Series.

MEASURING HEAD CIRCUMFERENCE IN PEDIATRICS

Head Circumference & Pediatric Growth Chart:-

- Using a measuring tape (paper or plastic) measure the circumference of the head from the most circumferential area of the skull. Compare the recordings with the growth chart to see the percentile range of the head circumference of the infants head.
- Same can be done for height and weight, once the results of the height and weight are obtained. Compare these results with the height and weight growth chart to check the percentile range.
- For infants, the height can be measured in a supine position on the infant scale and weight can be obtained by placing the infant on the infant weighing scale, the weight measured by the scale will be displayed on the device screen.

Important Note: Double check your work while recording the measurement for head circumference, height, and weight.

Reference: Information about circumference, height, and weight can be found on center for disease control and prevention website on the following link: http://www.cdc.gov/growthcharts/clinical_charts.htm.

PULMONARY FUNCTION TEST

Pulmonary function tests also are known as "**lung function tests**". It is a useful assessment tool used to assess the functional status of the respiratory system.

Lung function tests are based on the measurement of volume of air inhaled and exhaled in:-
a. **Quiet breathing (Static Lung Volume and Capacities)** and
b. **Forced breathing (Dynamic Lung Volume and Capacities)**.

Spirometer is the most commonly used instrument to perform the test.

Lung function tests can measure the following:

a. Amount of air the person can inspire (inspiration or inhale) into the lungs. This amount obtained is then compared with another individual of the same gender, age and height to check for normal ranges.
b. Amount of air the person can expire (expiration or exhale) out of the lungs, the time taken to do so.
c. Function of lungs.
d. Strength of inspiratory muscles.

UNDERSTANDING THE LUNG VOLUMES AND CAPACITIES

LUNG VOLUMES

TIDAL VOLUME
The volume of air inhaled and exhaled out of lungs in a single normal respiration.

INSPIRATORY RESERVE VOLUME
The additional volume of air that can be inhaled forcefully, after the end of the normal inhalation phase.

EXPIRATORY RESERVE VOLUME
The additional volume of air that can be exhaled forcefully, after normal exhalation phase.

RESIDUAL VOLUME
The volume of air that remains in the lungs after forced exhalation.

RESPIRATORY MINUTE VOLUME (RMV)
Is the volume of air inhaled and exhaled in every minute. It can be calculated as a product of tidal volume (TV) and respiratory rate (RR). (**TV x RR**)

FORCED EXPIRATORY VOLUME (FEV)
The volume of air exhaled forcefully in a given unit of time after deep inspiration. It is also known as timed vital capacity or forced expiratory vital capacity (FEVC).

LUNG CAPACITIES

INSPIRATORY CAPACITY
The maximum volume of air inhaled after normal expiration. It is a combination of tidal volume and inspiratory reserve volume.

VITAL CAPACITY (VC)
The maximum volume of air exhaled out of the lungs forcefully after maximal inhalation. It is a combination of inspiratory reserve volume, tidal volume, and expiratory reserve volume.

FUNCTIONAL RESIDUAL CAPACITY
The volume of air remaining in lungs after normal exhalation (tidal). It is a combination of expiratory reserve volume and residual volume.

TOTAL LUNG CAPACITY (TLC)
The volume of air present in lungs after a maximal inhalation. It is a combination of all volumes.

FORCED VITAL CAPACITY (FVC)
The volume of air exhaled forcefully and rapidly after maximal inhalation.

FORCED EXPIRATORY VOLUME IN 1 SEC (FEV1)
The amount of air exhaled during the 1st second of the FVC. For healthy adults, 70% of FVC is exhaled during this duration.

PEAK EXPIRATORY FLOW RATE (PEFR)
Peak expiratory flow rate (PEFR) is the maximum rate at which the air can be expired after a deep inspiration.

SPIROMETRY

Spirometry is the procedure used to measure the lung volumes and capacities. Instrument used for this procedure is called the **spirometer**, other devices used are

  i. Respirometer
  ii. Plethysmograph

PULMONARY FUNCTION TEST
OBJECTIVES

1. Adequate preparation for performing spirometry includes:
✓ Appropriate request for testing.
✓ Obtaining previous spirometry tests (if appropriate).
✓ Preparation of room in which the patient's spirometry procedure is to be performed (including suitability of performing in patient's home if appropriate).
✓ Preparation of equipment.
✓ Test required.
2. Ensuring it is appropriate to perform spirometry with the patient, including an explanation of when and when not, to perform spirometry.
3. Explanation and demonstration of procedure to the patient.
4. Correct positioning of the patient.
5. Correct performance of spirometry.
6. Understanding of when to stop or interrupt the test.
7. Correct recording and reporting of results.
8. Correct cleaning of equipment and disposal of waste.

PULMONARY FUNCTION TEST
STEPS

1. Check the indications and contraindications for the procedure to be performed.
2. Perform standard precautions (*Handwash &PPE*).
3. Perform patient identification.
4. Explain the procedure to the patient and gain informed consent.
5. Select proper equipment.
✓ Spirometry machine.
✓ Clean mouthpiece.
6. Collect and assemble equipment.
7. Next step would be to place the patient in a comfortable position.
8. Instruct the patient to get a good seal around the mouthpiece; next inhale deeply and exhale forcefully into the machine for as long as possible.

9. Attempt the same for at least 3 times to establish the best baseline.
10. Correlate results on the machine.
11. Examining the results can help in determining whether the disease is an **obstructive or restrictive pattern**.
12. Perform hand hygiene.
13. Record the patient's FEV1, FVC, FEV/FVC ratio. As per facility guidelines.
14. Clean the mouthpiece and the equipment.

POINTS TO CONSIDER:
Prior to the Procedure:-

1. Smokers are usually asked to refrain from smoking for a period of time.
2. Patient's height and weight shall be measured for the results to be accurately calculated.
3. The patient shall notify the doctor about prescribed and over-the-counter medications or any supplements he or she is consuming.
4. Specific preparation shall be made as per patient's condition.

During the Procedure:-

1. Patient will be asked:
✓ To loosen tight clothing, jewelry, or other objects that may interfere with the procedure.
✓ To empty urinary bladder before the procedure for comfort.
✓ To sit or stand during the procedure.
✓ To wear a soft nose clip so that all of the breaths go through mouth only.
2. The patient will be given a sterile mouthpiece that will be attached to the spirometer.
3. The patient will be instructed to use their lips to form a tight seal around the mouthpiece.
4. Different breathing activities will be instructed during the procedures.
✓ These activities may comprise of some inhalation and some exhalation activities.
✓ The activities may have to be performed several times before the test is completed.
5. The patient will be monitored carefully for any signs of distress.

Post-Procedure

1. The patient shall be given sufficient time to rest depending on the condition.

AUTOCLAVING AND STERILIZATION PROCEDURES

An autoclave is a device that sterilizes equipment and supplies in medical facility by means of:

- **High pressure** (saturated steam)
- **High temperature** (121 °C)
- **Specified Time:** As recommended. Example, 15-20 minutes.

Risks associated with autoclave:

1. Heat burns to the operator by high-temperature materials and accidental touching of the autoclave chamber walls and door.
2. Steam burns to the operator by residual steam coming out from autoclave and materials on the opening of the lid or door on completion of the cycle.
3. Scalds can occur by boiling liquids and spillage from the autoclave device.
4. Injury can occur if the device explodes.

Personal Protective Equipment for Safety:

1. Heat-insulating gloves that provide complete coverage of hands and forearms
2. Lab coat
3. Eye protection
4. Closed-toe footwear

Preparing the materials to be placed in autoclave:

a. Materials should be safe to use in autoclave:
   - ✓ Any substance that may cause toxic effect or damage should not be placed in the autoclave. If crack found, do not place the glassware in the autoclave.
b. If placing a glassware, make sure to check for any crack/s prior to autoclaving it.
c. Make sure to prepare and pack the materials as per recommended guidelines:
   - ✓ Loose dry materials must be wrapped or bagged in steam-penetrating paper or loosely covered with aluminum foil. Wrapping too tightly will impede steam penetration, decreasing the effectiveness of the process.
   - ✓ Loosen all lids to prevent pressure buildup. All containers must be covered by a loosened lid or steam-penetrating bung.
   - ✓ Containers of liquid must not exceed two-thirds (2/3) full, with lids loosened.
   - ✓ Glassware must be heat-resistant borosilicate.
   - ✓ Plastics must be heat-resistant, i.e., polycarbonate (PC), PTFE ("Teflon") and most polypropylene (PP) items.
   - ✓ Discarded sharps must be in a designated 'Sharps' container.
   - ✓ All items must be tagged with autoclave tape.
d. Use of secondary container
   - ✓ If you suspect chances of spills, make sure to secure the container so that it does not spill within the autoclave. Place the item in a special container rather than directly placing it in a potential spill container to be placed into the autoclave.

PHASE 1. Loading Autoclave

- Wear all appropriate personal protective equipment prior to starting the autoclave loading procedure.
- Next step after donning PPE, place material in an autoclave. Make sure that incompatible materials are not placed in the autoclave.
- While placing materials in the autoclave do not overload, leave some room for steam to circulate.
- Finally, close and lock the door.

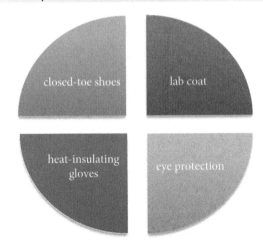

Figure 5.16a PPE for Autoclave

PHASE 2. Operating Autoclave

- Once confirmed that the door is locked and closed. Choose appropriate cycle for the material as per facility guidelines or check for instructions in the manufacturer instructions manual for "how to choose the cycle".

- Ensure use of proper temperature and time for autoclave cycles.
- Once the cycle has started, fill out the log sheet for information on autoclave as per facility guidelines.
- Avoid unlocking or opening of autoclave door while the machine is in operation.
- If a problem is detected, immediately stop the cycle and follow the facility reporting guidelines for problematic machines and devices.

PHASE 3. Unloading Autoclave

- Don personal protective equipment as mentioned in loading phase of the autoclave.
- Make sure to check that the autoclave cycle is complete.
- Double check to see if the pressure and temperature have returned to normal prior to opening the autoclave door.
- While opening the door ensure to stay away from it so that the steam does not come into contact with the body parts, wait for the pressure to normalize.
- Wait for an appropriate amount of time, so that the steam escapes the autoclave prior to removing the load.
- A specific area should be designated where loads are placed to cool down after their removal from the autoclave. Care should be taken to indicate the non-operators about the load temperature to avoid any injury. Post a sign that indicates (**"HOT MATERIAL" do not touch**) or something similar as per recommended guidelines.
- Once the load is removed close the door.

Spill Clean-up

- The autoclave should not be operated if there is a spill.
- The spill should be cleaned prior to its operation for the next load, clean the spill using a spill kit. Make sure that cleaning the spill is done when the temperature of the spilled material has returned to normal room temperature.
- Attempting to clean the autoclave spill right away may cause injuries to the operator due to the high temperature of the spillage.
- Follow recommended guidelines for disposal of materials.
- Record the spillage in an appropriate log book.

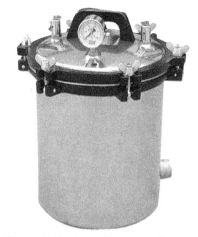

Figure 5.17a Autoclave Unit (Type 1)

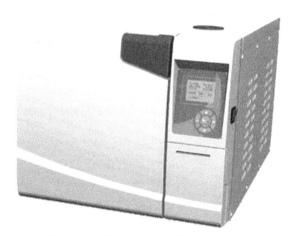

Figure 5.17b Autoclave Unit (Type 2)

Reference
1. www.cdc.gov
2. http://www.nhlbi.nih.gov/health/health-topics/topics/hbp/

CHAPTER 6
END OF CHAPTER REVIEW QUESTIONS

Question Set 1: Match the Following   10 points 1 point each

Answer	Column 1	Column 2
	1. EXPIRATORY RESERVE VOLUME	A. Volume of air inhales and exhaled out of lungs in a single normal respiration.
	2. RESPIRATORY MINUTE VOLUME (RMV)	B. Additional volume of air that can be inhaled forcefully, after the end of normal inhalation phase.
	3. TOTAL LUNG CAPACITY (TLC)	C. Additional volume of air that can be exhaled forcefully, after normal exhalation phase.
	4. INSPIRATORY RESERVE VOLUME	D. Volume of air that remains in the lungs after forced exhalation.
	5. VITAL CAPACITY (VC)	E. Is the volume of air inhaled and exhaled in every minute. It can be calculated as a product of tidal volume (TV) and respiratory rate (RR).
	6. TIDAL VOLUME	F. Volume of air which can be exhaled forcefully in a given unit of time after deep inspiration. It is also known as timed vital capacity or forced expiratory vital capacity (FEVC).
	7. RESIDUAL VOLUME	G. Maximum volume of air that is inhaled after normal expiration. It is a combination of tidal volume and inspiratory reserve volume.
	8. FORCED EXPIRATORY VOLUME (FEV)	H. Maximum volume of air that can be exhaled out of the lungs forcefully after maximal inhalation. It is a combination of inspiratory reserve volume, tidal volume and expiratory reserve volume.
	9. FUNCTIONAL RESIDUAL CAPACITY	I. Volume of air remaining in lungs after tidal exhalation. It is a combination of expiratory reserve volume and residual volume.
	10. INSPIRATORY CAPACITY	J. Volume of air present in lungs after a maximal inhalation. It is a combination of all volumes.

Question Set 2: Essay Questions   35 points 5 points each

1. Enlist the steps of recording blood pressure.
2. Enlist the steps of recording temperature.
3. Enlist the steps of recording pulse.
4. Enlist the steps of recording respiration.
5. Enlist the steps of recording height.
6. Enlist the steps of recording weight.
7. Explain phases of autoclave (loading, operating and unloading).

Question Set 3: Fill in the Blanks — 15 points 1 point each

1. Body temperature is >37.5–38.3 °C (99.5–100.9 °F) is known as _____

2. Body temperature greater than 100.4° F (38° C) indicates a fever and is known as _____

3. Body temperature reading greater than 104.0-106.7° F (40.0 - 41.5° C), is a serious condition, and a temperature greater than 109.4° F (43° C) is fatal and is known as _____

4. _____ pulse is the most easily accessible and commonly used pulse site. The radial pulse can be located by placing the index and middle finger at the base of the thumb over the wrist.

5. To locate the _____pulse, the chest piece of the stethoscope is placed gently and firmly over the apex of the heart, located in the fifth intercostal space (between the ribs) on the left side of the chest on the midclavicular line. The sound heard will be "lubb and dubb", this should be counted as one beat only.

6. _____ is a combination of hypoxia and hypercapnea, due to obstruction of the air passage.

7. _____ is known as difficulty in breathing.

8. _____ breathing is the periodic breathing characterized by rhythmic hyperpnea and apnea.

9. _____ is another form of periodic breathing characterized by a period of apnea and hyperpnea. After an apneic period, hyperpnea occurs abruptly.

10. _____ is known as a decrease in pulmonary ventilation caused by a decrease in rate or force of breathing. Thus, the amount of air moving in and out of lungs is reduced.

11. _____ is the difference between the systolic pressure and diastolic pressure.

12. _____ pressure is the average pressure existing in the arteries. Formula to calculate mean arterial blood pressure

13. _____ is the measurement of the force which the blood exerts on the walls of the arteries; this force is produced by the "systolic phase" of the cardiac cycle during which the left ventricle contracts to eject the blood out of the heart through the aorta

14. The _____pulse can be located by placing the index and middle finger at the base of the little finger over the wrist, the reason for checking this pulse is to find out the circulation status of the hand

15. The _____pulse is located in temple area of the forehead.

Question Set 4: True and False — 40 points 2 points each

1. Palpation is a method of visual assessment of the patient.
   Answer: True or False

2. Inspection is a method of using one's hands to examine the patient's body.
   Answer: True or False

3. Percussion is a method of tapping on a surface of the human body to determine the underlying structure.

   Answer: True or False

4. Auscultation is a method of listening to the internal sounds of the body, mostly using a stethoscope.

   Answer: True or False

5. Hyperthermia: body temperature less than 95° F (35° C).

   Answer: True or False

6. Normal temperature: body temperature is 36.5–37.5 °C (97.7 – 99.5 °F)

   Answer: True or False

7. The radial pulse can be located in the antecubital space, which is the space located at the inner aspect of the elbow. This site is most commonly used to obtain blood pressure.

   Answer: True or False

8. The carotid pulse is located between the larynx and sternocleidomastoid on the anterior side of the neck, slightly to one side of the midline (trachea).

   Answer: True or False

9. The popliteal pulse is in the mid-groin region and should be firmly compressed to assess the pulse.

   Answer: True or False

10. The femoral pulse can be located on the posterior aspect of the knee and can be felt easily if the knee is slightly flexed.

    Answer: True or False

11. The posterior tibial pulse is located on the posterior aspect of the ankle joint.

    Answer: True or False

12. Dorsalis Pedis: Pulse is located on the superior surface of the foot, usually found between the first and second metatarsal bones.

    Answer: True or False

13. Eupnea: Rate 12-20, rhythm: even and regular, depth: normal.

    Answer: True or False

14. Hyperpnea is a decrease in pulmonary ventilation due to increase in rate and force of respiration (occurs mainly due to insufficient oxygen supply and increase in carbon dioxide in the blood).

    Answer: True or False

15. Hypopnea is a decrease in rate and depth of breathing (shallow and slow).

    Answer: True or False

16. Hyperventilation is an abnormal fast and increased depth of breathing, may lead to dizziness, discomfort and chest pain. Large amount of air moves in and out of lungs.

    Answer: True or False

17. Liver function tests also known as "lung function tests". It is a useful assessment tool used to assess the functional status of the respiratory system.

    Answer: True or False

18. Advantages of using an automated oscillometric blood pressure device are automatic recording, automatic inflation, no skills required for listening sounds and time saving.

    Answer: True or False

19. Spirometry is the procedure that can be used to measure the lung volumes and capacities.

    Answer: True or False

20. At the same BMI, older people, on an average, tend to have more body fat than younger adults.

    Answer: True or False

SECTION 2

CHAPTER 7: PATIENT POSITIONING & BED MOBILITY TECHNIQUES

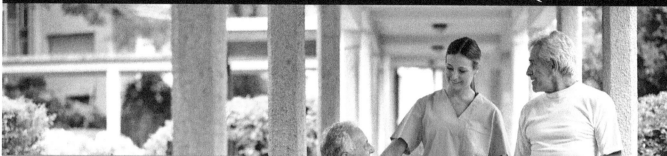

Learning Objectives: At the end of this chapter the student will be able to describe

Patient Positioning

1) Positioning patients: why is turning and positioning of patient-important?
2) Positioning patients: Goals
3) Positioning patients: how to prevent skin breakdown?
4) What are different patient positions?
   - i) Supine
   - ii) Sidelying
   - iii) Prone
   - iv) Semifowler
     - (1) Low Fowler
     - (2) High Fowler
   - v) Lithotomy
   - vi) Trendelenburg
   - vii) Reverse Trendelenburg
   - viii) Sims
   - ix) Sitting
   - x) Long Sitting
5) How to turn a patient (competency checklist)?
6) Changing position from supine to prone
7) Changing position from prone to supine

Bed Mobility Techniques

1) Bed Mobility
   a) Supine to sidelying
   b) Supine to sit
2) Patient positioning: post position techniques
   a) While in supine position
   b) While in semi-supine position
   c) While in prone position
   d) While in right lateral position
   e) While in fowlers position
   f) While in orthopneic position
   g) While in sitting position

PATIENT CARE INTERVENTION: PATIENT POSITIONING

Positioning patients: why is turning and positioning of a patient important?

Proper positioning is a necessary tool to maintain patient function. Determining the most optimal position for patients is very crucial. For patients who are unable to change positions independently, proper positioning is essential for increasing function and preventing complications. Bedsores also known as decubitus ulcer can occur if the patient stays in one position for a prolonged period of time, decubitus ulcer is increasing in patients admitted to healthcare facilities. Hence special care should be taken to change the patient position more frequently.

POSITIONING PATIENTS: GOALS

- Maintain comfort level of the patient.
- Maintain joint flexibility of the patient.
- Prevent skin breakdown and pressures on bony surfaces.
- Prepare or expose body surfaces for treatment or evaluation purposes.

POSITIONING PATIENTS: HOW TO PREVENT SKIN BREAKDOWN:

1. Frequent mobilizing of a patient with activities such as walking or changing positions.
2. Frequent position change schedule at least every two hours.
3. The introduction of basic techniques to reduce edema.
4. Provide proper nutrition.

Note: Use of special mattresses or equipment for patients who are unable to move.

WHAT ARE DIFFERENT PATIENT POSITIONS?

1. **Supine**: patient is lying on his or her back.

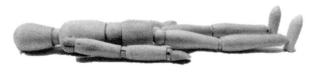

Figure 7.1 Supine

2. **Side-Lying**: patient is lying on his or her side.

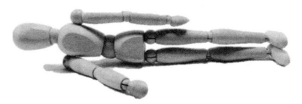

Figure 7.2 Side-Lying

3. **Prone**: patient is lying on his or her stomach.

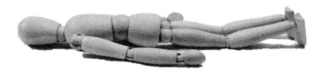

Figure 7.3 Prone

4. **Semifowler:**

a. **Low Fowler**: patient is sitting on his or her back with the head of the bed elevated.

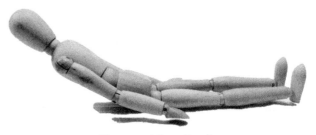

Figure 7.4 Low Fowler

b. **High Fowler**: patient is sitting upright on his or her back.

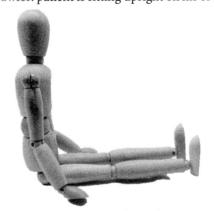

Figure 7.5 High Fowler

5. Lithotomy: patient is lying in a supine position with hip and knee bend at approximately between 60-90 degrees.

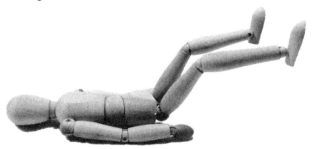

Figure 7.6 Lithotomy

6. Trendelenburg: patient is lying on his or her back, with the bed in a declined position (foot up and head down).

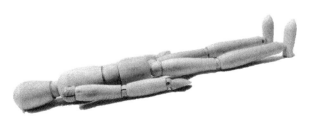

Figure 7.7 Trendelenburg

7. Reverse Trendelenburg: opposite of Trendelenburg.

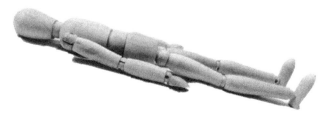

Figure 7.8 Reverse Trendelenburg

8. Sims position:

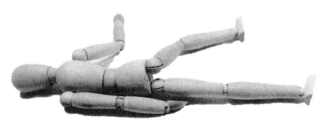

Figure 7.9 Sims Position (lateral recumbent position)

9. Sitting: sitting upright with hip and knee flexion at 90 degrees.

10. Long Sitting: sitting with hip at 90-degree flexion and knee extended.

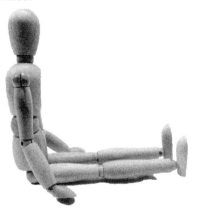

Figure 7.10 Long Sitting

HOW TO TURN A PATIENT: COMPETENCY CHECKLIST

Step 1. Check patient status and double check the position of the patient.

Step 2. Make sure to move the patient far enough towards one side of the bed.

Step 3. Determine the type of turning to be performed:
   a. Logrolling: turn the whole body in one stage
   b. Segmental rolling: turn body in segments (e.g. lower trunk followed by upper trunk)

Step 4. More than one person may be required for turning the patient.

CHANGING PATIENT POSITION FROM SUPINE TO PRONE

1. Instruct the patient about what will take place and prepare them prior to performing the position change.

2. Move patient's head and upper trunk.

3. Next move patients lower trunk then move the lower extremities.

4. Hold the right lower extremity and cross it over the left lower extremity.

5. The right ankle will rest over the left ankle.

6. The caregiver should be on the side to which the patient is to be turned.

7. To prevent the patient from falling during the process of changing positions, use enough pillows or towels.

8. Position the right upper extremity is such a way that the palm is placed on the right hip.

9. Head position during turning or changing position can be controlled by the patient; assistance might be required if the patient has lost head control.

10. While initiating the position change, the caregivers, hands are on the patient's back.

11. Make sure to control the movement during the shift in position. Avoid any sudden or jerky movements during this technique.

CHANGING PATIENT POSITION FROM PRONE TO SUPINE

1. Starting with patient in prone position. The patient is initially placed far enough to one side of the bed to allow a full turning movement to the supine position.
   - If using log rolling technique turn lower and upper extremities together (as on unit) into a supine position.
   - If using the segmental technique, the patient is moved in stages. Move the head and upper trunk, and then move the lower trunk. Finally, move the lower extremities.
2. Cross the uppermost leg over the lowermost leg and tuck the lowermost upper extremity under the patient. Stand on the far side of the bed, next roll the patient toward you to a sidelying position. Determine if there is enough space to continue. Guide the patient from sidelying to supine by resisting at the posterior shoulder and pelvis. Make sure to control the movement during the change of position, avoid any sudden or jerky movements.

BED MOBILITY TECHNIQUES

a. **Supine to sidelying**: position patient close to the far edge of the bed (with a person, bedrail or wall protecting the patient from falling). Stand facing the patient, place the uppermost lower extremity over the lowermost lower extremity, place the uppermost upper extremity on the chest & the lowermost upper extremity in abduction. Roll the patient towards you by pulling gently on the posterior aspect of the scapula and pelvis.

b. **Supine to sit**: move the patient close to the edge of the bed (EOB). Roll the patient into the sidelying position facing the edge of the bed (EOB). Simultaneously
   - **Elevate the trunk by lifting under the shoulders.**
   - **Lower the feet and lower extremities off of the EOB.**

PATIENT POSITIONING: POST POSITION TECHNIQUES

After the patient has been placed into a comfortable position, place pillows and other supportive devices to help the patient comfortably maintain the position.

WHILE IN SUPINE POSITION

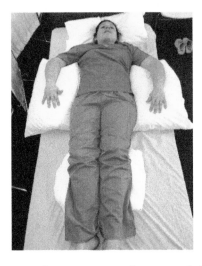

1. Patient lying in supine with bed flat, and head raised about 2-3 inches with the use of the pillow.
2. The pillow used should extend a couple of inches below the shoulder blades.
3. A sheet rolled and placed on the lateral side of the legs to prevent external rotation of the hip joint. The approximate location of placement of this rolled sheet can be from hip to just above the knee. Make sure to check if the leg is stable and not externally rotated.
4. Next, place pillow under patient's knees.
5. Pillow placed under the knees can also reach the ankle to prevent the ankle from rubbing onto the bed sheet.
6. Another set of pillows can be placed under the forearm (elbow to wrist).

WHILE IN SEMI-SUPINE POSITION

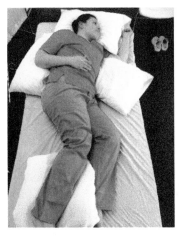

While the patient is in supine position. Turn the patient's trunk and shoulder backward leaving a 45° angle between the patient's back and the bed.
1. Properly position a pillow for appropriate head and back support.
2. Left arm should be flexed forward with elbow flexed.
3. Right arm should also be flexed at the elbow and the forearm should be brought across the chest with palm down.

4. With both legs extended. Position right leg a little behind the left leg. Use pillow to support the right leg.

WHILE IN PRONE POSITION

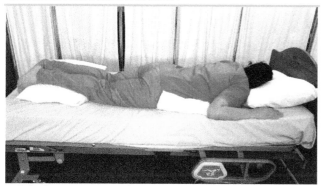

While the patient is in the prone position (on the abdomen) with head turned to either side and legs extended.

1. Position a pillow underneath the patient's head such that it should be able to extend below the patient's shoulders.
2. Position another pillow under the abdomen; this will relieve pressure on the patient's back and in females will reduce pressure on the breast tissues. Instead of using pillow a sheet or towel can be rolled and placed under patient's shoulders.
3. The arm on the side of the head turned should be placed (supported) on a pillow from elbow to wrist. The opposite arm should be kept extended or flexed depending on the comfort of the patient.
4. A pillow should be placed under the lower legs such that the knees are minimally flexed; this will prevent pressure on the toes.

WHILE IN RIGHT LATERAL POSITION

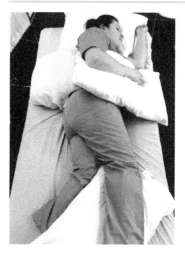

While patient is in right lateral position:
Position a pillow underneath the patient's head such that it should be able to extend below the patient's shoulders.

1. Flex the left shoulder of the patient, next flex elbow with the palm of the hand facing up.
2. For right shoulder: if flexed, position it on the pillow. If in extension, place it on the patient's lateral side of the hip.
3. Next place a pillow underneath the patient's right leg.
4. If required, place a pillow behind the patient's back to maintain the position.

WHILE IN FOWLER'S POSITION

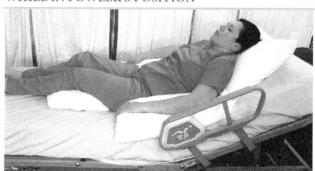

This position, or a variation of it, is used for feeding patients in bed, for the patient's comfort, for certain treatments and procedures and for those who have trouble breathing.

1. Position the head of the bed according to the desired fowler position:
    a. **30° for Semi-Fowler's**
    b. **45° to 60° for Fowler's**
    c. **90° for High Fowler's**
2. Position a pillow underneath the patient's head such that it should be able to extend four to five inches below the patient's shoulders.
3. Flex elbows and place a pillow under both the arms.
4. Place a pillow underneath both legs (preferably under the knees).

WHILE IN ORTHOPNEIC POSITION

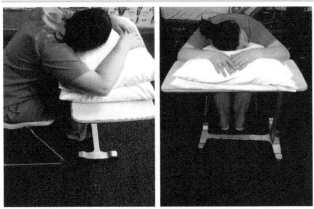

Figure 7.11 ORTHOPNEIC POSITION

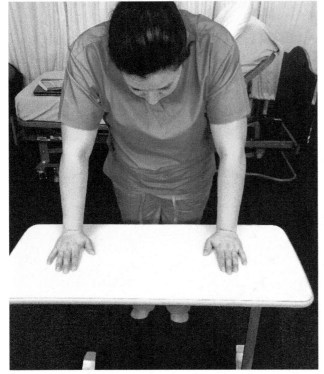

Figure 7.11a ORTHOPNEIC POSITION (ALTERNATE)

1. If the patient is:
   - in bed, position the bed at 90° angle.
   - sitting on a chair or bedside table across the bed.
2. In both scenarios (bed or chair) place one or two pillows on top of the bedside table or table.
3. Ask the patient to lean forward across the bedside table or table with arms and head, rest on the pillows.

Note: if the patient is standing, he or she should lean forward on the table as shown in figure 7.11a.

WHILE IN SITTING POSITION

The patient is in sitting position on a chair with head and spine in properly aligned position, make sure to check that the patients back and buttocks are against the backrest of the chair, whereas the feet are flat on the floor.

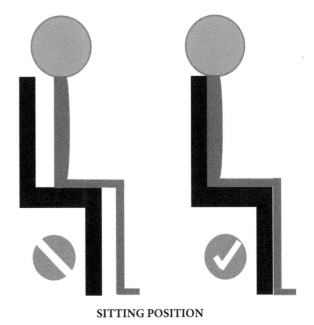

SITTING POSITION

CHAPTER 7
END OF CHAPTER REVIEW QUESTIONS

Question Set 1: Match the Following
20 point: 2 points each

Answer		Column 1	Column 2
	1.	Trendelenburg	patient is lying on his or her back
	2.	Reverse Trendelenburg	patient is lying on his or her side
	3.	Sitting	patient is lying on his or her stomach
	4.	Proper Positioning	patient is sitting on his or her back with the head of the bed elevated
	5.	Lithotomy	patient is sitting upright on his or her back
	6.	High fowler	patient is lying in a supine position with hip and knee bend at approximately between 60-90 degrees
	7.	Supine	patient is lying on his or her back, with the bed in a declined position, foot up and head down.
	8.	Side-Lying	opposite of Trendelenburg
	9.	Prone	sitting upright with hip and knee at 90 degrees
	10.	Low fowler	is a necessary tool to maintain patient function

Question Set 2: Essay Questions
36 point: 6 points each

1. Enlist the goals for patient positioning.
2. How to prevent skin breakdown?
3. List the steps required to turn a patient.
4. How to change patient position from prone to supine?
5. List types of different fowler positions.
6. Explain in brief about changing a patient position from supine to prone.

Question Set 3: Describe in Brief
10 point: 5 points each

Bed mobility techniques of

a. Supine to sidelying
b. Supine to sit

Question Set 4: Describe in Brief
35 point: 5 points each

After the patient has been placed into a comfortable position place pillows and other supportive devices to help the patient comfortably maintain the position. Discuss in brief about **pillow placement/s** of the following positions:-

a. While in supine position
b. While in semi-supine position
c. While in prone position
d. While in right lateral position
e. While in fowler's position
f. While in orthopneic position
g. While in sitting position

SECTION 2

CHAPTER 8: RANGE OF MOTION

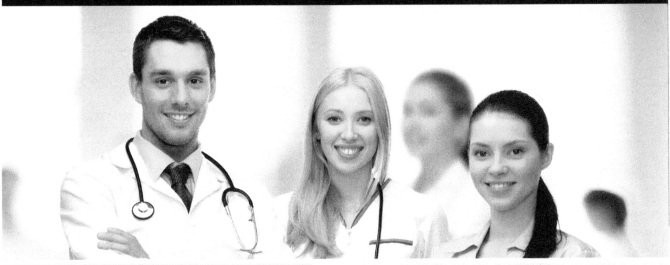

LEARNING OBJECTIVES

At the end of this chapter the student will be able to describe:

1) Evaluation of range of motion
2) Parts of goniometry
3) Placement of goniometer
4) Types of range of motion exercises
   a. Passive
   b. Active
   c. Active assisted
5) Range of motion goals
6) Effect of joint immobilization
7) Causes of decreased range of motion
8) Contraindications of range of motion
9) Precautions for performing ROM on patients with specific conditions
10) General precautions
11) Few factors that affect body alignment and mobility

12) Range of motion: specific to joints
   a. Spinal Column (Vertebral Column) Movements
   b. Shoulder Joint Movements
   c. Elbow Joint Movements
   d. Wrist Joint Movements
   e. Metacarpophalangeal Joint Movements
   f. Distal Interphalangeal Joint Movements
   g. Proximal Interphalangeal Joint Movements
   h. Hip Joint Movements
   i. Knee Joint Movement
   j. Ankle Joint Movement
13) Performing range of motion
14) Key principles while performing range of motion exercises
15) Types of range of motion
16) Illustrations of joint movements
17) Illustrations of performing joint range of motion on each joint
18) Range of motion flow sheet (practice skills sheet)

PATIENT CARE INTERVENTION:

RANGE OF MOTION

The range of motion (ROM) is done to maintain the flexibility and mobility of the joint. It helps in decreasing the stiffness of joints and muscle wasting thereby helping joints from undergoing deterioration. The range of motion is the amount of range that a joint can freely go through without any restrictions. Every joint has a normal range of motion and due to condition, disease, injury, disorder or immobility, the joint may undergo reduction of its normal range thereby limiting the joint range. The range of motion if performed on a regular basis can preserve the joint range of motion.

EVALUATION OF RANGE OF MOTION (ROM)

GONIOMETRY

(Greek word {GONIO: ANGLE} {METERY: MEASURE})
The goniometer is an instrument used to measure joint range of motion. The technique involves placing the goniometer on the joint to be evaluated for a range of motion, followed by moving the joint through a range of motion actively or passively. Care must be taken to place the goniometer in the right location for accurate results.

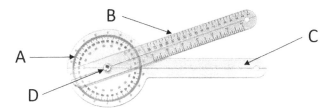

Figure 8.1 GONIOMETER
A: BODY B: MOVABLE ARM C: FIXED ARM
D: FULCRUM OR AXIS

Placement of the goniometer:

1. Fulcrum should be placed on the joint axis.
2. Fixed arm should be placed on the fixed body segment.
3. Movable arm should be placed on the movable body segment (body segment to be moved).

For e.g. performing goniometry on the elbow joint
FULCRUM: place fulcrum of the goniometer laterally on the elbow joint.
FIXED ARM: placed laterally on the upper arm.
MOVABLE ARM: placed laterally on the forearm.
Move the joint through the available range of motion and check for the range in the goniometer.

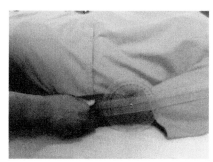

INITIAL PLACEMENT

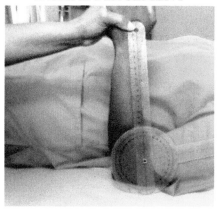

MIDRANGE PLACEMENT

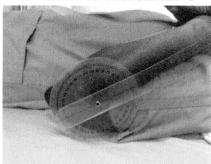

FINAL PLACEMENT

Elbow flexion: range of motion measurement using goniometer
Figure 8.2 USING GONIOMETER

TYPES OF RANGE OF MOTION EXERCISES

Passive range of motion (or PROM)

a. Performed by a caregiver.
b. No effort from the patient, since the patient is unable to perform the range of motion independently.
c. It may involve performing range of motion throughout the body in series.

Active range of motion (or AROM)

a. Performed by the patient.

b. No effort from the caregiver is required, since the patient is able to perform the range of motion independently.

c. It may involve performing range of motion throughout the body in series.

Active assisted range of motion (or AAROM)

a. Performed by the patient and caregiver.

b. Active effort from patient and assistance from the caregiver is provided when necessary. Assistance from the caregiver is required since the patient is only able to perform an incomplete or partial range of motion independently.

c. It may involve performing range of motion throughout the body in series.

Range of Motion: Goals

1. To prevent muscle contractures.
2. To prevent joint stiffness and freezing or adhesions of joints.
3. To prevent muscle wasting and maintain elasticity of muscle.
4. To provide circulation.
5. To provide sensory stimulation.
6. To prevent osteoporosis.

Range of Motion: Effect of Joint Immobilization

Joint immobilization may lead to:

- Joint stiffness and adhesion
- Disuse muscle atrophy and muscle weakness
- Articular surface degeneration
- Muscle and soft tissues shortening
- Bone changes (Osteoporosis)

Range of Motion: Causes of decreased ROM

- Prolonged immobilization
- Prolong bed rest
- Trauma (bones, joints or soft tissues)
- Muscle weakness or paralysis
- Post-surgery
- Joint conditions, disease or disorder
- Neuromuscular conditions, disease or disorder

Range of Motion: Contraindication of ROM

1. Dislocated joints
2. Unhealed fracture

3. Immediately after surgery on musculoskeletal and integumentary system

Range of Motion: Precautions for performing ROM on patients with specific conditions

1. Joint infection
2. Joint inflammation
3. Patients on pain medication
4. Patients suffering from osteoporosis
5. Patients suffering from arthritis

Range of Motion: General Precautions

The caregiver should

- provide appropriate support to the limbs during movement.
- grasp the part to be moved in a gentle manner. The grasp should be maintained as close as possible towards the joint, and finally, the grasp should be comfortable for the patient.
- movements performed should be slow and in an appropriate rhythm, maintain the speed of motion.
- check for patient's facial expression, as it might be an indication of pain experienced by the patient during the movements being performed. If a patient complains of pain, stop the movement immediately.

Range of Motion: Some factors that affect body alignment and mobility

1. Age
2. Physical Status: Health
3. Musculoskeletal Conditions (e.g. osteoarthritis)
4. Nervous System Conditions (e.g. stroke)
5. Cardiovascular System Conditions (e.g. thrombosis)
6. Pulmonary System Conditions (e.g. pneumonia)
7. Metabolic Conditions
8. Integumentary System Conditions (e.g. burns)
9. Mental Status (e.g. depression)

RANGE OF MOTIONS

1. Complete Range
2. Partial Range

RANGE OF MOTION: SPECIFIC TO JOINTS

Spinal Column (Vertebral Column) Movements

Movement 1.   Flexion
Movement 2.   Extension
Movement 3.   Lateral Flexion
Movement 4.   Rotation

Shoulder Joint Movements

Movement 1.   Flexion
Movement 2.   Extension
Movement 3.   Adduction
Movement 4.   Abduction
Movement 5.   Medial Rotation
Movement 6.   Lateral Rotation

Elbow Joint Movements

Movement 1.   Flexion
Movement 2.   Extension
Movement 3.   Pronation
Movement 4.   Supination

Wrist Joint Movements

Movement 1.   Flexion
Movement 2.   Extension
Movement 3.   Adduction (Ulnar Deviation)
Movement 4.   Abduction (Radial Deviation)
Movement 5.   Circumduction

Metacarpophalangeal Joint Movements

Movement 1.   Flexion
Movement 2.   Extension

Distal Interphalangeal Joint Movements

Movement 1.   Flexion
Movement 2.   Extension

Proximal Interphalangeal Joint Movements

Movement 1.   Flexion
Movement 2.   Extension

Hip Joint Movements

Movement 1.   Flexion
Movement 2.   Extension
Movement 3.   Adduction
Movement 4.   Abduction
Movement 5.   Medial Rotation

Movement 6.   Lateral Rotation

Knee Joint Movement

Movement 1.   Flexion
Movement 2.   Extension

Ankle Joint Movement

Movement 1.   Plantar Flexion
Movement 2.   Dorsi Flexion
Movement 3.   Inversion
Movement 4.   Eversion

PERFORMING RANGE OF MOTION

Performing range of motion at shoulder joint

Range of Motion (Movement)
1.   Flexion and Extension
2.   Abduction & Adduction
3.   External & Internal Rotation

Performing range of motion at elbow joint

Range of Motion (Movement)
1.   Flexion and Extension
2.   Supination & Pronation

Performing range of motion at wrist joint

Range of Motion (Movement)
1.   Flexion and Extension
2.   Abduction & Adduction

Performing range of motion at hip joint

Range of Motion (Movement)
1.   Flexion and Extension
2.   Abduction & Adduction
3.   External & Internal Rotation

Performing range of motion at knee joint

Range of Motion (Movement)
1.   Flexion and Extension

Performing range of motion at ankle joint

Range of Motion (Movement)
1.   Dorsiflexion and Plantar Flexion

Key principles while performing range of motion exercises

Principle 1.   Stabilize the joints carefully
Principle 2.   Pain-free range of motion

TYPES OF RANGE OF MOTION	
ROM Type 1.	Passive: Complete assistance for movement
ROM Type 2.	Active: No assistance required for the movement
ROM Type 3.	Active Assisted: Active movement but assistance provided as per need

JOINT MOVEMENTS

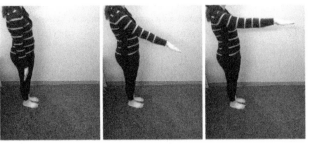

Neutral　　　Shoulder Flexion
Figure 8.6 Shoulder Joint Movements

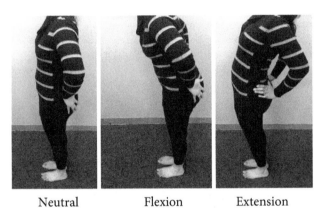

Neutral　　　Flexion　　　Extension
Figure 8.3 Lumbar Joint Movements

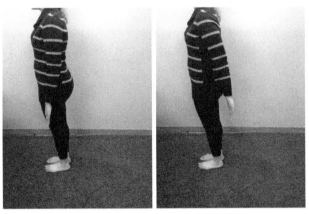

Neutral　　　Shoulder Extension
Figure 8.7 Shoulder Joint Movements

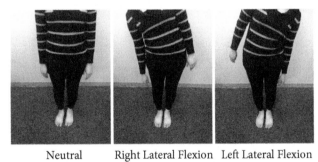

Neutral　Right Lateral Flexion　Left Lateral Flexion
Figure 8.4 Lumbar Joint Movements

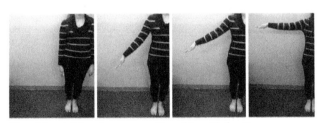

Shoulder Adduction　　Shoulder Abduction
Figure 8.8 Shoulder Joint Movements

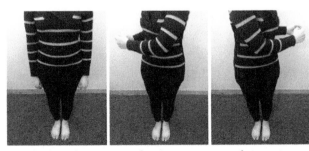

Neutral　　　Right Rotation　　Left Rotation
Figure 8.5 Lumbar Joint Rotations

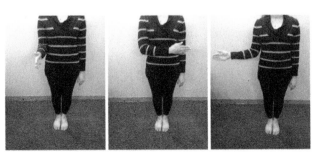

Neutral　　Internal Rotation　External Rotation
Figure 8.9 Shoulder Joint Movements

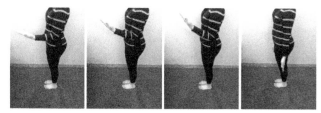

Elbow Flexion　　　Elbow Extension

Figure 8.10 Elbow Joint Movements

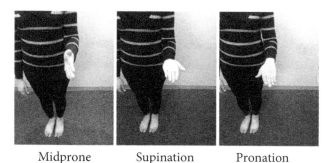

Midprone　　　Supination　　　Pronation

Figure 8.11 Elbow Joint Movements

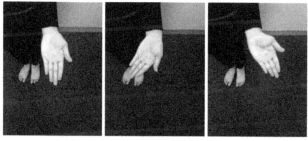

Neutral　　　Adduction　　　Abduction

Figure 8.12 Wrist Joint Movements

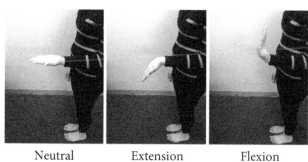

Neutral　　　Extension　　　Flexion

Figure 8.13 Wrist Joint Movements

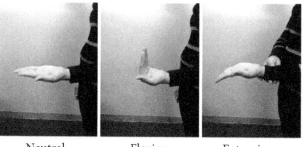

Neutral　　　Flexion　　　Extension

Figure 8.14 Metacarpo-Phalangeal Joint Movements

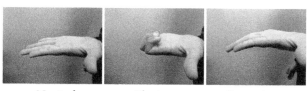

Neutral　　　Flexion　　　Extension

Figure 8.15 Phalangeal Joint Movements

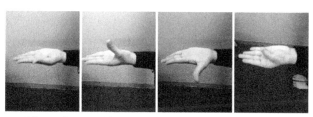

Neutral　　Flexion　　Extension　　Opposition

Figure 8.16 1st Metacarpo-Phalangeal Joint Movements

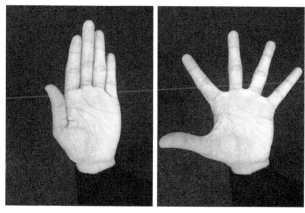

Adduction　　　Abduction

Figure 8.17 Metacarpo-Phalangeal Joint Movements

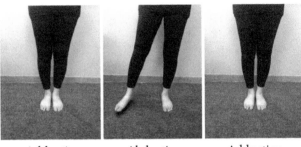

Adduction   Abduction   Adduction

Figure 8.18 Hip Joint Movements

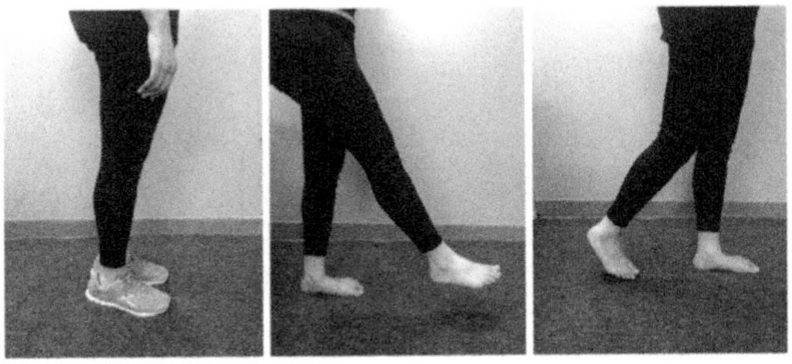

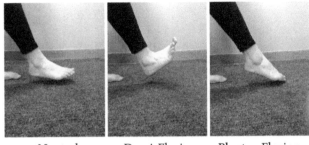

Neutral   Dorsi-Flexion   Plantar-Flexion

Figure 8.22 Ankle Joint Movements

Neutral   Flexion   Extension

Figure 8.19 Hip Joint Movements

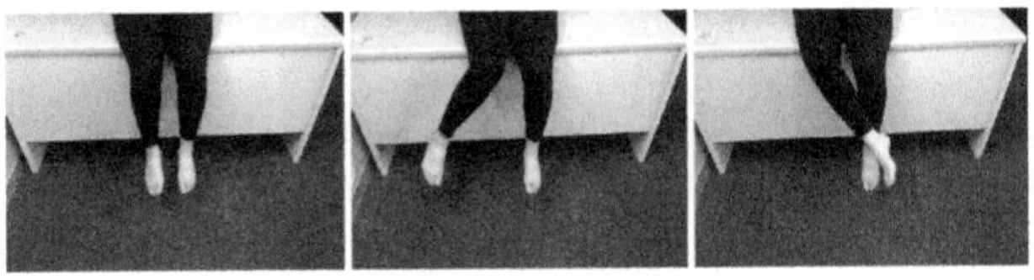

Neutral   Internal Rotation   External Rotation

Figure 8.20 Hip Joint Movements

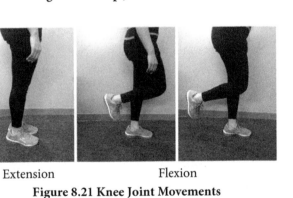

Extension   Flexion

Figure 8.21 Knee Joint Movements

PERFORMING RANGE OF MOTION

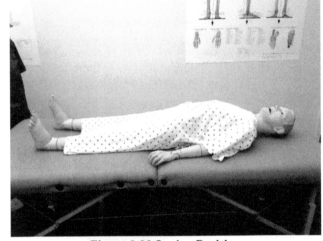

Figure 8.23 Supine Position

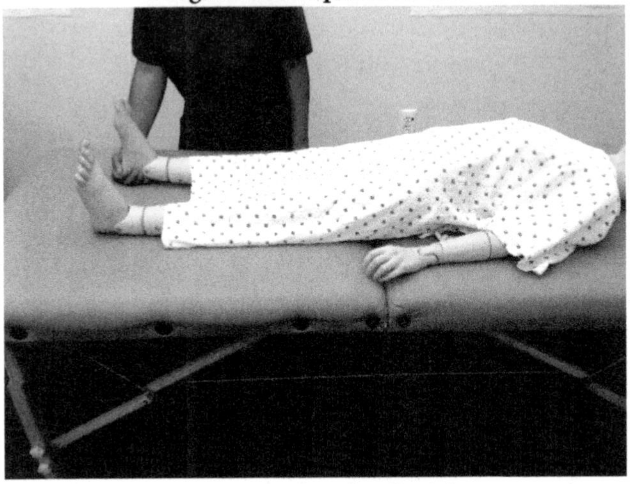

Figure 8.23a Starting Position

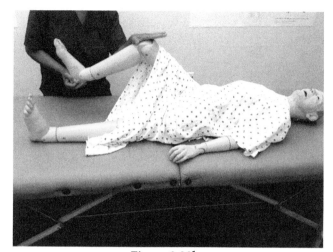

Figure 8.23b

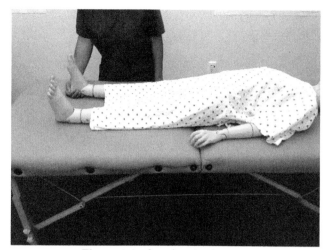

Figure 8.24 Starting Position

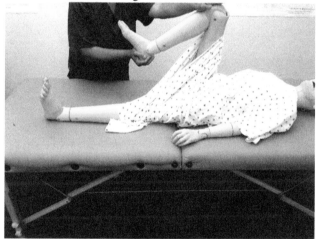

Figure 8.23c

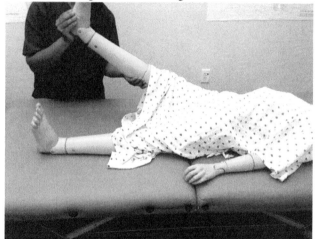

Figure 8.24a

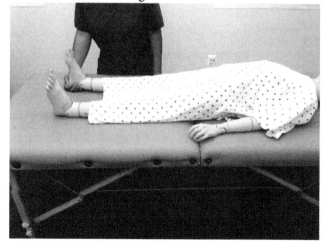

**Figure 8.23d Hip and knee flexion and extension
(Patient: Supine Position)**

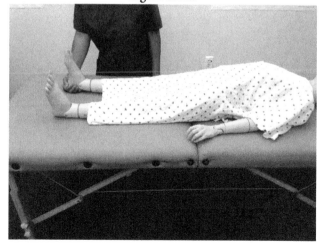

**Figure 8.24b Hip flexion
(Patient: Supine Position)**

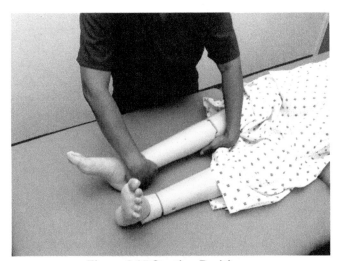

Figure 8.25 Starting Position

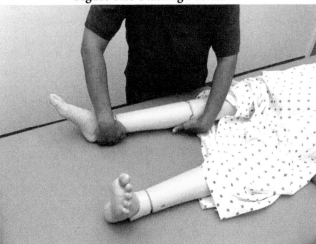

Figure 8.25a

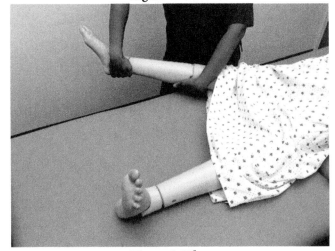

Figure 8.25b

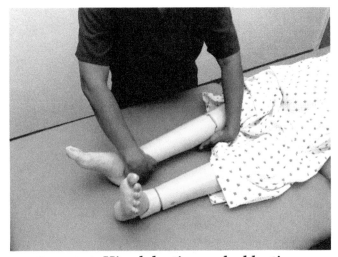

Figure 8.25c Hip abduction and adduction (Patient: Supine Position)

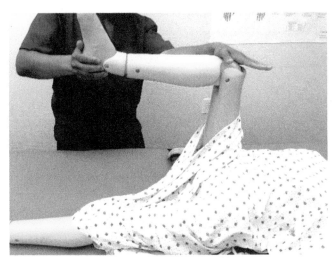

Figure 8.26 Starting Position

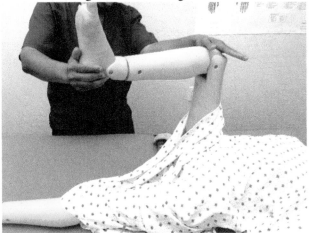

Figure 8.26a

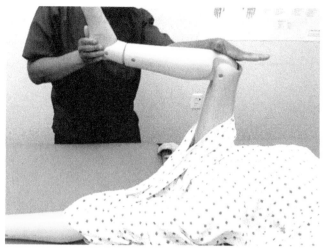

Figure 8.26b Hip external and internal rotation
(Patient: Supine Position)

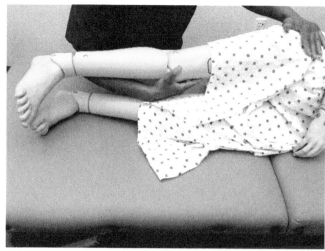

Figure 8.27b Hip abduction and adduction
(Patient: Side-lying Position)

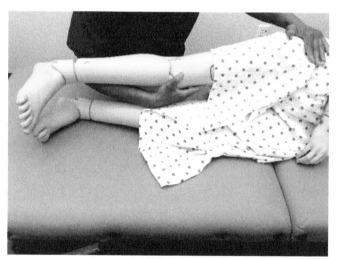

Figure 8.27 Starting Position

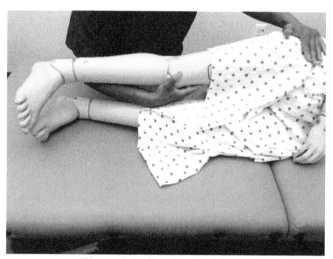

Figure 8.28 Starting Position

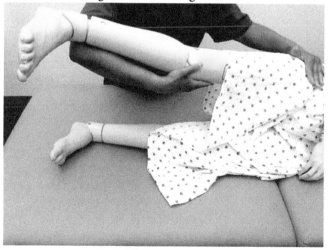

Figure 8.27a

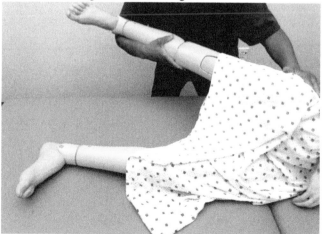

Figure 8.28a

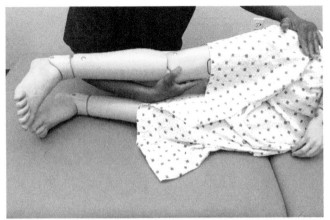

Figure 8.28b Hip extension
(Patient: Side-lying Position)

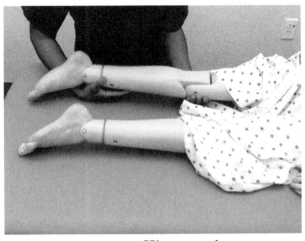

Figure 8.29b Hip extension
(Patient: Prone Position)

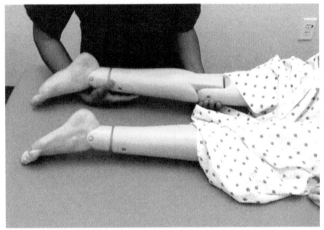

Figure 8.29 Starting Position

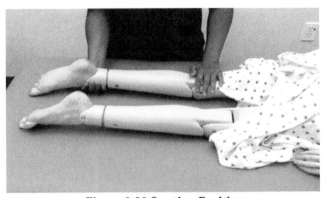

Figure 8.30 Starting Position

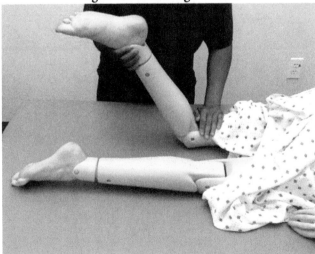

Figure 8.30a

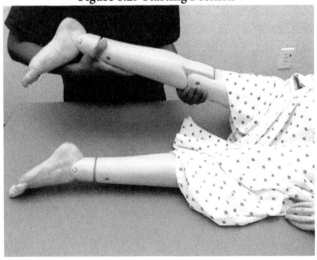

Figure 8.29a

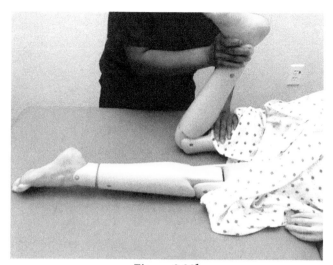

Figure 8.30b

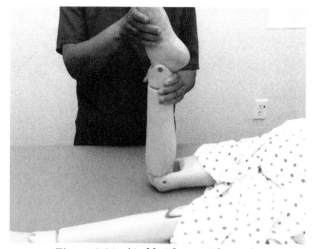

Figure 8.31a (Ankle Plantar-Flexion)

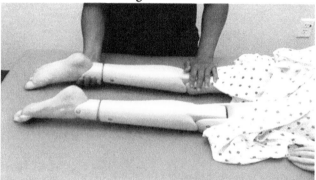

Figure 8.30c Knee flexion and extension
(Patient: Prone Position)

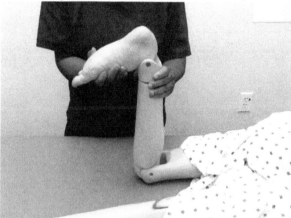

Figure 8.31b (Ankle Dorsi-Flexion) Alternate hand
placement on plantar surface may also be used.

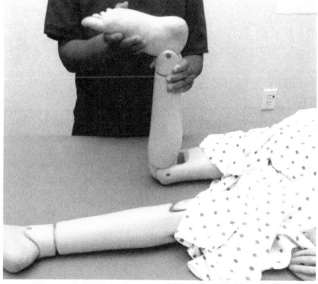

Figure 8.31 Starting Position (Ankle Neutral)

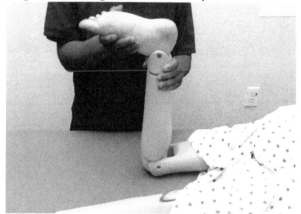

Figure 8.31c Back to starting position
(Patient: Prone Position)

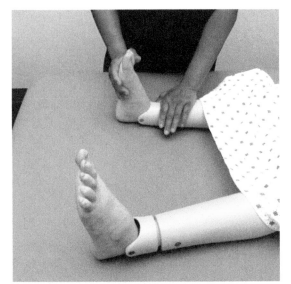

Figure 8.32 Starting Position

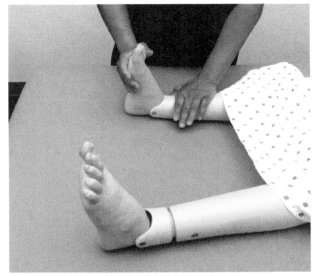

Figure 8.32c Back to starting position
(Patient: Supine Position)

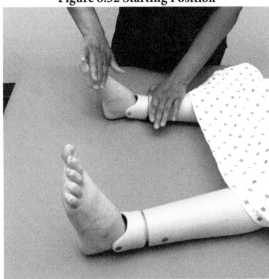

Figure 8.32a (Ankle Plantar-Flexion)

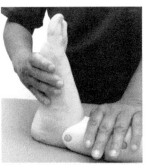 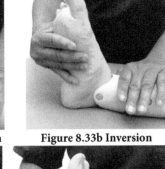

Figure 8.33a Start Position   Figure 8.33b Inversion

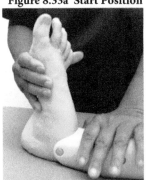 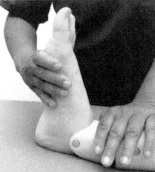

Figure 8.33c Eversion   Figure 8.33d Neutral
Ankle inversion and eversion
(Patient: Supine Position)

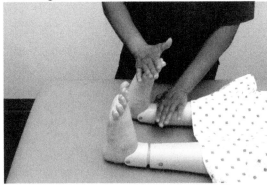

Figure 8.32b (Ankle Dorsi-Flexion)

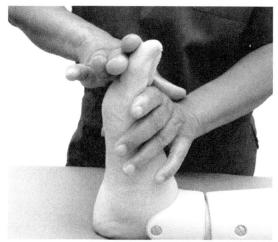

Figure 8.34a Phalangeal Extension

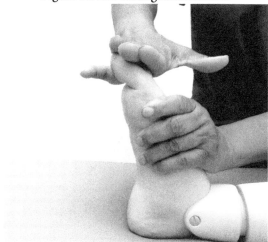

Figure 8.34b Phalangeal Flexion

Phalanges and big toe extension and flexion
(Patient: Supine Position)

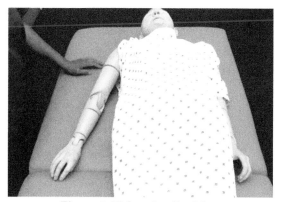

Figure 8.35 Starting Position

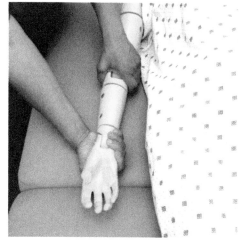

Figure 8.35a

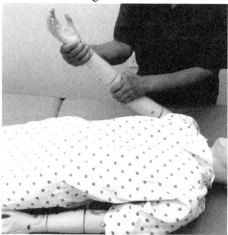

Figure 8.35b

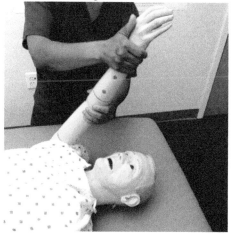

Figure 8.35c Shoulder flexion supine
(Patient: Supine Position)

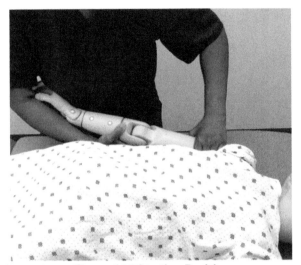

Figure 8.36 Starting Position

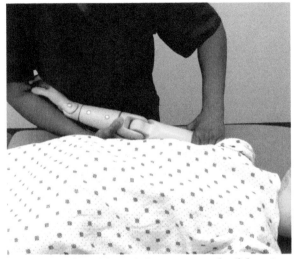

Figure 8.36c Shoulder abduction and adduction
(Patient: Supine Position)

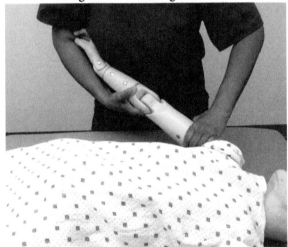

Figure 8.36a

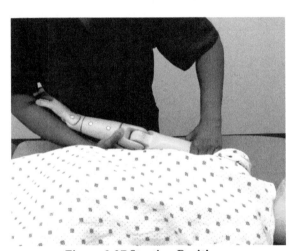

Figure 8.37 Starting Position

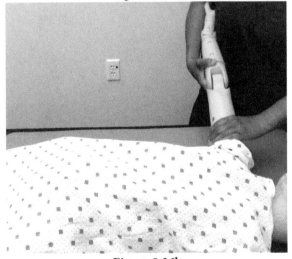

Figure 8.36b

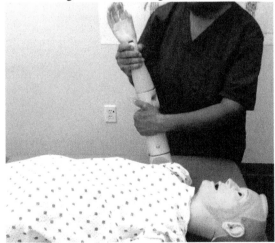

Figure 8.37a

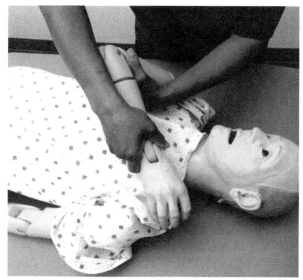

Figure 8.37b Shoulder horizontal adduction (Patient: Supine Position)

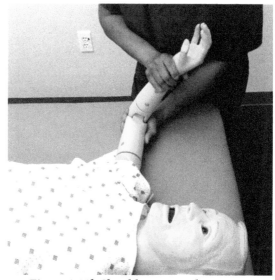

Figure 8.38b Shoulder External Rotation

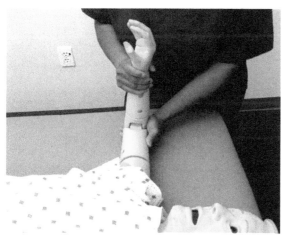

Figure 8.38 Starting Position

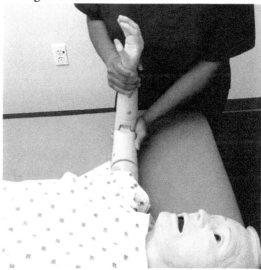

Figure 8.38c
Shoulder internal and external rotation (Patient: Supine Position)

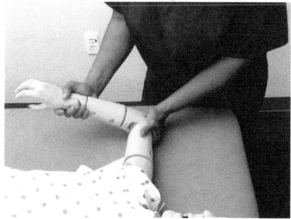

Figure 8.38a Shoulder Internal Rotation

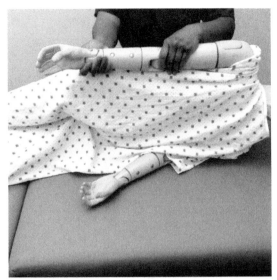

Figure 8.39 Starting Position

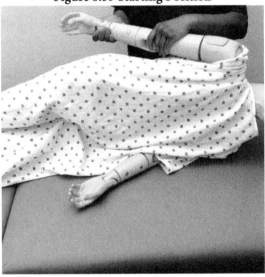

Figure 8.39a
Shoulder extension
(Patient: Side-lying Position)

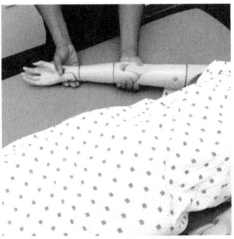

Figure 8.40 Starting Position

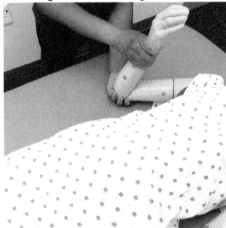

Figure 8.40a

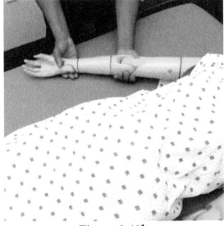

Figure 8.40b
Elbow flexion and extension
(Patient: Supine Position)

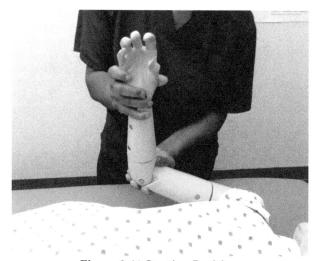

Figure 8.41 Starting Position

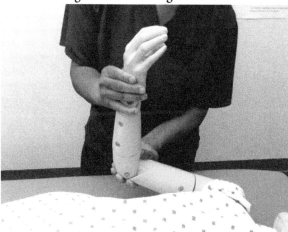

Figure 8.41a Supination

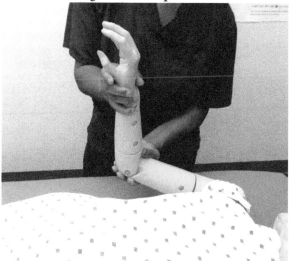

Figure 8.41b Pronation

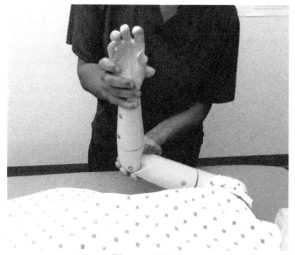

**Figure 8.41c
Forearm supination and pronation
(Patient: Supine Position)**

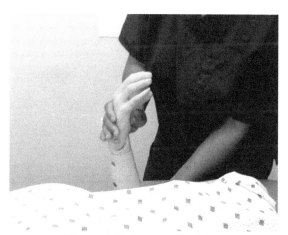

Figure 8.42 Starting Position

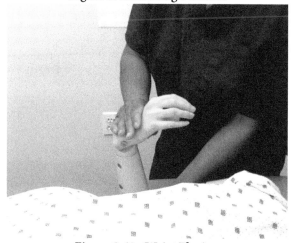

Figure 8.42a Wrist Flexion

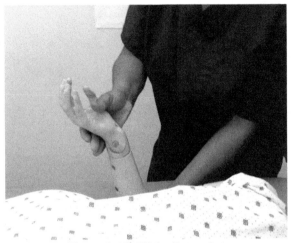

Figure 8.42b Wrist Extension

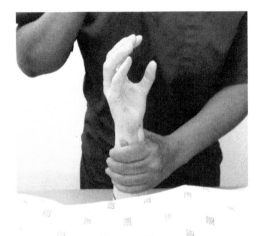

Figure 8.43 Starting Position

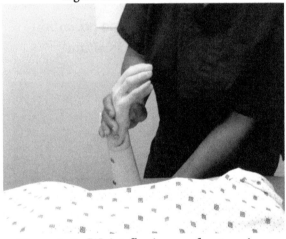

**Figure 8.42c Wrist flexion and extension
(Patient: Supine Position)**

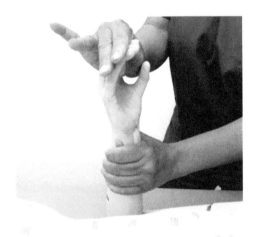

Figure 8.43a

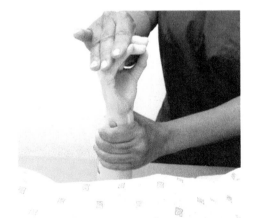

Figure 8.43b

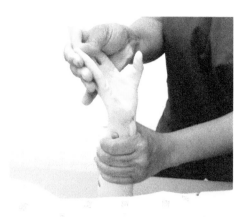

Figure 8.43c
Phalangeal joint flexion and extension
(Patient: Supine Position)

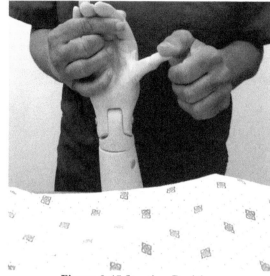

Figure 8.45 Starting Position

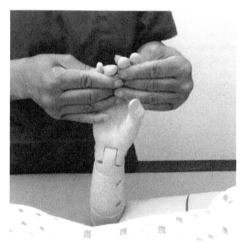

Figure 8.44 Starting Position (adduction)

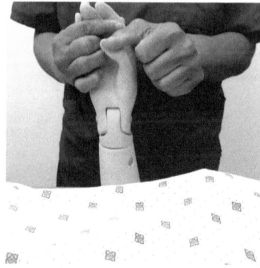

Figure 8.45a Starting Position
Thumb extension and flexion
(Patient: Supine Position)

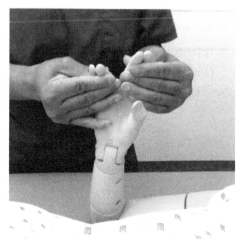

Figure 8.44a Phalangeal joint adduction and
abduction (Patient: Supine Position)

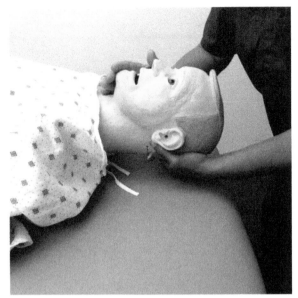

Figure 8.46 Starting Position

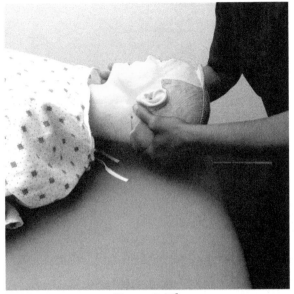

Figure 8.46b

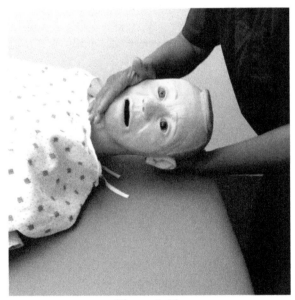

Figure 8.46a

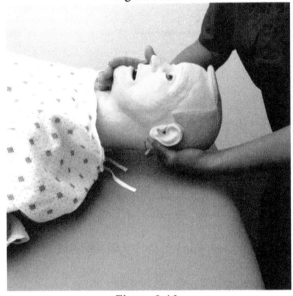

Figure 8.46c

**Neck rotation left and neck rotation right
(Patient: Supine Position)**

Note: Perform procedures only if within your scope of
practice.

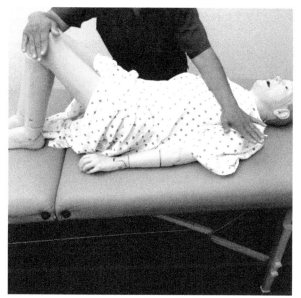

Figure 8.47 Starting Position

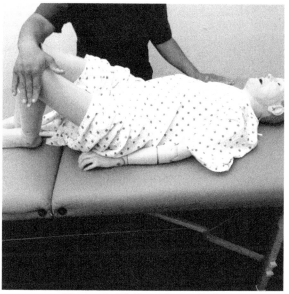

Figure 8.47b Rotation to Left

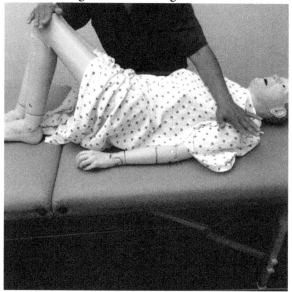

Figure 8.47a Rotation to Right

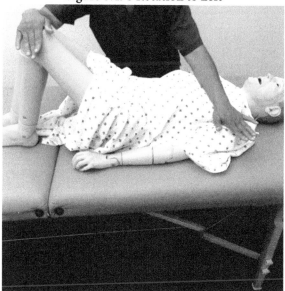

Figure 8.47c
Lumbar and pelvic rotations
(Patient: Supine Position)

RANGE OF MOTION FLOW SHEET (Practice Skills Sheet)

Joints	Right Side		Left Side	
	REPETITIONS	SUBJECT POSITION	REPETITIONS	SUBJECT POSITION
Hip Joint				
Flexion				
Extension				
Abduction				
Adduction				
Internal rotation				
External rotation				
Knee Joint				
Flexion				
Extension				
Ankle Joint				
Dorsi flexion				
Plantar flexion				
Shoulder Joint				
Flexion				
Extension				
Abduction				
Adduction				
Internal rotation				
External rotation				
Elbow Joint				
Flexion				
Extension				
Wrist Joint				
Flexion				
Extension				
Radial				
Ulnar				
MCP Joint				
Flexion				
Extension				
PIP Joint				
Flexion				
Extension				
DIP Joint				
Flexion				
Extension				

CHAPTER 8
END OF CHAPTER REVIEW QUESTIONS

Question Set 1: Multiple Choice
20 point: 2 points each

1. Spinal Column (Vertebral Column) movements include all the following except:
   a) Movement 1.   Flexion
   b) Movement 2.   Extension
   c) Movement 3.   Lateral Flexion
   d) Movement 4.   Circumduction

2. Shoulder Joint movements include all the following except:
   a) Movement 1.   Flexion
   b) Movement 2.   Extension
   c) Movement 3.   Inversion
   d) Movement 4.   Abduction
   e) Movement 5.   Medial Rotation
   f) Movement 6.   Lateral Rotation

3. Elbow Joint movements include all the following except:
   a) Movement 1.   Flexion
   b) Movement 2.   Extension
   c) Movement 3.   Adduction
   d) Movement 4.   Supination

4. Wrist Joint movements include all the following except:
   a) Movement 1.   Flexion
   b) Movement 2.   Extension
   c) Movement 3.   Adduction(Ulnar Deviation)
   d) Movement 4.   Abduction (Radial Deviation)
   e) Movement 5.   Eversion

5. Metacarpophalangeal Joint movements include all the following except:
   a) Movement 1.   Flexion
   b) Movement 2.   Circumduction

6. Distal Interphalangeal Joint movements include all the following except:
   a) Movement 1.   Hyper-flexion
   b) Movement 2.   Extension

7. Proximal Interphalangeal Joint movements include all the following except:
   a) Movement 1.   Hyper-flexion
   b) Movement 2.   Extension

8. Hip Joint movements include all the following except:
   a) Movement 1.   Flexion
   b) Movement 2.   Extension
   c) Movement 3.   Adduction
   d) Movement 4.   Abduction
   e) Movement 5.   Medial Rotation
   f) Movement 6.   Radial Deviation

9. Knee Joint movements include all the following except:
   a) Movement 1.   Hyper-flexion
   b) Movement 2.   Extension

10. Ankle Joint movements include all the following except:
   a) Movement 1.   Plantar Flexion
   b) Movement 2.   Dorsi Flexion
   c) Movement 3.   Ulnar Rotation
   d) Movement 4.   Eversion

Question Set 2: Essay Questions   20 point: 5 points each

1. Explain the types of range of motion exercises.
2. List the parts of a goniometer and briefly describe its use.
3. List the key principles while performing range of motion exercises.
4. List the contraindications of range of motion exercises.

Question Set 3: Identity Range of Motions   42 point: 2 points each

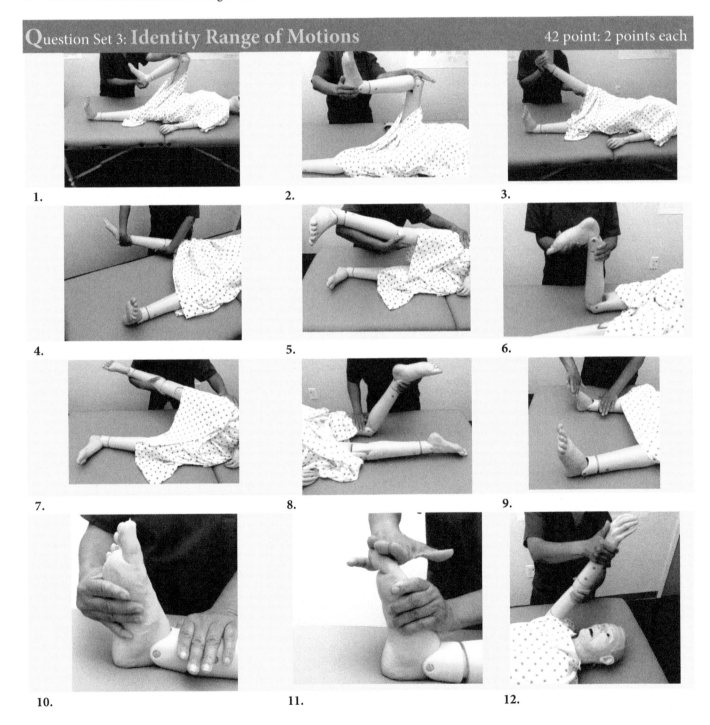

1.

2.

3.

4.

5.

6.

7.

8.

9.

10.

11.

12.

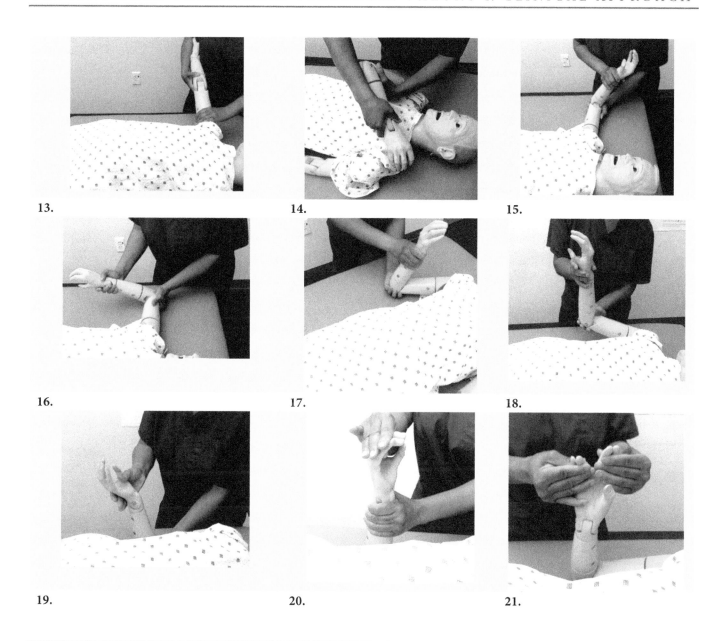

13.

14.

15.

16.

17.

18.

19.

20.

21.

Question Set 4: Identity Joint Movements

20 point: 2 points each

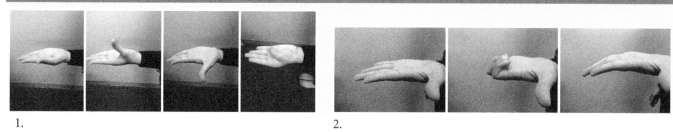

1.

2.

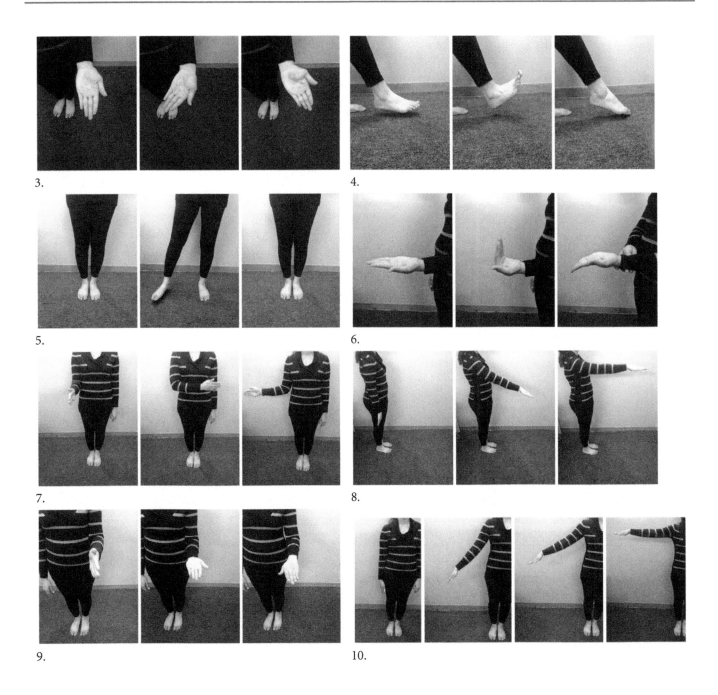

3.

4.

5.

6.

7.

8.

9.

10.

SECTION 2
CHAPTER 9: THERAPEUTIC EXERCISES

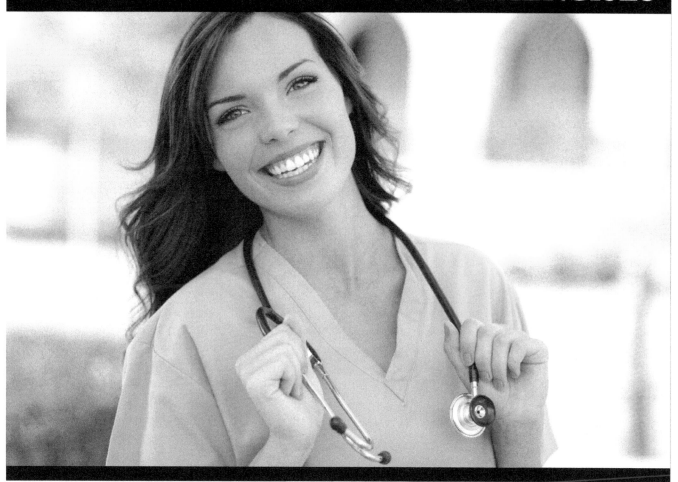

Learning Objectives

At the end of this chapter the student will be able to describe:

1. Manual muscle testing
2. Steps in performing manual muscle testing
3. Types of therapeutic exercises
   a. Active exercises
   b. Active assisted exercises
   c. Resisted exercises
4. General steps in performing therapeutic exercises
5. Illustration of therapeutic exercise

PATIENT CARE INTERVENTION: THERAPEUTIC EXERCISES

Therapeutic exercises are mainly designed to improve patient's mobility and strengthen affected area of the body. Key components involve performing the exercises regularly, with appropriate sets and repetitions.

Types of therapeutic exercises can be divided as follows:

1. **Active**
2. **Passive**
3. **Active Assisted**
4. **Resisted**
   a. **Isotonic**
      i. **Concentric**
      ii. **Eccentric**
   b. **Isometric**

Manual Muscle Testing

Manual muscle testing is a procedure used to evaluate the function and strength of an individual muscle or muscle groups.

MMT Grading Scale Range: 0 to 5		
0	None	No visible or palpable contraction
1	Trace	Visible or palpable contraction with no motion (Flicker)
2	Poor	Full ROM in a gravity eliminated plane
3	Fair	Full ROM against gravity
4	Good	Full ROM against gravity, with moderate resistance
5	Normal	Full ROM against gravity, with maximal resistance

STEPS IN PERFORMING MANUAL MUSCLE TESTING (MMT):
1. Explain the procedure to the patient.
2. Position the patient in a comfortable position.

3. Stabilize the body part and select the muscle to be evaluated.
4. Start from grade 2:
   a. If unable to perform a shift to grade 1.
   b. If able to perform a shift to grade 3.
5. Record the grade.

TYPES OF THERAPEUTIC EXERCISES	
Active Exercises	Actively performed by the patient with minimum or no resistance.
Active Assisted Exercises	Actively performed by the patient and may be assisted when required during a specific range.
Resisted Exercises	Actively performed by the patient and resistance is applied against the active movement.
1) Isotonic Muscle Contraction: meaning "same tension"	Isotonic muscle contractions are the muscle contractions that enable humans to move around with the desired movements. There are mainly two types of isotonic muscle contractions: • Concentric muscle contraction, and • Eccentric muscle contraction.
Concentric Muscle Contraction	Muscle **shortens** in length as tension within the muscle increases; this occurs in response to **lifting** a weight.
Simplification:	**Muscles shorten as muscle fibers contract.** When lifting a dumbbell in your hand and flexing your elbow, this occurs as a result of shortening of the muscle, thereby causing the weight to move in an upward direction due to concentric contraction of the biceps muscle.

Eccentric Muscle Contraction	Muscle **lengthens** in length as tension within the muscle increases; this occurs in response to *lowering* a weight.
Simplification:	When lifting a dumbbell in your hand and flexing your elbow, this occurs as a result of shortening of the muscle, thereby causing the weight to move in an upward direction due to concentric contraction of the biceps muscle. However, when lowering the dumbbell slowly while controlling the movement leads to eccentric contraction.
2) Isometric Muscle Contraction meaning "same length"	Muscle **maintains the same (iso) length (metric)** as tension within the muscle increases; this occurs as a result of holding a contraction in a muscle without moving a joint in a static position.
Simplification:	In this type of contraction, the muscle contracts. However, while the muscle is in a state of contraction the length of the overall muscle remains the same. This type of contraction can be seen when holding an object, it occurs as a result of the increase muscle contraction without much change in the overall length of the muscle to grip or hold the object.

Comparing isotonic with isometric contractions

TYPES OF CONTRACTION	Joint Movement (resulting from muscle contraction)	Change in overall length of muscle
Isotonic (muscle contraction) There are 2 types of isotonic muscle contraction: • Concentric • Eccentric	**MOVEMENT** occurs (direction of movement depends on type of contraction, i.e. concentric or eccentric)	**Length of muscle changes** concentric contraction = muscle shortens eccentric contraction = muscle lengthens
Isometric (muscle contraction)	**MINIMAL TO NO MOVEMENT**	No change in muscle length

GENERAL STEPS IN PERFORMING THERAPEUTIC EXERCISES:

1. Explain the procedure and give instructions.
2. Position the patient comfortably.
3. Select the muscle to be exercised.
4. Stabilize the joints as per requirements.
5. Select the type of exercise to be performed.
6. Appropriate sets and repetitions must be selected.

EXERCISE FOR MUSCLES

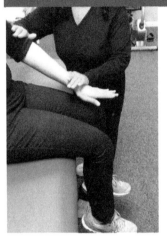 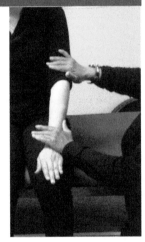

Side view   Front view

Figure 9.1a Anterior Fibers of Deltoid

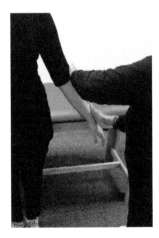 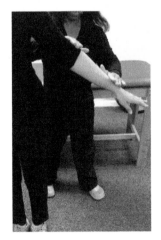

From Front   From Back

Figure 9.1b Middle Fibers of Deltoid

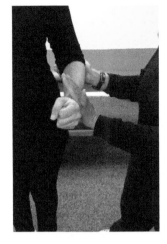 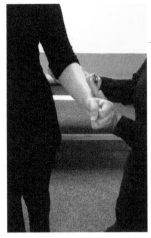

Initial Position   Final Position

Figure 9.2 External Rotators

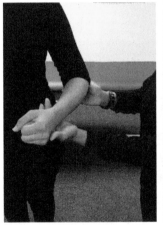 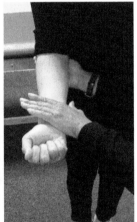

Figure 9.3 Internal Rotators   **Figure 9.4 Biceps**

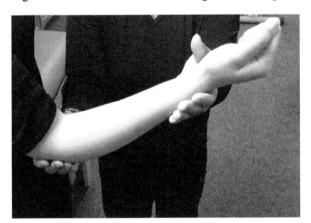

Figure 9.5a Triceps (Initial Range)

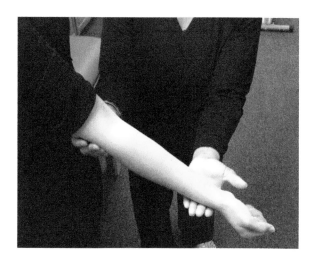

Figure 9.5b Triceps (Final Range)

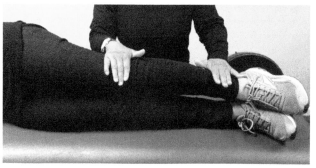

Figure 9.7a Abductors (Initial Range)

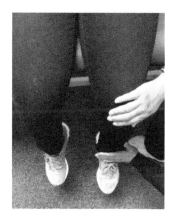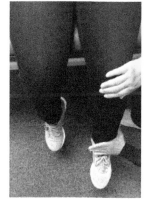

Figure 9.6a Quadriceps (Initial Range)

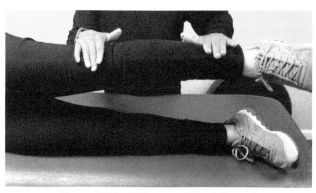

Figure 9.7b Abductors (Final Range)

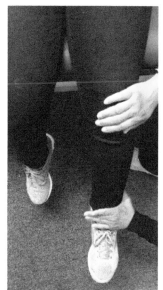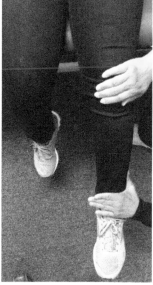

Figure 9.6b Quadriceps (Final Range)

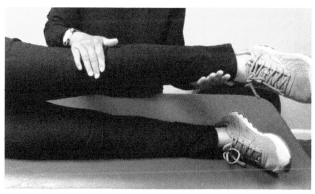

Figure 9.8a Adductors (Initial Range)

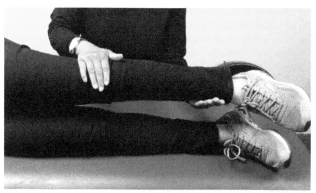

Figure 9.8b Adductors (Final Range)

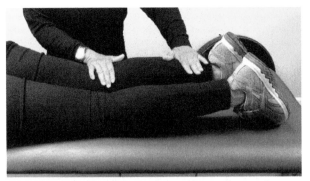

Figure 9.9a Knee Flexors (Initial Range)

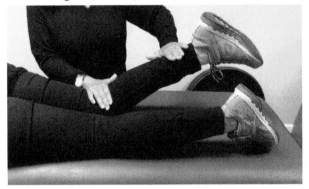

Figure 9.9b Knee Flexors (Mid-Range)

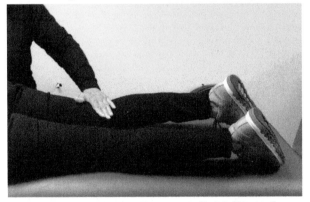

Figure 9.10a Hip Extensors (Initial Range)

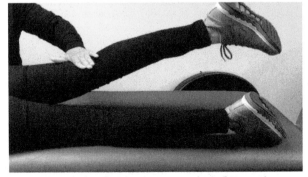

Figure 9.10b Hip Extensors (Final Range)

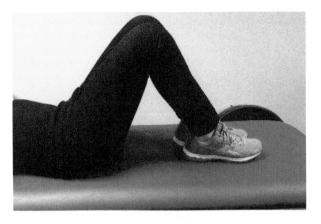

Figure 9.11a Bridging (Initial Position)

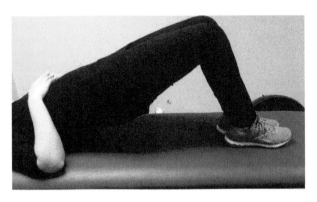

Figure 9.11b Bridging (Final Position)

CHAPTER 9
END OF CHAPTER REVIEW QUESTIONS

Question Set 1: Match the following (Manual Muscle Testing)   12 point: 2 points each

Answer	Column 1	Column 2
	Fair	a. No visible or palpable contraction
	Good	b. Visible or palpable contraction with no motion (Flicker)
	None	c. Full ROM in a gravity eliminated plane
	Normal	d. Full ROM against gravity
	Trace	e. Full ROM against gravity, with moderate resistance
	Poor	f. Full ROM against gravity, with maximal resistance

Question Set 2: Essay Questions   40 point: 5 points each

1. Explain the steps involved in performing manual muscle testing?

2. Explain the types of therapeutic exercises?

3. What is the difference between isotonic and isometric exercises?

4. Explain in detail about concentric exercises, provide an example for the same?

5. Explain in detail about eccentric exercises, provide an example for the same?

6. Enlist the steps in performing therapeutic exercises?

7. Identify 5 activities of daily life that involves isometric muscle contractions?

8. Identify 5 activities of daily life that involves isotonic (concentric or eccentric) muscle contractions?

Instructions: Identify the name of the muscle(s) on which resistive exercise are being performed.

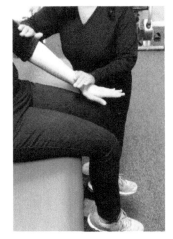

1.

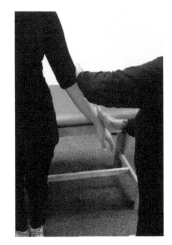

2.

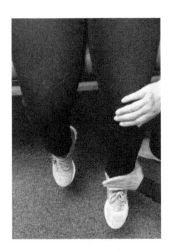

3.

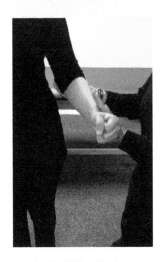

4.

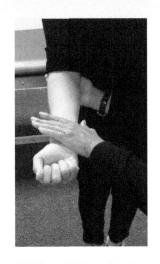

5.

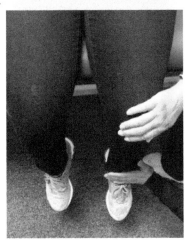

6.

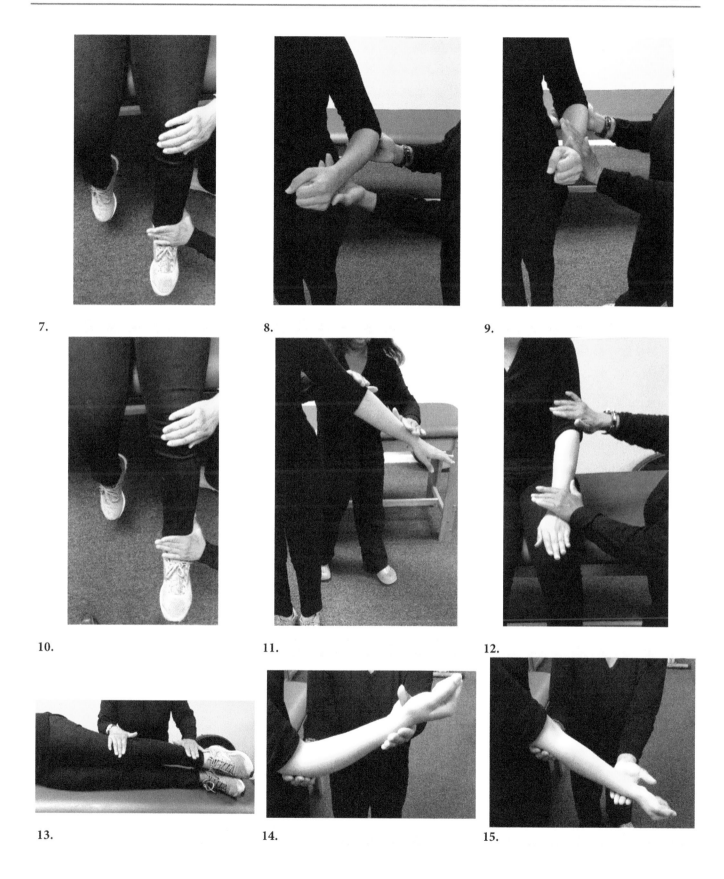

7.

8.

9.

10.

11.

12.

13.

14.

15.

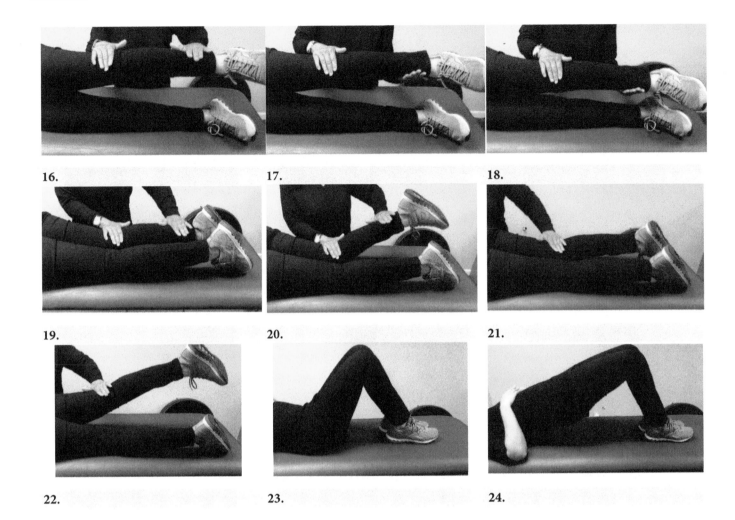

16.

17.

18.

19.

20.

21.

22.

23.

24.

177

SECTION 3

CHAPTER 10: GAIT

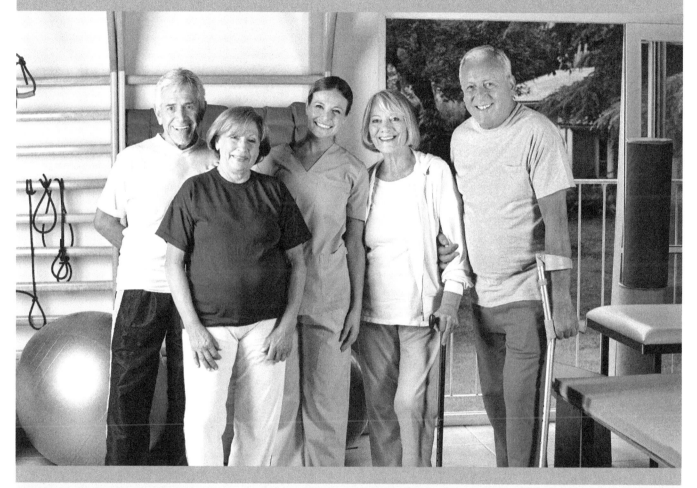

Learning Objectives

At the end of this chapter the student will be able to describe:

- Gait Terminologies
- Gait Cycle
  - Stance phase
  - Swing phase
- Illustration of Gait Cycle

GAIT TERMINOLOGIES

- **Gait cycle:** heel strike to heel strike of the same leg.
- **Stride length:** distance between heel strike of one leg to next heel strike of the same leg.
- **Step length:** distance between heel strike of one foot to heel strike of opposite foot.
- **Cadence:** measure of walking speed; steps per minute (normal is 80-120).
- **Velocity:** distance per time.
- **Stride duration:** time in seconds for one gait cycle.
- **Width of walking base:** normal is 2-4 inches.
- **Single support:** one foot is in contact with the ground while the other leg is not.
- **Double support:** both feet are in contact with the ground at once.
- **Non-support:** neither foot is in contact with the ground (does not occur with walking).

GAIT CYCLE

Stance phase: makes up 60% of the gait cycle.

In this phase, the foot is in constant contact with the floor.

1. **Heel strike:** Only heel of the foot comes in contact with the floor. (Figure 10.1 & Figure 10.2)

2. **Foot flat:** Foot comes in contact with the floor, but no weight bearing. (Figure 10.1 & Figure 10.2)

3. **Midstance:** Foot in contact with the floor, weight bearing takes place. (Figure 10.1 & Figure 10.2)

4. **Heel off:** Only the heel of the same foot comes off the floor (heel raises from the floor). (Figure 10.1 & Figure 10.2)

5. **Toe off:** Last phase of stance phase in which the toe of the same foot leaves contact with the floor. (Figure 10.1 & Figure 10.2)

Swing phase: makes up 40% of the gait cycle.

In this phase, the foot is not in constant contact with the floor.

1. **Acceleration:** Next phase after toe off, the foot is off the floor trying to progress in a forward direction. (Figure 10.1 & Figure 10.2)

2. **Midswing:** The leg has now swung and has crossed the midrange and progresses further ahead. (Figure 10.1 & Figure 10.2)

3. **Deceleration:** Last phase in the swing phase when the leg is proceeding towards slowing down for its subsequent contact with the floor, the next phase after deceleration would be the heel strike which would mark the beginning of stance phase. (Figure 10.1 & Figure 10.2)

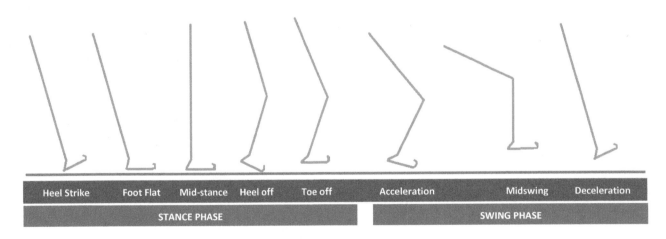

Figure 10.1 Gait Phases

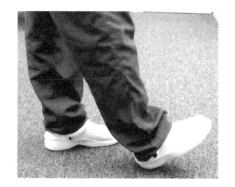

HEEL STRIKE

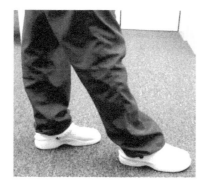

FOOTFLAT

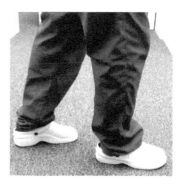

MIDSTANCE

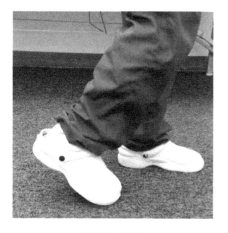

HEEL OFF

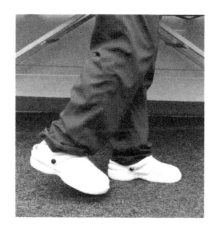

TOE OFF

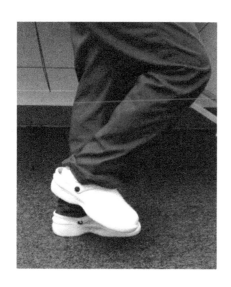

ACCELERATION

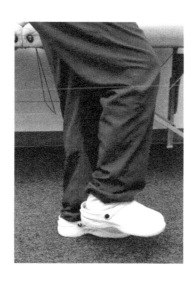

MIDSWING

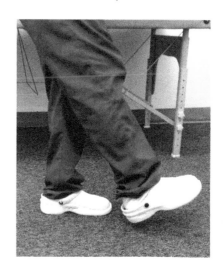

DECELERATION

Figure 10.2 Gait Cycle

Phase	ROM Requirements	Muscle Action
Heel Strike	1. Neutral dorsi flexion 2. Knee slightly flexed 3. 25-30 degrees of hip flexion	1. Concentric/eccentric dorsi flexion 2. Ankle eversion 3. Eccentric quadriceps 4. Eccentric/isometric hip extensors 5. Isometric hip adductors 6. Eccentric erector spinae
Foot Flat	1. 15 degrees of plantar flexion 2. 15-20 degrees knee flexion 3. 25-30 degrees of hip flexion	1. Eccentric dorsi flexion 2. Eccentric quadriceps 3. Concentric extensors 4. Isometric abductors
Mid-stance	1. Up to 10 degrees of dorsi flexion 2. Slight (5 degrees) knee flexion 3. Slight (5 degrees) hip flexion	1. Eccentric plantar flexion (soleus) 2. Ankle pronation (slight) 3. Quadriceps relatively inactive 4. Hamstrings relatively inactive 5. Concentric extensors
Heel-off	1. 15 degrees of dorsi flexion 2. Nearly full knee extension 3. 10 degrees hip extension	1. Concentric plantar flexion 2. Sub-talar neutral before heal off 3. Knee is inactive 4. Eccentric hip flexors
Toe-off	1. 20 degrees plantar flexion 2. About 40 degrees knee flexion 3. 10 degrees hip extension to neutral (moving toward flexion)	1. Concentric plantar flexion 2. Knee is relatively inactive 3. Hip flexors begin to concentrically contract
Acceleration	1. 10 degrees plantar flexion (moving toward neutral) 2. Knee moves into more flexion 3. Hip is neutral & moving into flexion	1. Concentric dorsi flexion 2. Concentric knee flexion 3. Concentric hip flexion
Mid-swing	1. Neutral dorsi flexion, up to 10 degrees plantar flexion 2. 65 degrees of knee flexion 3. Continues to flex up to 30 degrees	1. Concentric dorsi flexion 2. Quadriceps begin to extend knee: Hamstrings keep it flexed prior to this 3. Hip extensors begin to contract eccentrically
Deceleration	1. Ankle is neutral 2. Knee moves towards full extension 3. 25-30 degrees of hip flexion until just before heel strike, then will begin to extend	1. Concentric dorsi flexion 2. Knee is fixed once quads have extended the knee 3. Eccentric hip extension to prepare for heel strike

Table 10.1 Gait Cycle with Joint Movement and Muscle Actions

CHAPTER 10

END OF CHAPTER REVIEW QUESTIONS

Question Set 1: Match the following   45 point: 3 points each

Answer	Column 1	Column 2
	Double support	1. heel strike to heel strike of the same leg
	Non-support	2. distance between heel strike of right leg to next heel strike of right leg
	Heel off	3. distance between heel strike of one foot to heel strike of opposite foot
	Foot flat	4. measure of walking speed; steps per minute (normal is 80-120)
	Midstance	5. distance per time
	Toe off	6. time in seconds for one gait cycle
	Single support	7. normal is 2-4 inches
	Gait cycle	8. one foot is in contact with the ground while the other leg is not
	Stride length	9. both feet are in contact with the ground at once
	Step length	10. neither foot is in contact with the ground (does not occur with walking)
	Cadence	11. Only heel of the foot comes in contact with the floor.
	Velocity	12. Foot comes in contact with the floor, but no weight bearing.
	Stride duration	13. Foot in contact with the floor, weight bearing takes place.
	Width of walking base	14. Only the heel of the same foot comes off the floor (heel raises from the floor).
	Heel strike	15. Last phase of stance phase in which the toe of the same foot leaves contact with the floor.

Question Set 2: Essay Questions   10 point: 5 points each

1. Explain about the swing phase of the gait cycle.
2. Explain about the stance phase of the gait cycle.

Question Set 3: Identify illustrations *Gait Phases*   20 point: 2 points each

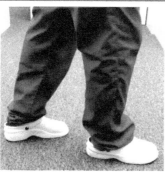

1.

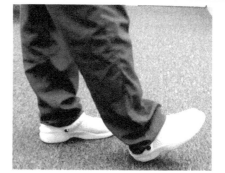

2.

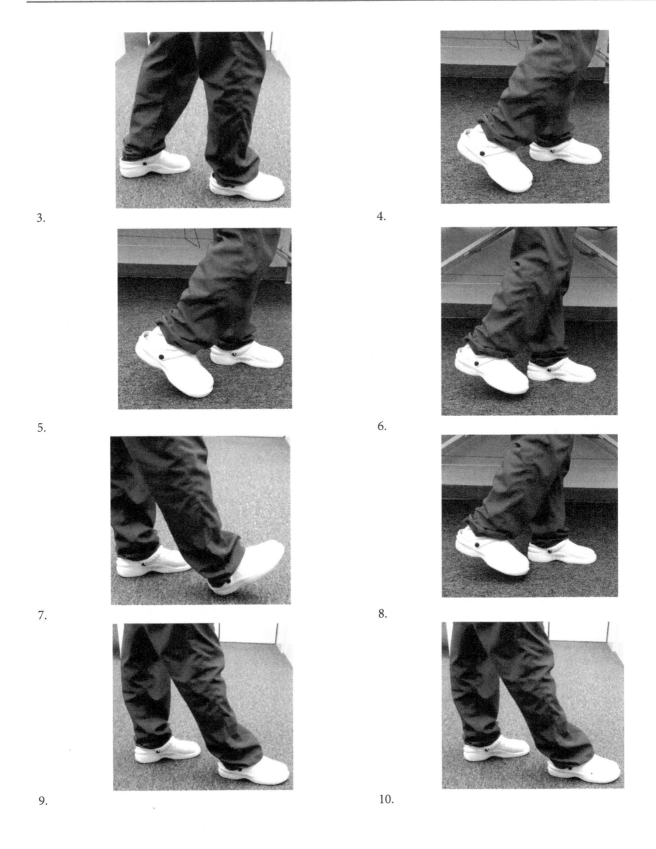

3.

4.

5.

6.

7.

8.

9.

10.

Question Set 4: Fill in the Missing Information — 25 point: 1 point each

Phase	ROM Requirements	Muscle Action
Heel Strike	1. Neutral dorsi_____ 2. Knee slightly_____ 3. 25-30 degrees of hip_____	1. Concentric/eccentric_____ 2. Ankle eversion 3. Eccentric quadriceps 4. Eccentric/isometric hip_____ 5. Isometric hip_____ 6. Eccentric erector spinae
Foot Flat	1. 15 degrees of_____ 2. 15-20 degrees knee_____ 3. 25-30 degrees of hip_____	1. Eccentric _____ 2. Eccentric quadriceps 3. Concentric extensors 4. _____ abductors
Mid-stance	1. Up to 10 degrees of _____ 2. Slight (5 degrees) knee flexion 3. Slight (5 degrees) _____ flexion	1. Eccentric plantar flexion (soleus) 2. Ankle pronation (slight) 3. Quadriceps relatively inactive 4. Hamstrings relatively inactive 5. _____ extensors
Heel-off	1. 15 degrees of _____ 2. Nearly full knee _____ 3. 10 degrees _____ extension	1. Concentric _____ 2. Sub-talar neutral before heal off 3. Knee is inactive 4. Eccentric hip _____
Toe-off	1. 20 degrees _____ 2. About 40 degrees _____ flexion 3. 10 degrees hip extension to neutral (moving toward flexion)	1. Concentric plantar flexion 2. Knee is relatively inactive 3. Hip flexors begin to concentrically contract
Acceleration	1. 10 degrees plantar flexion (moving toward neutral) 2. Knee moves into more towards flexion 3. Hip is neutral & moving into flexion	1. Concentric _____ 2. Concentric _____ flexion 3. Concentric hip flexion
Mid-swing	1. Neutral dorsi flexion, up to 10 degrees plantar flexion 2. 65 degrees of knee _____ 3. Continues to flex up to 30 degrees	1. Concentric dorsi flexion 2. Quadriceps begin to extend knee: Hamstrings keep it flexed prior to this 3. Hip _____ begin to contract eccentrically

SECTION 3

CHAPTER 11: ASSISTIVE DEVICES

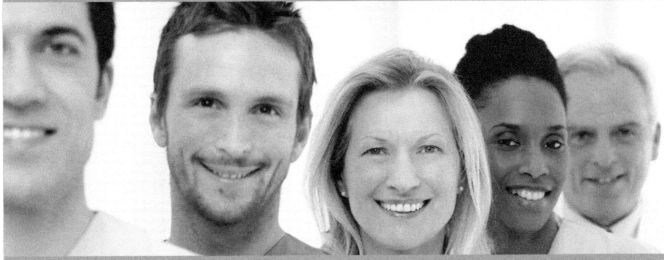

LEARNING OBJECTIVES

At the end of this chapter the student will be able to describe the following:

1. Uses and general principles of assistive devices
2. Types of weight-bearing patterns (ambulation):
   a. Non-weight bearing (NWB)
   b. Touch-down weight bearing (TDWB)
   c. Partial weight bearing (PWB)
   d. Weight bearing as tolerated (WBAT)
   e. Full weight bearing (FWB)
3. Types of assistive gait devices for:
   a. Partial weight bearing assistive devices
   b. Non-weight bearing assistive devices
4. Points to consider prior to choosing assistive devices.
5. Crutches
   a. Disadvantages of axillary crutches
   b. Measurement of axillary crutches
   c. Types of gait patterns with axillary crutches
6. Canes
   a. Disadvantages of a cane
   b. Measurement of a cane
   c. Types of gait patterns with canes
7. Forearm crutches
   a. Disadvantages of forearm crutches
   b. Measurement of forearm crutches
8. Walkers

   a. Disadvantages of using walkers
   b. Measurement of a walker
9. Illustration: 4-point crutch walking gait
10. Illustration: 2-point crutch walking gait
11. Illustration: 3-point crutch walking gait
12. Illustration: Swing-through gait
13. Illustration: Swing-to gait
14. Ascending stairs and curbs
15. Descending stairs and curbs

PATIENT CARE INTERVENTION: ASSISTIVE DEVICES

An assistive device can be used for the following reasons:

1. Patient with decreased balance, stability and coordination.
2. Patient with the inability to bear weight on a lower extremity (fracture or another injury).
3. Patient suffering from paralysis (one or both lower extremities).
4. Patient with amputation of a lower extremity.
5. Patient with neurological deficits.
6. Patient with new prosthetics or orthotics.
7. Patient with decreased mobility and body functions.

General Principles

1. The patient should be carefully evaluated, to select the appropriate assistive device to meet the patient's specific needs. The evaluator should be aware of the patient's total medical condition and weight-bearing status of the involved extremity when considering the type of assistive device to be used for the patient.
2. Range of motion of the extremities and the strength of the primary muscles (manual muscle testing) required for ambulation must be evaluated by the evaluator.

NOTE: The primary muscles required for ambulation with axillary crutches, using a three-point (non-weight bearing on one lower extremity) crutch gait pattern, are:

a. shoulder depressors
b. shoulder extensors
c. scapula stabilizers
d. elbow extensors and
e. finger flexors of the upper extremity

NOTE: The primary lower-extremity muscles in the weight-bearing lower extremity are:

a. hip extensors
b. hip abductors
c. knee extensors
d. knee flexors and
e. ankle dorsiflexors

Types of weight-bearing patterns (ambulation)

Non-weight bearing (NWB): Non-weight bearing on affected leg. Affected leg must be kept off the floor. Do not touch the floor with affected leg while standing or walking.

Touch-down weight bearing (TDWB), or toe-touch weight bearing (TTWB): Touch the floor with the affected leg for balance only without placing weight on the affected leg.

Partial weight bearing (PWB): A percentage of body weight is placed on the affected leg while walking or standing.

Weight bearing as tolerated (WBAT), or weight bearing to tolerance (WBTT): Weight bearing while walking or standing as per tolerated by the patient.

Full weight bearing (FWB): Complete body weight is placed on the affected leg while walking or standing.

Types of weight-bearing patterns with assistive devices
Partial Weight Bearing Assistive Devices
- Parallel Bars
- Walker
- Axillary Crutches (One or Two)
- Cane (One or Two)
- Lofstrand Crutches (forearm crutches)

Non-Weight Bearing Assistive Devices
- Parallel Bars
- Walker
- Two Axillary Crutches

Assistive devices: in the order of most to least stability and support

1. Parallel Bars
2. Walker
3. Axillary Crutches
4. Forearm Crutches (Lofstrand)
5. Two Canes
6. One Cane

Assistive devices: in the order of requiring least coordination to most coordination by the patient

1. Parallel Bars
2. Walker
3. One Cane

4. Two Canes
5. Axillary crutches
6. Forearm (Lofstrand) crutches

Points to consider prior to choosing assistive devices:
1. The amount of support the patient needs.
2. Patient's ability to manipulate the device.
3. Patient's disability, coordination, and stability status.

The main function of an assistive gait devices is to improve the patient's stability by increasing the base of support.

CRUTCHES

Axillary crutches are used to
1. Increase patient's base of support.
2. Provide lateral stability.
3. Reduce weight bearing on injured extremity.
4. Ambulate at a faster pace.
5. Provide a variety of gait patterns that can be used.

Disadvantages of axillary crutches:
1. Less stable than a walker.
2. Improper use of axillary crutches can cause injury to the axillary nerve.
3. Require good standing balance by the patient.
4. Upper body strength is required to use axillary crutches.

MEASUREMENT OF AXILLARY CRUTCHES:
Have the patient stand while wearing shoes
Equipment Adjustment
To adjust height:
Position axillary pad 2 inches or 3-5 finger widths below the axilla.

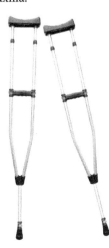

If patient is in standing position:
Starting from the axilla measure to a point (4-6 inches) anterior and (2-4 inches) lateral to the foot (tip of crutch).

If the patient is in supine position:
Starting from the axilla, measure to a point 6-8 inches away from the heel.

To position hand grip:
Should be adjusted in such a way that the patient has 15 to 25 degrees of elbow flexion.

Types of gait patterns with axillary crutches:-
- 2 Point Gait
- 3 Point Gait
- 4 Point Gait
- Swing Through Gait
- Swing To Gait

CANES

Canes are used to compensate for impaired balance or to increase balance and stability while walking.

Disadvantages of cane:
1. Provide limited support due to its small base of support.
2. Cannot be used for partial weight bearing ambulation.

MEASUREMENT OF A CANE
Equipment Adjustment
To adjust height:
To fit a patient with a cane, have the patient stand and measure from the patient's greater trochanter to a point 6 inches lateral to the patient's toes.
To position hand grip:
The hand grip of the cane should be adjusted in such a way that the patient has 15 to 25 degrees of elbow flexion.

Cane is a mostly used for patients with balance problem; **canes are of 3 types**
Cane Type 1. **One tip end**
Cane Type 2. **Tripod tip end**
Cane Type 3. **Quadruped tip end**

Types of gait patterns with canes
- 2 Point Gait
- 3 Point Gait

FOREARM CRUTCHES

- Forearm crutches are also called as **Loftstrand crutches**.
- Unlike axillary crutches, the forearm crutches do not have an axillary pad; this prevents the damage of axillary nerve.

Disadvantages of forearm crutches:

1. Forearm crutches are less stable.
2. The patient should have the stability and coordination to use this form of an assistive device.
3. The patient should have the upper-body strength to use the forearm crutches.

MEASUREMENT OF FOREARM CRUTCHES

Equipment Adjustment

To adjust height:

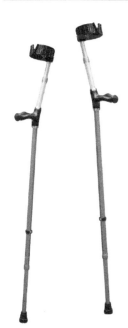

If patient is in standing position
Place the crutch parallel to the lateral aspect of the leg.

To position hand grip:
Handpiece should be at the level of the wrist crease or ulnar styloid process; this places the elbow at a 15 to 25 degrees of elbow flexion.

To position the forearm cuff:
The top of the forearm cuff should be adjusted so that it is located 1 to 1.5 inches distal to the olecranon process of the elbow, while the patient is grasping the headpiece of the crutch with the wrist in neutral position.

WALKERS

Walkers provide maximum stability and support, allowing the patient to be mobile. Walkers are designed in many styles, but all have four legs. Some walkers may have two or four wheels. Wheels allow the patient to gently push the walker forward, as opposed to picking the walker up to move it forward. Another variation in the design of the walker is the ability to fold the walker when it is not being used; this feature allows for easier transportation in a car and for storage.

Disadvantages of using walkers:

1. Walkers are cumbersome and difficult to store and transport.
2. Walkers are very difficult to use on stairs.
3. Walkers reduce the speed of ambulation.
4. The patient is unable to use a normal gait pattern by using a walker.

MEASUREMENT OF WALKER:

Equipment Adjustment

To adjust height and width:
If the patient is in standing position:

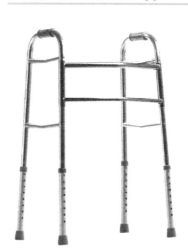

Adjust the height of the walker so that the patient has between 15 and 25 degrees of elbow flexion when grasping the hand grips on the walker.

The walker tips should be placed approximately 2 to 4 inches lateral and approximately 4 to 5 inches anterior to the forefoot to enhance the ease.

GAIT PATTERNS USING: ASSISTIVE DEVICES

4-POINT GAIT

1. Advance the right crutch forward.
2. Advance the left foot forward.
3. Advance the left crutch forward.
4. Advance the right foot forward.

Advantages:

Provides excellent stability as there are always three points in contact with the ground.

Disadvantages:

Slow walking speed.

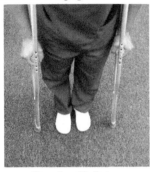
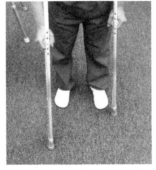

Starting Point

Right Crutch Forward

Point 1

Figure 11.1a

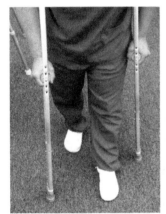
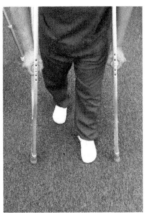

Left Foot Forward

Point 2

Left Crutch Forward

Point 3

Figure 11.1b

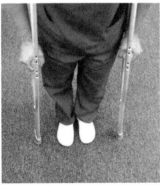

Right Foot Forward

Point 4

Figure 11.1c 4 POINT GAIT

2-POINT GAIT

1. Advance the right crutch and left foot forward simultaneously.
2. Advance the left crutch and the right foot forward simultaneously.

Advantages:

Faster than four point gait. Good support and stability from two opposing points of contact.

Disadvantages:

Can be difficult to learn the pattern.

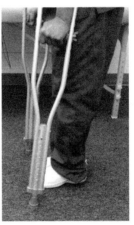
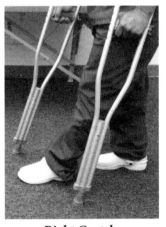

Starting Point

Right Crutches & Left Foot Forward

Point 1

Figure 11.2a

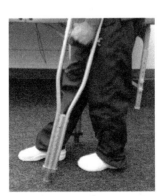

Left Crutches & Right Foot Forward

Point 2

Figure 11.2b 2 POINT GAIT

3-POINT GAIT

1. Advance both crutches and the affected (WBAT) or (TTWB) foot forward simultaneously.
2. Advance the unaffected foot forward.

USES

Used when patient has one full weight bearing (FWB) lower extremity and one (WBAT) or (TTWB) lower extremity.

Advantages:

Eliminates all weight-bearing on the affected leg. Usually indicated for use with involvement of one extremity only.

Disadvantages:

Good balance is required.

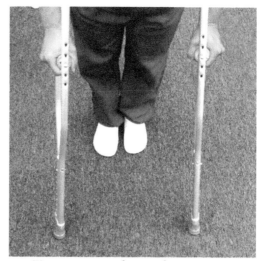

Figure 11.4a Both Crutches Forward

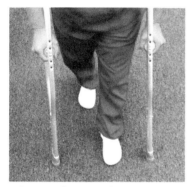

Figure 11.3a Both Crutches & Left Foot Forward (WBAT) or (TTWB)

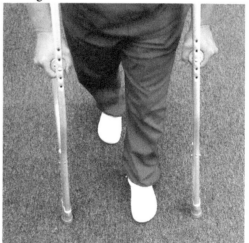

Figure 11.4b Left Foot Forward

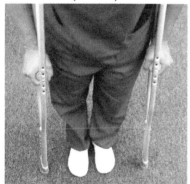

Figure 11.3b Right Leg Forward (FWB)

MODIFIED 3-POINT GAIT

1. Advance both crutches forward simultaneously.
2. Advance the affected (WBAT) foot forward.
3. Advance the unaffected foot.

USES

Used when the patient has one full weight bearing (FWB) lower extremity and one partial weight bearing (WBAT) lower extremity.

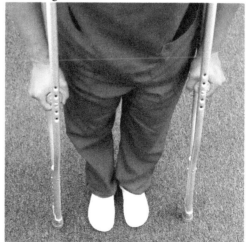

Figure 11.4b Left Foot Forward
MODIFIED 3 POINT GAIT

SWING-THROUGH GAIT

1. Advance both crutches forward simultaneously.
2. Advance both legs forward simultaneously past the crutches.

Advantage:

Fastest gait pattern.

Disadvantage:

Energy consuming and requires good upper extremity strength.

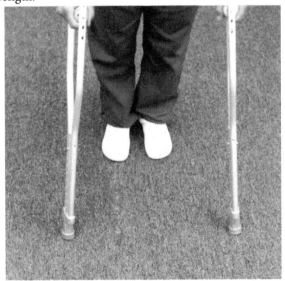

Figure 11.5a Both Crutches Forward

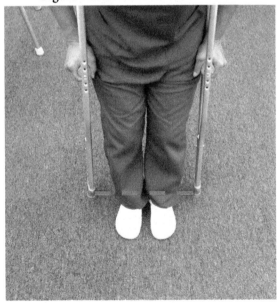

Figure 11.5b Swing Both Legs
Crossing the line of crutches (red line)
SWING-THROUGH GAIT

SWING-TO GAIT

1. Advance both crutches forward simultaneously.
2. Advance both legs forward simultaneously without passing the line of crutches.

Advantage:

Easy to learn. Usually indicated for patients with limited use of lower extremities, and trunk instability.

Disadvantage:

Requires good upper extremity strength.

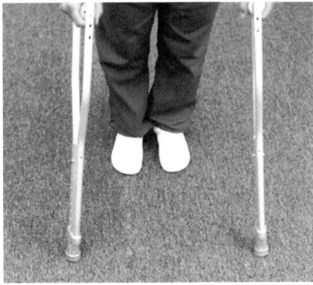

Figure 11.6a Both Crutches Forward

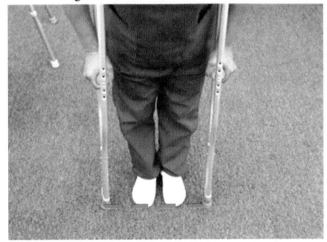

Figure 11.6b Both Legs Forward in line with crutches
(red line)
SWING-TO GAIT

ASCENDING STAIRS AND CURBS

Progression towards going upstairs should be done by progressing the non-injured leg followed by crutches and the injured leg together.

Guarding during ascending stairs

Stand behind and slightly to the involved side of the patient.

DESCENDING STAIRS AND CURBS

Progression towards going downstairs should be done by progressing the injured leg and the crutches together followed by non-injured.

Guarding during descending stairs

Stand in front and slightly to the involved side of the patient.

CHAPTER 11
END OF CHAPTER REVIEW QUESTIONS

Question Set 1: True or False   46 points: 2 points each

1. An assistive device is used by patients with decreased balance, increase stability and coordination.
   Answer: True or False

2. An assistive device is used by patients with new prosthetics or orthotics.
   Answer: True or False

3. An assistive device is used by patients with decreased mobility and body functions.
   Answer: True or False

4. An assistive device is used by patients with amputation of a lower extremity.
   Answer: True or False

5. Patients with neurological deficits use an assistive device.
   Answer: True or False

6. An assistive device is used by patients suffering from paralysis (one or both lower extremities).
   Answer: True or False

7. An assistive device is used by patients with the ability to bear weight on a lower extremity.
   Answer: True or False

8. Canes are used to compensate for impaired balance or to increase balance and decrease stability while walking.
   Answer: True or False

9. The disadvantage of a cane is to provide limited support due to its large base of support. It cannot be used for partial weight bearing ambulation.
   Answer: True or False

10. Forearm crutches are also called as axillary crutches.
    Answer: True or False

11. Axillary crutches and forearm crutches cause damage to axillary nerve due to the presence of an axillary pad.
    Answer: True or False

12. Forearm crutches are the most stable assistive device.
    Answer: True or False

13. The patient should have the stability and coordination to use forearm crutches.
    Answer: True or False

14. Patients should have the upper-body strength to use the forearm crutches.
    Answer: True or False

15. The advantage of a 2 point gait is that it provides excellent stability as there are always three points in contact with the ground.
Answer: True or False

16. Fast walking speed is a disadvantage of 4 point gait pattern.
Answer: True or False

17. Swing through gait is energy consuming and requires good lower extremity strength.
Answer: True or False

18. Swing to gait is easy to learn. Usually indicated for patients with limited use of upper extremities, and trunk instability
Answer: True or False

19. Swing to gait requires good lower extremity strength.
Answer: True or False

20. While ascending stairs, progress the injured leg following by crutches and the involved leg together.
Answer: True or False

21. Guarding during ascending stairs must be done by standing in front and slightly to the involved side of the patient.
Answer: True or False

22. While ascending stairs progress the uninvolved leg and the crutches followed by the involved leg.
Answer: True or False

23. Guarding during descending stairs must be done by standing in front and slightly to the involved side of the patient.
Answer: True or False

Question Set 2: Fill in the Blanks   10 points: 1 point each

1) The primary muscles required for ambulation with axillary crutches, using a three-point (non-weight bearing on one lower extremity) crutch gait pattern, are:

   a. shoulder _____

   b. shoulder _____

   c. scapula _____

   d. elbow _____ and

   e. finger _____ for the upper extremity

2) The primary lower-extremity muscles in the weight-bearing lower extremity are:

   a. hip _____

   b. hip _____

   c. knee _____

   d. knee _____ and

   e. ankle _____

Question Set 3: Match the Following
5 points: 1 point each

Answer	Column 1	Column 2
	Full weight bearing (FWB)	a. Affected leg must be kept off the floor. Do not touch the floor with affected leg while standing or walking.
	Weight bearing as tolerated (WBAT), or weight bearing to tolerance (WBTT)	b. Touch the floor with the affected leg for balance only without placing weight on the affected leg.
	Non-weight bearing (NWB)	c. A percentage of body weight is placed on the affected leg while walking or standing.
	Touch-down weight bearing (TDWB), or toe-touch weight bearing (TTWB)	d. Weight bearing while walking or standing as per tolerated by the patient.
	Partial weight bearing (PWB)	e. Complete body weight is placed on the affected leg while walking or standing.

Question Set 4: Essay Questions
50 points: 5 points each

1. List assistive devices which can assist in partial weight bearing while walking.
2. List assistive devices which can assist in non-weight bearing while walking.
3. List assistive devices in order of most to least stability and support.
4. List assistive devices in order of requiring minimum coordination to maximum coordination by the patient.
5. Describe in brief axillary crutch measurement for patients customized fit.
6. Describe in brief cane measurement for patients customized fit.
7. Describe in brief forearm crutch measurement for patients customized fit.
8. Describe in brief the difference between swing-to and swing-through gait.
9. List steps required to accomplish 3 point gait.
10. List steps required to accomplish 4 point gait.

Question Set 5: Multiple Choice
9 points: 3 points each

1) **Axillary crutches are used for the following purposes except:**
   a) Decreases patient's base of support.
   b) Provide lateral stability
   c) Reduce weight bearing on injury extremity.
   d) Ambulate at a faster pace.

2) **Which of the following statement below is not true while using an axillary crutch?**
   a) More stable than a walker.
   b) Improper use of axillary crutches can cause injury to the axillary nerve.
   c) Requires good standing balance by the patient.
   d) Upper body strength is required to use axillary crutches.

3) **Which of the following is not true while using a walker?**
   a) Walkers are cumbersome and difficult to store and transport.
   b) Walkers are very easy to use on stairs.
   c) Walkers reduce the speed of ambulation.
   d) Patient is unable to use a normal gait pattern while using a walker.

SECTION 3

CHAPTER 12: ORTHOSIS AND PROSTHESIS

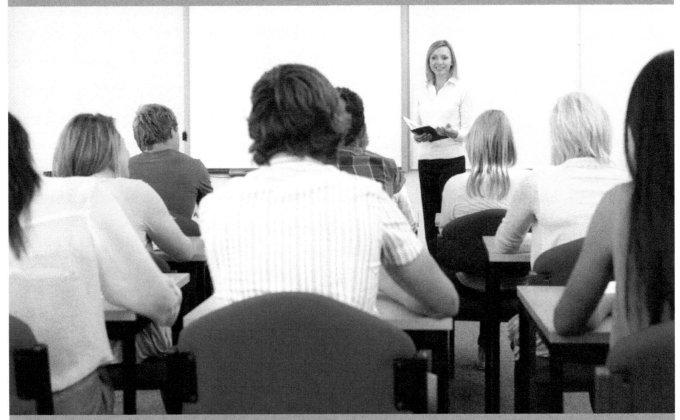

LEARNING OBJECTIVES

At the end of this chapter the student will be able to describe the following:

1) Orthosis
    i) Functions of an orthosis
        (1) Lower limb (LL) orthosis
        (2) Spinal orthosis
        (3) Upper limb (UL) orthosis
2) Prosthesis
    i) Functions of a prosthesis device
    ii) An ideal prosthesis
3) Patient care for orthosis and prosthesis

PATIENT CARE INTERVENTION: ORTHOSIS AND PROSTHESIS

Orthosis is a device used to support the body part. It may be temporary or permanent. **Mainly two functional types:**

Static: device does not allow movement.

Dynamic: device allows movement.

LOWER LIMB (LL) ORTHOSIS			
FO	Foot Orthosis	AFO	Ankle-Foot Orthosis
KO	Knee Orthosis	KAFO	Knee-Ankle-Foot Orthosis
HO	Hip Orthosis	HKAFO	Hip-Knee-Ankle-Foot Orthosis
		RGO	Reciprocal Gait Orthosis
SPINAL ORTHOSIS			
CO	Cervical Orthosis	CTO	Cervical-Thoracic Orthosis
TO	Thoracic Orthosis	CTLSO	Cervical-Thoraco-Lumbo-Sacral Orthosis
SO	Sacral Orthosis	TLSO	Thoraco-Lumbo-Sacral Orthosis
SIO	Sacroiliac Orthosis	LSO	Lumbosacral Orthosis
UPPER LIMB (UL) ORTHOSIS			
HO	Hand Orthosis	WHO	Wrist-Hand Orthosis
WO	Wrist Orthosis	EWHO	Elbow-Wrist-Hand Orthosis
EO	Elbow Orthosis	SEO	Shoulder-Elbow Orthosis
SO	Shoulder Orthosis	SEWHO	Shoulder-Elbow-Wrist-Hand Orthosis

TABLE 12.1 ORTHOSIS

Functions of an orthosis:

1) Prevents and corrects deformity.
2) Relieves pain and weight bearing.
3) Helps in ambulation.
4) Controls instability by restricting joint movement.

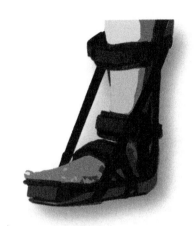

Figure 12.1 FOOT ORTHOSIS

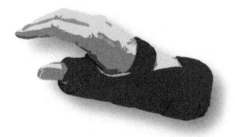

Figure 12.2 WRIST AND HAND ORTHOSIS

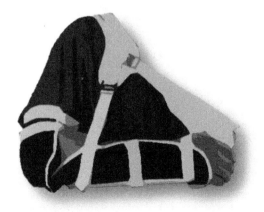

Figure 12.3 SHOULDER ORTHOSIS

Prosthesis is a device used to replace a part of the body which has beeen removed, absent or amputated.

Functions of a prosthesis:

Restores shape and function: Prosthesis are usually prescribed based on the level of amputation. All prosthesis usually contain a socket and terminal device.

An ideal prosthesis:

1. Should be functional
2. Should fit well
3. Should be light in weight
4. Should be easy to use
5. Should be cosmetically acceptable
6. Able to easily maintain
7. Able to easily repair

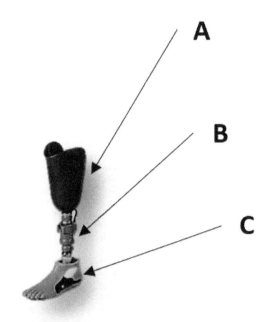

A: SOCKET   B: PLYON   C: FOOT (GRIP)
Figure 12.4a Parts of a Below Knee Prosthesis

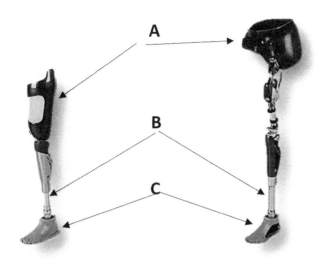

A: SOCKET   B: PLYON   C: FOOT (GRIP)

Figure 12.4b Parts of an Above Knee Prosthesis

CHAPTER 12
END OF CHAPTER REVIEW QUESTIONS

Question Set 1: Essay Questions
20 points: 5 points each

1. Describe orthosis and its functions.
2. Describe prosthesis and its functions.
3. Describe the patient care for orthosis and prosthesis.
4. Describe an ideal prosthesis.

PATIENT CARE FOR ORTHOSIS AND PROSTHESIS:

Provide proper care, maintenance and documentation of orthosis and prosthesis:

1. An appropriate weekly scheduling must be provided to patients that wear orthosis and prosthesis.
2. Educate patients on wearing and removing the orthosis and prosthesis.
3. Instruct on daily or scheduled cleaning on orthosis and prosthesis as required.
4. Inform the patient to check regularly on the skin or part of the body on which the orthosis or prosthesis is worn for any discomfort or skin color change.
5. Get a feedback from the patient on how comfortable is the orthosis or prosthesis.
6. Check the pressure bearing areas of the body while the orthosis or prosthesis are worn or onto the body part.
7. Instruct patient on chances of skin damage, application of orthosis must be properly applied to avoid the friction against the skin.

NOTE: Qualified professionals perform prosthesis and orthosis care. Assistant(s), Technician(s), and Aid(s) may assist the qualified professionals.

SECTION 3

CHAPTER 13: TRANSFER TECHNIQUES

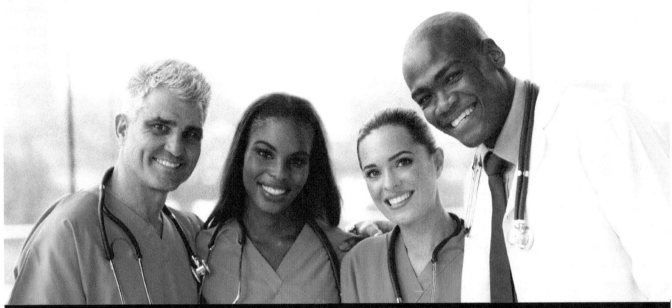

LEARNING OBJECTIVES

At the end of this chapter the student will be able to describe the following:

1) Levels of assistance
2) Types of Transfer
   - Dependent transfer
   - Assisted transfer
   - Independent transfer
3) Safety consideration (transfer)
4) Sit to stand transfer
5) Stand to sit transfer
6) Preventing falls
7) Assisting a fallen patient
   - Identifying fall risk
   - Managing the fallen patient
   - To assess the fallen patient
   - Transferring a patient from another lying surface to lying surface

8) Transferring a patient from lying surface to another lying surface using equipment
9) Illustration: Wheelchair to bed
10) Illustration: Bed to wheelchair
11) Illustration: Wheelchair to chair
12) Illustration: Chair to wheelchair
13) Illustration: Wheelchair to floor
14) Illustration: Wheelchair to bed
15) Illustration: Floor to Bed
16) Illustration: Floor to wheelchair
17) Illustration: Floor to wheelchair (independent)
18) Illustration: Wheelchair to floor (independent)
19) Illustration: Sit to stand
20) Illustration: Stand to sit

PATIENT CARE INTERVENTION: TRANSFER

Transfer techniques are the procedure for moving a patient from one surface to another or moving the patient from one position to another. Care should be taken while performing these techniques as improper transfer techniques may result in injury to the person being transferred and/or the carer involved in transferring the patient. The carer should be aware of the type of assistance needed and the type of transfer that is to be performed. Determine the number of carers that will be required during the transfer (one or two) for an individual patient.

Levels of Assistance

1. **Stand-by assist**: Assistance is provided if needed by the patient.
2. **Minimal assist**: Patient performs maximum activity.
3. **Moderate assist**: Patient performs at least 50% of the activity.
4. **Maximal assist**: Patient performs minimum activity.

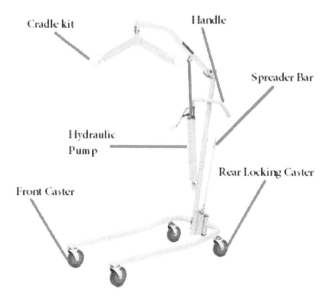

Figure 13.1 Hoyer Lift Unit

Labels: Cradle kit, Handle, Spreader Bar, Hydraulic Pump, Rear Locking Caster, Front Caster

Three types of transfer

1. **Dependent Transfer**: patient is unable to transfer on their own.
2. **Assisted Transfer**: patient needs assistance during transfer.
3. **Independent Transfer**: patient can transfer on their own without assistance.

Safety Consideration

I. Know your patient's ability and level of assistance that might be required during transfer.
II. Check to see if the equipment necessary are available for use, inspect your equipment.
III. Surfaces should be leveled as much as possible.
IV. Wheelchair should always be in locked position.
V. Try to put the chair against a secure wall or surface to avoid sliding away.
VI. Leg rest and arm rest should be removed as per requirement of your transfer.
VII. Patient must have appropriate clothing and shoes on (non-skid shoes).
VIII. Plan the transfer by preparing the patient and yourself:
    a. Instruct the patient and explain the procedure.
    b. Demonstrate the technique to be performed.
IX. Check to see if there are any obstructions in the environment.
X. Use of proper body mechanics:
    a. Feet apart with a wide base of support to get stability.
    b. Keep your back straight and knees bend while lifting the object.
    c. Position yourself (center of gravity) as close as possible to the patient.
    d. Keep your feet pointed in the direction of the transfer to avoid twisting injuries.
XI. Perform transfer in parts if applicable.

SIT TO STAND

Independent sit to stand

1. Ask the patient to put their hands on the armrests of the chair, or the firm surface of the furniture on which they are sitting.
2. Ask the patient to put their feet flat on the floor. The feet should be apart and tucked back under the chair.
3. Ask the patient to lean forward in the chair and shuffle their bottom to the edge of the seat.
4. Ask the patient to lean forward while still sitting, so their upper body is above and over the top of their feet.
5. If needed, gently rock the patient back and forth to build up momentum to help them stand.
6. The patient pushes themselves up to a standing position using the armrests or surface on which they were sitting. Note: Hand or Bed blocks may provide support for a patient who is standing up from a bed or other firm surface.

STAND TO SIT

Independent stand to sit

1. Check to see if the patient can feel the edge of the seat or bed on the backs of their legs or knees.
2. If the patient is seated on a bed before lying down, ensure they sit near the head of the bed, so they do not have to be repositioned after they lie down.
3. Ask the patient to reach behind and take hold of the armrests or feel for the firm surface of the furniture on which they are about to sit.
4. Ask the patient to lean forward and, at the same time, bend at the knees and hips to lower themselves onto the furniture.

Note: All movements should be slow and controlled by the patient.

PREVENTING FALL

If the patient slips forward in a chair, they may be at risk of falling to the floor.

Here are some risk factors to check for:

- Does the patient have sufficient balance or trunk control to sit unsupported?
- Is the patient wearing slippery clothes?
- Is the seat surface slippery or does the seat slope forwards?
- Has the patient been sitting for too long? If yes, they may be trying to move because they are uncomfortable.
- Is the chair suitable for the patient? It may not be a suitable depth, size or shape.
- Are the patient's feet unsupported? Feet should reach the floor or be supported by a footstool.
- If a hoist is used, is the patient positioned appropriately (back supported in the chair).

ASSISTING A FALLEN PATIENT

IDENTIFYING FALL RISK

Preventing falls are far more effective than trying to manage a fall in progress or managing the after-effects of a fall. The main goal is to prevent falls by identifying risk factors and then implementing controls to eliminate, isolate or minimize them from occurring.

MANAGING THE FALLEN PATIENT

Carers should never try to lift a fallen patient off the floor unless it is an emergency or life-threatening situation. Give the patient time to get calm and then either assist them to get up or help them with a hoist, or a powered device. If you find a fallen patient, you need to assess the situation carefully to ensure that the patient is not injured further while you are trying to assist them getting up.

TO ASSESS THE FALLEN PATIENT:

- Make sure the area around the patient is safe and that no further harm can occur, for instance, clear any spills or objects away.
- Call for help.
- Assess the patient's circulation, airway, and breathing. Maintain according to CPR guidelines and the patient's care plan.
- Continue the assessment as needed, using approved First Aid procedures.
- If the patient is injured, do not move them, make them comfortable on the floor and seek further medical advice.
- Have the patient stay calm and relaxed.

- Choose the right technique to help them up. Explain the procedure and communicate with them throughout the procedure to provide feedback and assurance.

TRANSFERRING A PATIENT FROM LYING SURFACE TO ANOTHER LYING SURFACE

If you are transferring a patient from a bed to a trolley, for example, you need to use a large transfer board to bridge the two surfaces. Some transfer boards can be used with a slide sheet. It is best if the slide sheet has long handles.

Extra measures may be required for patients who:

- are attached to medical equipment, such as drains
- have poor skin integrity or pressure sores
- are obese
- have suspected or confirmed fractures
- have fragile bones

TRANSFERRING A PATIENT FROM LYING SURFACE TO ANOTHER LYING SURFACE USING EQUIPMENT

You can use a large transfer board with full-length slide sheet, or a roller board, for this technique. You will need at least three carers – two to pull the slide sheet and one to push the patient from the other side. Other carers may be required to control the patient's head or feet, or to manage attached medical equipment.

1. Roll the patient into sidelying position.
2. Position the transfer board and slide sheet under the patient. Follow the manufacturer's instructions.
3. Position the second lying surface (bed) next to the bed on which the patient is lying. It should be of the same height or slightly lower than the surface on which the patient is lying.
4. Make sure both beds/trolleys have their brakes on.
5. Create a bridge between the two surfaces with the transfer board.
6. Caregivers take up their positions with feet shoulder distance apart and one foot forward:
   a. Two caregivers are required to perform this task.
7. The lead carer gives the "Ready, steady, slide" command.
8. On the "slide" command carers smoothly move the patient in the direction of the transfer.
9. Remove the slide sheet and transfer board.

MOST COMMON TYPE OF TRANSFERS PERFORMED

I. Wheelchair to bed
II. Bed to wheelchair
III. Wheelchair to chair
IV. Chair to wheelchair
V. Wheelchair to floor
VI. Wheelchair to bed
VII. Floor to wheelchair
VIII. Floor to wheelchair (independent)
IX. Wheelchair to floor (independent)
X. Sit to stand
XI. Stand to sit

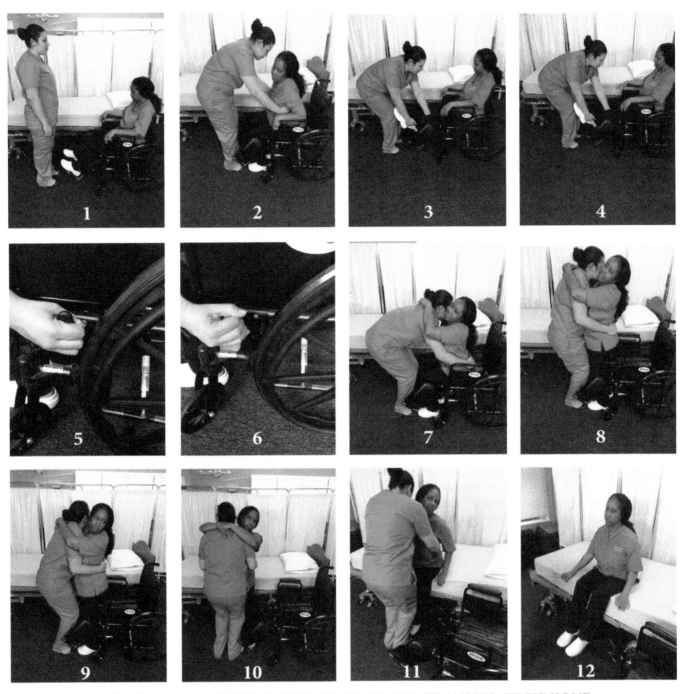

ONE PERSON: ASSISTED WHEELCHAIR TO BED TRANSFER TECHNIQUE

Figure 13.2

Note: locking the wheelchair using its brake's is recommended at the start of a transfer technique involving a wheelchair.

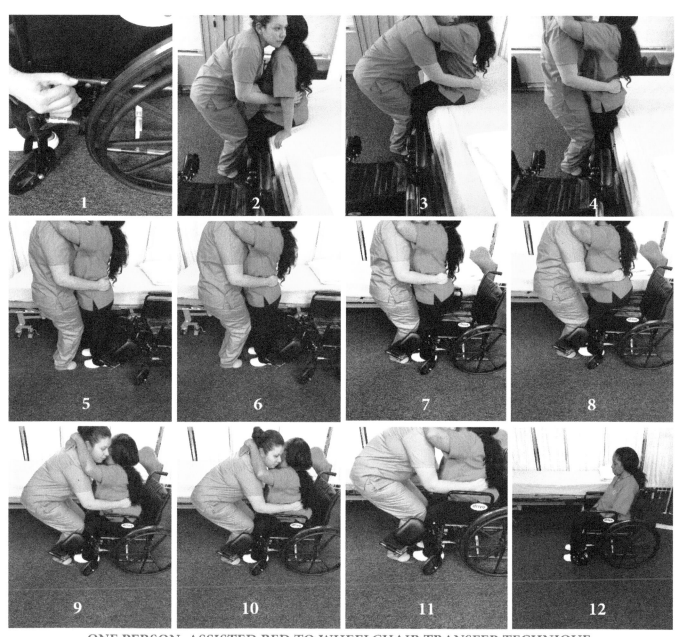

ONE PERSON: ASSISTED BED TO WHEELCHAIR TRANSFER TECHNIQUE

Figure 13.3

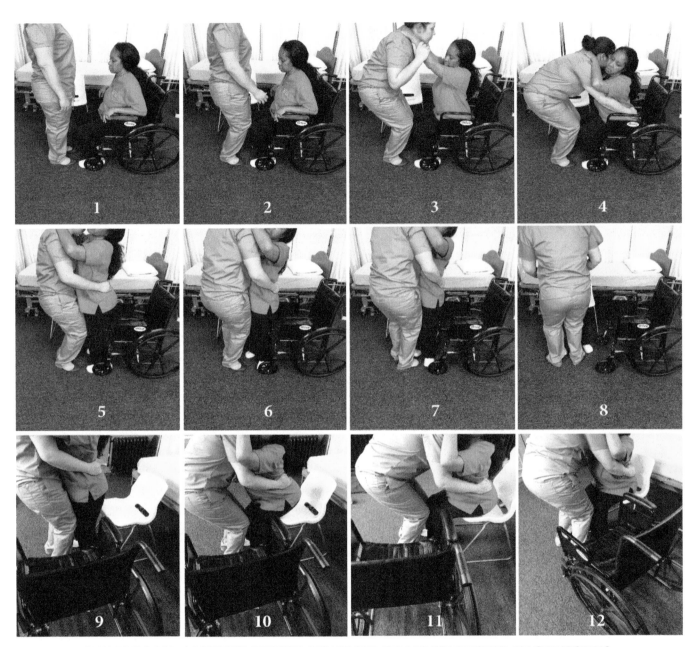

ONE PERSON: ASSISTED WHEELCHAIR TO CHAIR TRANSFER TECHNIQUES

Figure 13.4

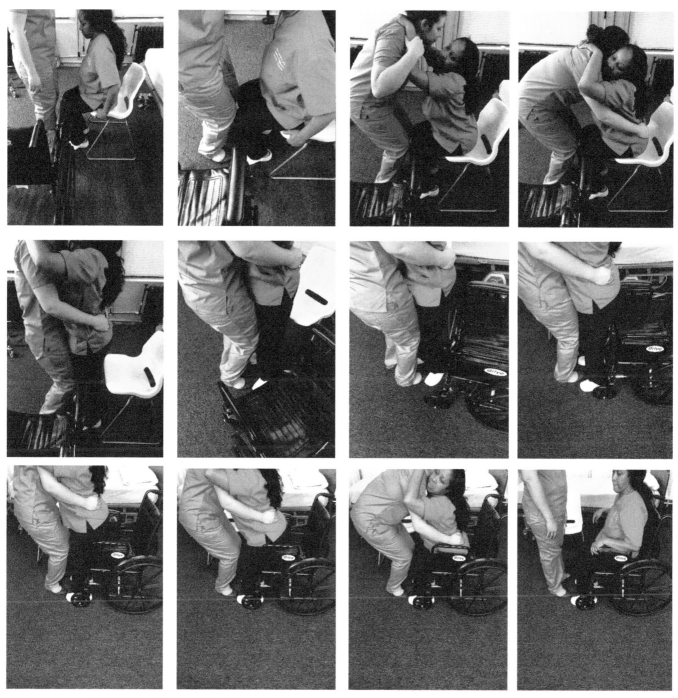

ONE PERSON: ASSISTED CHAIR TO WHEELCHAIR TRANSFER TECHNIQUE

Figure 13.5

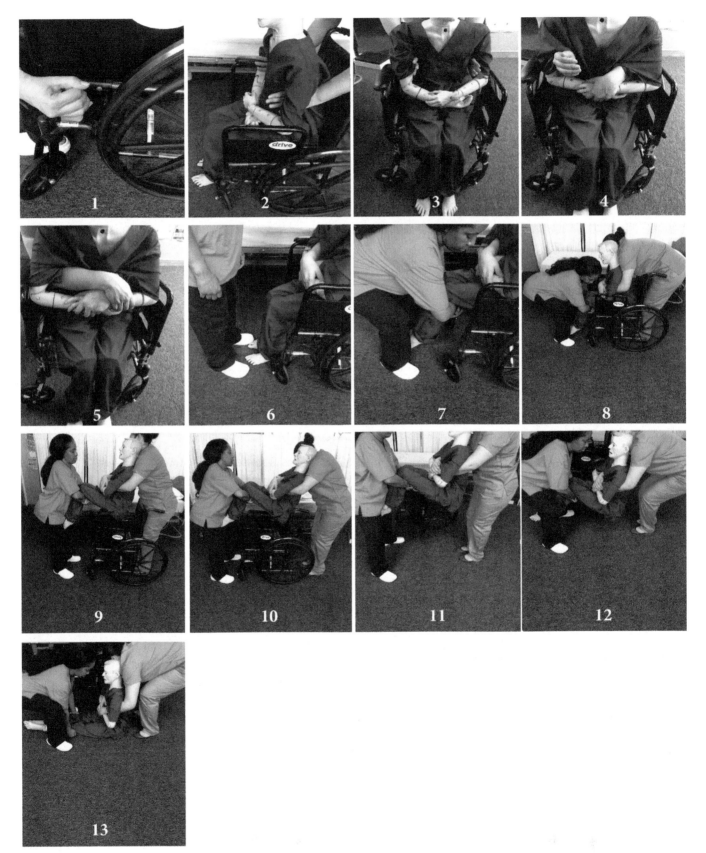

Figure 13.6 TWO PERSON: WHEELCHAIR TO FLOOR TRANSFER TECHNIQUE

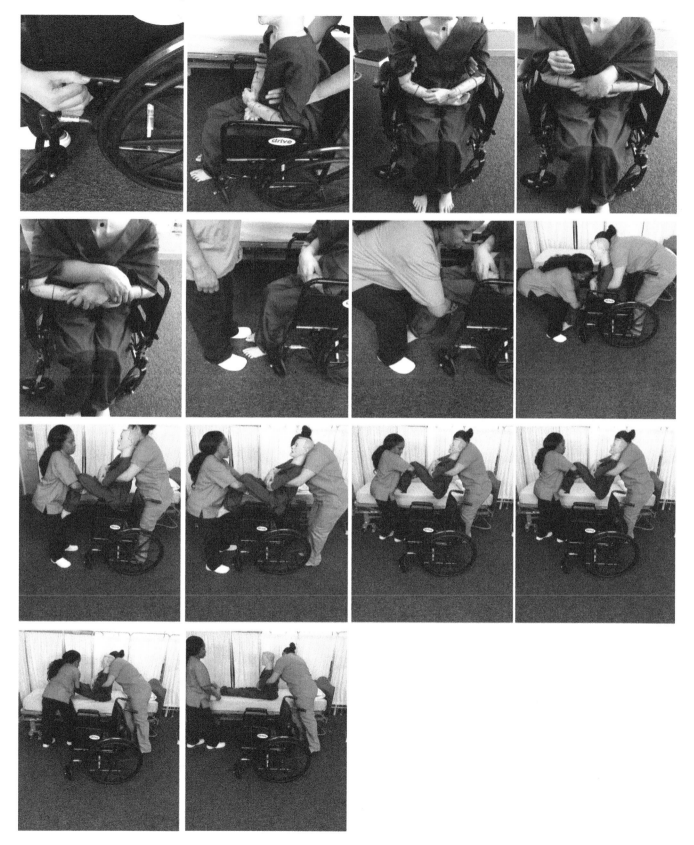

Figure 13.7   TWO PERSON: WHEELCHAIR TO BED TRANSFER TECHNIQUE

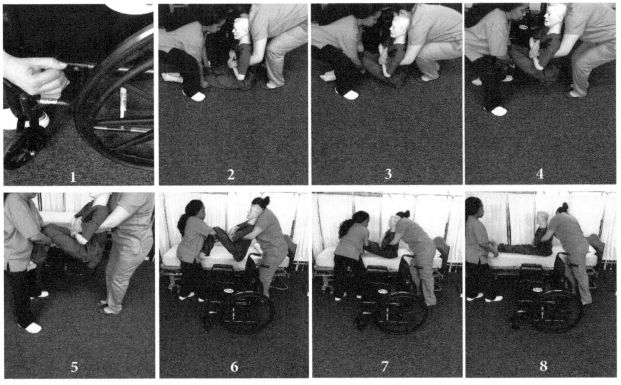

Figure 13.8a TWO PERSON: FLOOR TO BED TRANSFER

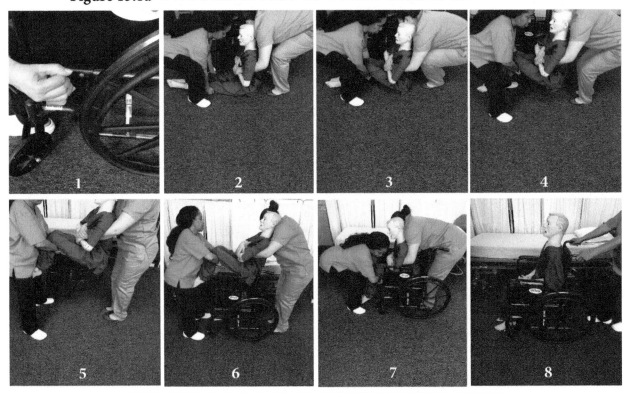

TWO PERSON: FLOOR TO WHEELCHAIR TRANSFER

Figure 13.8b

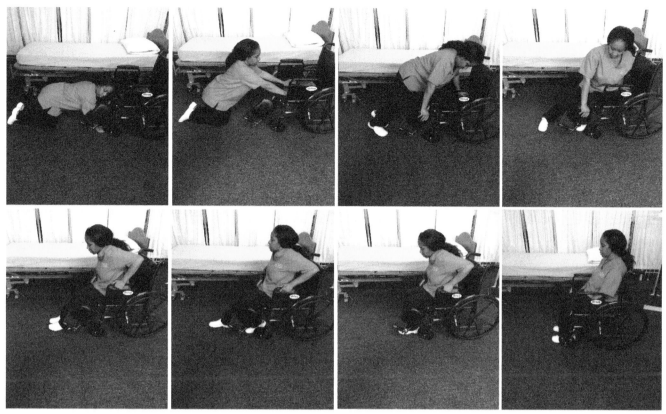

Figure 13.9a INDEPENDENT: FLOOR TO WHEELCHAIR TRANSFER

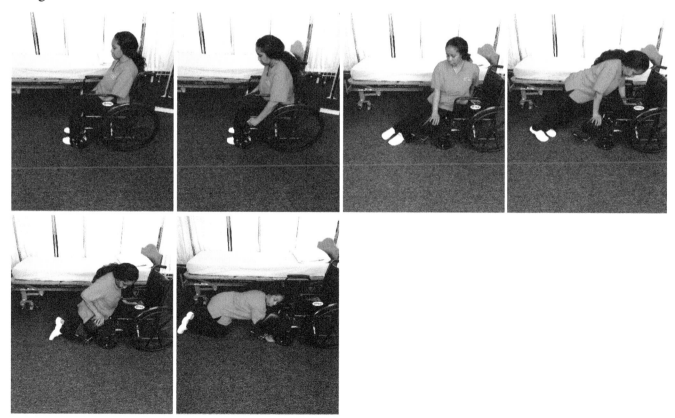

Figure 13.9b INDEPENDENT: WHEELCHAIR TO FLOOR TRANSFER

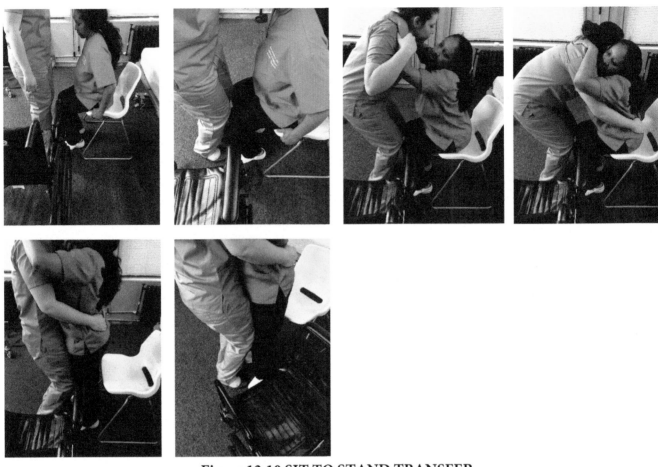

Figure 13.10 SIT TO STAND TRANSFER

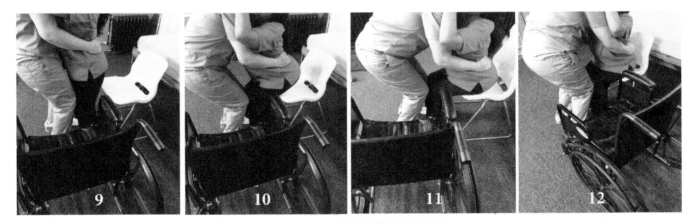

Figure 13.11 STAND TO SIT

CHAPTER 13
END OF CHAPTER REVIEW QUESTIONS
Question Set 1: Essay Questions
50 points 5 point each

1. Describe 3 main types of transfers.

2. Describe safety considerations for transfer techniques.

3. List the levels of assistance during transfer technique.

4. Enlist the steps involved for independent sit to stand transfer technique.

5. Enlist the steps involved for sit to stand transfer with one or two carers.

6. How can a patient fall be prevented?

7. Describe about assisting a fallen patient.

8. List most common types of transfers performed in a healthcare setting.

9. Describe the techniques of transferring a patient from lying surface to another lying surface using the equipment.

10. Summarize floor to bed and floor to wheelchair transfer.

SECTION 4

CHAPTER 14: WOUND CARE AND PRESSURE SORES

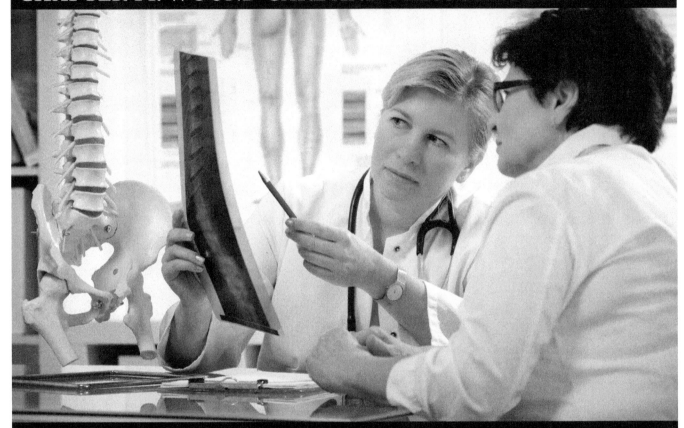

LEARNING OBJECTIVES

At the end of this chapter the student will be able to describe the following:

1) Factors causing pressure sore
2) Wound description
3) Phases of wound healing
4) Introduction to pressure ulcer
5) Pressure ulcer stages/categories
6) Brief wound examination and assessment
7) Types of wound debridement
   a. Autolytic debridement
   b. Enzymatic debridement
   c. Mechanical debridement
   d. Surgical debridement
8) Dressings
   a. Gauze

   b. Film dressing
   c. Hydrogel
   d. Foam
   e. Alginates
   f. Composite
   g. Hydrocolloid
9) Skincare & preventing bed sores
10) Venous & arterial ulcer comparison

PATIENT CARE INTERVENTION: WOUND CARE AND PRESSURE SORES

EXTERNAL AND INTERNAL FACTORS: CAUSING PRESSURE SORES

A. External Factors

- **P**ressure: decreases the blood flow to the area of the skin causing hypoxia. The pressure points are the areas which are compressed between the outer surface and the bone.
- **F**riction: occurs if the skin is rubbed against the non-moving surface of the bed when moving the patient in an opposite direction.
- **S**hear: this is caused by pulling effect on the skin in a direction.
- **T**hermal damage: occurs if the temperature is too low or too high to tolerate.
- **I**atrogenic: healthcare related.
- **D**rugs: some drugs like anti-inflammatory (cortico-steroids).
- **M**alnutrition: poor nutrition status.

Remember: P, MD, FITS

B. Internal Factors

- **S**ystemic: coexisting disease.
- **A**ging: decrease in skins ability to produce elastin and collagen making it thinner and less elastic.
- **O**besity: decrease in blood supply to resist bacterial infection and deliver nutrients.
- **I**nfection: causes increase in duration of the inflammatory phase, thereby delaying collagen synthesis, preventing epithelialization and may result in further tissue destruction.

Remember: SOAI

C. Internal/External Factors

- **Body Fluids**: Fluids like urine, feces, and perspiration can cause tissue damage.
- **Allergic Reactions**: This occurs due to the development of contact dermatitis that triggers an allergic response.

WOUND DESCRIPTION

A wound can be:

- **Acute** – A wound that shows a progress of healing in a timely manner.
- **Chronic** – A wound that does not show progress of healing in a timely manner. The anatomical structure may not be restored back to its normal shape.
- **Superficial** – Shallow and partial thickness wound that extends through the epidermis but not through the dermis. Examples: abrasions, blisters, and stage 2 ulcers.
- **Deep** – Deep and full thickness wound that extends through the dermis and subcutaneous tissue, sometimes may extend to underlying fascia. Examples: stage 3 and 4 pressure ulcers as well as deep lacerations.

PHASES OF WOUND HEALING:

Inflammatory Phase

Hemostasis:-

- Usually takes 0 to 2 days in length.
- The thrombin converts into fibrinogen.
- Coagulation takes place due to dilation of blood vessels.

Inflammation:-

- Usually takes 2 to 4 days in length.
- This stage is characterized by pain, redness, heat, swelling and loss of function at the site of injury.

Proliferative Phase

Usually takes 4 to 21 days in length.

Granulation:-

- In this stage there is filling of the wound with new tissues. Hence this phase is also called the "rebuilding phase". This is caused by granulation, which is a tissue that grows from the base of the wound.

Angiogenesis:-

- New blood vessels are formed called as angiogenesis.

Contraction:-

- Wound contraction takes place to close the wound by bringing the wound edges closer. The mechanism of the contraction is that it causes shrinking of the wound that leads to the generation of forces in the contractile elements of the fibroblast towards the center of the wound, this results in wound contraction.

Epithelialization

- Epithelial cells migrate across the new tissue to form a barrier between the wound and the environment.

Maturation Phase

- Can take up to 2 years in length.
- In this phase of wound healing the wound gains tensile strength and appears to be healed.

INTRODUCTION TO PRESSURE ULCER

A pressure ulcer is an injury that results in the breakdown of the skin and underlying tissue of a specific area. The breakdown of the skin occurs when a section of the skin is placed under pressure or shear force.

PRESSURE ULCER STAGES/CATEGORIES

CATEGORY/STAGE I:
NON-BLANCHABLE ERYTHEMA

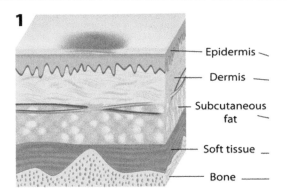

Figure 14.1

- Intact skin with non-blanchable erythema (redness).
- Skin temperature may be warm or cold.
- Tissue may be firm or non-firm.
- Found on localized area, mostly on the body prominence.
- Sensation of the area may be painful and/or itchy.

CATEGORY/STAGE II:
PARTIAL THICKNESS SKIN LOSS

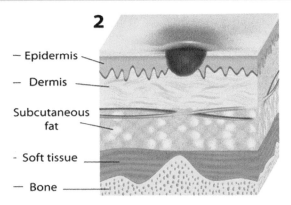

Figure 14.2

- Loss of partial thickness skin tissue.
- Involves epidermis or dermis, or may involve both.
- Ulcer found in this stage is superficial.
- Ulcer found are open and shallow.
- Abrasions and blisters may be present.

CATEGORY/STAGE III:
FULL THICKNESS SKIN LOSS

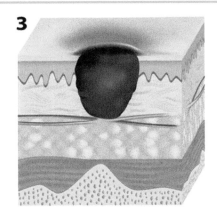

Figure 14.3

- In this stage, there is a full thickness tissue loss.
- Subcutaneous tissue may be damaged or may have undergone necrosis.
- Present as a deep crater.
- Subcutaneous tissue may be visible.

CATEGORY/STAGE IV:
FULL THICKNESS TISSUE LOSS

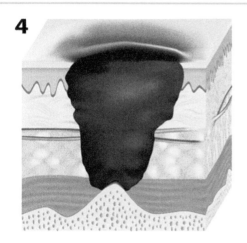

Figure 14.4

- Loss of full thickness tissue.
- Bones, muscles, and other tissues may be exposed.
- Necrotic damage of the tissue.
- Undermining and tunneling (sinus tract) may be present.

BRIEF WOUND EXAMINATION & ASSESSMENT
Wound Location

Check anatomical locations as per the anatomical landmarks. For example heel, ankle, sacrum and coccyx.

Etiology of Pressure Sores

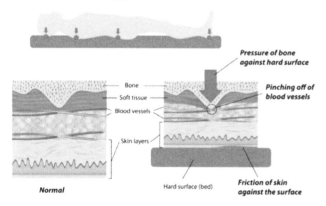

Figure 14.5

Wound Size (Length x Width x Depth)

- Check for wound length (head to toe [edge to edge]). see figure 14.6

- Check for wound width (side to side [edge to edge]). see figure 14.6
- Check for wound depth (from the base of the wound to the surface). see figure 14.7
- Check for wound girth (circumferential or volumetric). see figure 14.7

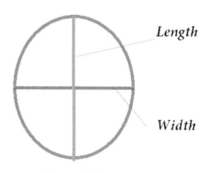

Figure 14.6

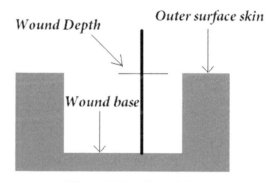

Figure 14.7

Undermining and tracts

Presence or absence of tunneling or sinus tract.

Wound Exudate (Drainage)

Serous: clear, amber, thin and watery.

Fibrinous: cloudy and thin, with strands of fibrin.

Serosanguineous: clear, pink, thin and watery.

Sanguineous: reddish, thin and watery.

Seropurulent: yellow or tan, cloudy and thick.

Purulent: opaque, milky; sometimes green.

Hemopurulent: reddish, milky and viscous.

Hemorrhagic: red and thick.

Exudate (drainage) may be light, moderate or heavy

Color and Involved Tissue

Red: healthy granulation tissue.

Yellow: necrotic tissue.

Black/brown: eschar necrotic tissue (dried).

Surface Temperature

Check surface temperature using appropriate equipment.

Other components of wound examination are

- condition of peri-wound tissue
- sensory integrity
- presence or absence of infection in the wound
- wound odor

WOUND CARE

1. Infection Control
2. Wound Debridement
3. Wound Dressing (Types)
4. Skin Care

INFECTION CONTROL

Wound cultures provide information about the presence or absence of infection in the wound. Based on the wound culture results a treatment is prescribed.

Some important points to remember are:-

- *Hand washing must always be practiced.*
- *Techniques performed must be sterile.*

WOUND DEBRIDEMENT

A technique that aims at removal of unhealthy tissue from a wound for promoting the process of healing. This can be done in various ways which include **autolytic** (using your body's processes) debridement, **chemical** debridement, **mechanical** debridement or **surgical** debridement to remove the unhealthy tissue.

Remember: CAMS

TYPES OF WOUND DEBRIDEMENT

Debridement Techniques

Autolytic Debridement:

Description:

- Autolysis is a process in which the bodies own enzymes and moisture is used to re-hydrate, soften and liquefy hard eschar and slough.
- It is a selective technique in which only the necrotic tissue is liquefied.
- It causes little to no pain.
- It causes no damage to the surrounding tissues.
- It can be achieved by using occlusive or semi-occlusive dressings, which can maintain wound fluid in contact with the necrotic tissue.
- It can be achieved with other dressings like hydrocolloids, hydrogels and transparent films.

Enzymatic Debridement:

Description:

Enzymes are used to perform debridement of the wound tissue. These enzymes will cause the necrotic tissue to slough. This technique is ideal to use on large necrotic debris. It is fast acting and with minimal to no damage of the healthy tissue if performed appropriately. It is considered a selective technique. Can be used for individuals who cannot tolerate surgical debridement technique. Should not be performed on dry gangrene and clean granulated tissue.

Mechanical Debridement:

Description:

- This technique uses mechanical means of removing the necrotic debris.
- Used for moist necrotic tissues.
- For example allowing the dressing to proceed from wet to dry, then manually removing the dressing.
- While removing the dressing, the healthy tissue may also get traumatized.
- It may be painful to the patients and hence considered a non-selective debridement technique.

- Another example of this technique would be the use of hydrotherapy, dextranomer or pulsatile lavage with suction.

Surgical Debridement:

Description:

- In this technique surgical instruments are used for removing the necrotic tissue, this can be performed under anesthesia.
- This is considered a very selective technique because the person performing the surgical procedure will only remove the necrotic tissue and not the healthy tissue.

WOUND DRESSINGS

GAUZE DRESSING

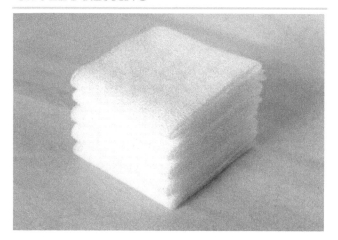

Figure 14.8

- Gauze wound dressings are made of:-
  - cotton (woven or nonwoven) or
  - other synthetic material.
- Permeable to water and oxygen.
- Non-occlusive in nature.
- Absorbs water.
- Can be used in different ways (wet, moist, dry or with another topical agent like antiseptics).
- Readily available in different sizes and shapes.
- Inexpensive type of dressing.
- Provides mechanical debridement.

USES

- Can be used as a primary or secondary wound dressing.
- Can be used on infected wounds.

- Can be used to keep the wound moist.
- Can be used for large wound exudates (drainage).
- Can be used for wound that consists of sinus tract or tunneling.

Points to remember

- Must be changed appropriately.
- If the gauze dressing is used as a primary dressing, a secondary dressing may be required to secure the gauze dressing in place.
- May cause pain while removing it.
- Gauze dressing application must be done by following the proper application procedure.

FILM DRESSING

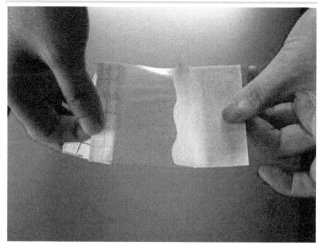

Figure 14.9

- Film dressings are thin, adhesive and flexible in nature.
- It is permeable to oxygen and impermeable to water and other elements like (bacteria), this minimizes the risk of wound getting infected.
- It is transparent, which means the wound can be seen through the dressing, without removing it.
- It does not absorb water.
- Fits the surface due to its flexibility.
- Provides autolytic debridement.

USES

- Can be used as a primary or secondary wound dressing.
- Can be used for stage 1 and stage 2 pressure ulcers.

- Can be used when a barrier is required to separate the internal and external environment for preventing wound infection.

Points to remember

- Should not be used with heavy wound exudate (drainage).
- Wrinkling of the dressing may occur.
- Avoid the use of this dressing with infected wounds.

HYDROGEL DRESSING

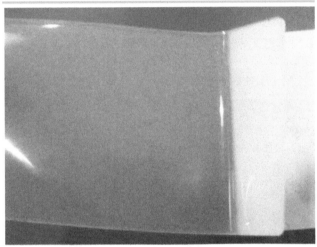

Figure 14.10

- Hydrogel wound dressings are water or glycerin-based wound dressings that are available in different forms like sheets, amorphous gels, or impregnated gauzes.
- Hydrogels are insoluble in water.
- It can provide minimum absorption.
- Fits the surface due to its flexibility.
- Adherent or non-adherent (majority) types available.
- Provides autolytic debridement.

USES

- Can be used to fill dead space in the wound.
- Can be used for partial to full thickness wounds.
- Can be used for necrotic tissue with slough.
- Can be used to rehydrate wound bed.
- Can be used with infected wounds (amorphous form).

Points to remember

- Should not be used on wounds with heavy exudates.
- May require a use of secondary dressing.

- Hydrogels have low temperature (cool in nature), this may help in reducing wound pain.

FOAM DRESSING

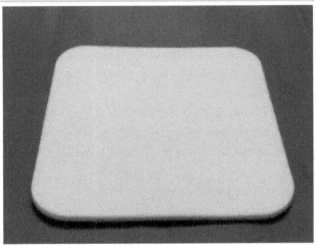

Figure 14.11

- Foam wound dressings are available in different shapes and forms.
- They are hydrophilic (tendency to mix with water).
- The absorption depends on the type of foam dressing used.
- It can provide minimum to moderate absorption.
- Adherent or non-adherent (majority) types available.

USES

- Can be used for partial to full thickness wounds.
- Can be used as a secondary wound dressing.
- Can be used for wound protection and insulation.
- Can be used for deep wounds.

Points to remember

- Frequent change of dressing may be required.

ALGINATE DRESSING

- Alginate wound dressings are made from soft, absorbent seaweed.
- Alginate when placed in wound bed forms a gel, this provides a moist environment for wound healing.
- Available in different forms for appropriate use.
- This dressing may require secondary dressing.
- Permeable and non-occlusive in nature.

USES

- Can be used for moderate to maximum exudate.
- Can be used for wounds with exudate and necrosis.
- Can be used with non-infected and infected wound with exudate.
- Can be used to fill dead space.

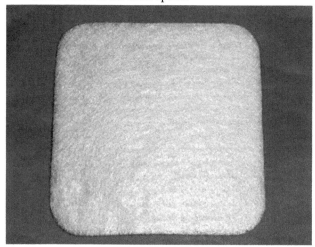

Figure 14.12

Points to remember

- Do not use on dry wounds.

COMPOSITE DRESSING

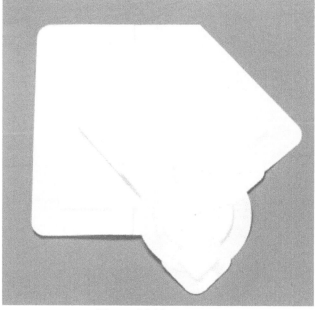

Figure 14.13

3 layer dressing

- **Outer layer**: bacterial barrier; film dressing.

- **Middle layer**: absorbs moisture; foam, hydrocolloid and hydrogel.
- **Inner layer**: trauma protection to wound bed: non-adherent dressing.

  Because composite dressings are prepackaged, they have less flexibility in terms of indications for use, and buying and storing these dressings can be quite costly.

HYDROCOLLOID DRESSING

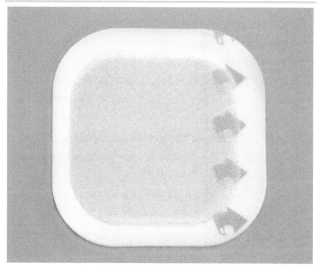

Figure 14.14

- Hydrocolloid wound dressings contain a hydrophilic component which when comes in contact with the wound fluid converts into a gelatinous mass; this provides a moist environment for wound healing.
- This type of dressing may be occlusive or semi-occlusive.
- Provides autolytic debridement.
- Lower infection rate.
- Available in different shapes and sizes.

USES

- Can be used to protect partial thickness wound.
- Can be used for mild to moderate absorption.
- Impermeable to external contaminants like oxygen or water.

Points to remember

- A yellow color drainage residue with or without odor may be seen on dressing removal; this is due to the gelatinous mass formation as a result of the reaction between the hydrocolloid dressing and the wound fluids.

Skin Care & Preventing Bed Sores

- Skin inspection must be done daily to check for pressure loading areas over the anatomical bony prominences.
- If an area appears to be red due to pressure loading, ensure that the patient is not turned to the side of the reddened area. Have the patient in a position that would keep the pressure off the reddened area.
- Avoid applying pressure or shear force that can damage the skin.
- Keep the skin hydrated to prevent skin damage, as dry skin is prone to get damaged, which may lead to the development of ulcers.
- The skin should not be excessively moistened.
- Avoid having the patient in one position for a long time.
- Have patient practice pressure relieve by weight shifting and lifts.
- If patient unable to move, use of support surface is recommended along with passive positioning techniques.
- Use of transfer aids is recommended to avoid pressure and friction force on skin.
- Always lift the patient, never drag the patient against any surface while changing positions.
- Always ensure that the patient is not lying on a body prominence with erythema.
- While sitting on the bed, the patient might tend to slide forward in the bed placing pressure on sacrum and coccyx.
- While sitting in a chair or wheelchair. If the patient's feet are not able to touch the floor, place a tool (foot). Since the inability of the patients foot to reach the floor will lead to sliding of the patient in a forward direction placing pressure on the bony prominences.
- Wheelchair push-ups should be performed every 15 minutes or as recommended.
- When in bed, the position should be changed every 2 hours or as recommended according to the patient's condition and/or health status.

- Repositioning techniques should be discussed with all the members involved in taking care of the patient at risk of developing pressure ulcers.

VENOUS & ARTERIAL ULCER COMPARISON

ULCER	ARTERIAL	VENOUS
Pain	Leg Elevated	Comfortable with leg elevated
Location	Anterior Tibia Lateral Malleolus Lower leg (toes & feet)	Medial Malleolus Lower leg
Appearance	Deep & Irregular	Shallow & Irregular
Drainage	No to Minimal	Moderate to large
Gangrene	Present (Maybe)	Absent
Pedal Pulse	Absent or Decrease	Present
Temperature	------------------	Part Cool to Touch

Table 14.1
Venous & Arterial Ulcer Comparison

CHAPTER 14
END OF CHAPTER REVIEW QUESTIONS

Question Set 1: Essay Questions
35 points: 5 points each

1. Describe external factors that cause pressure sores.

2. Describe internal factors that cause pressure sores.

3. Explain the phases of wound healing.

4. List and explain types of wound debridement techniques.

5. Describe the pressure ulcer stages/categories.

6. Explain in brief about how a pressure sore can be prevented.

7. Describe in brief different types of wound dressings.

Question Set 2: Match the Following
8 points: 2 points each
Note: Wound Description

Answer	Column 1	Column 2
	Deep	a. A wound that has a predictable course for healing (it precedes through the three phases in a timely manner).
	Chronic	b. A wound that does not progress in a timely manner; it may not restore the anatomical structure.
	Superficial	c. A shallow, partial thickness wound that extends through the epidermis but not through the dermis; will heal by the process of regeneration; superficial wounds include abrasions, blisters, and stage 2 ulcers.
	Acute	d. A full thickness wound that extends through the dermis and subcutaneous tissue; May extend to underlying fascia; Heal by tissue repair; Include stage 3 and 4 pressure ulcers as well as deep lacerations.

SECTION 4

CHAPTER 15: WHEELCHAIR MEASUREMENT

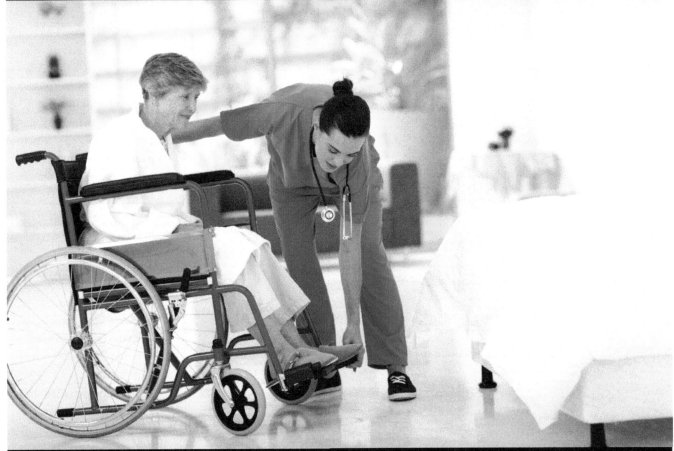

LEARNING OBJECTIVES

At the end of this chapter the student will be able to describe the following:

1) Wheelchair management goals
2) Types of wheelchair
3) Wheelchair measurement for customized fit (illustrations of measurement)
4) Wheelchair component measurements for customized fit:
    (1) Leg length
    (2) Seat depth
    (3) Seat width
    (4) Seat height
    (5) Armrest height
5) Wheelchair parts
6) Wheelchair: going up a curb
7) Wheelchair: going down a curb
8) Wheelchair: performing wheelie
9) Muscles to be trained for wheelchair maneuver

PATIENT CARE INTERVENTION: WHEELCHAIR MANAGEMENT

Wheelchair can be considered as an orthosis which can be used by the patient for personal transport and provides appropriate support to allow maximum function.

Wheelchair management goals

1. To maintain independence and safety of the patient.
2. To maintain and improve the posture of the patient.
3. To prevent the development of pressure sores.
4. To maximize and optimize comfort and function.

Types of Wheelchair

1. Standard wheelchair
2. Standard lightweight wheelchair
3. Ultra-lightweight transport wheelchair
4. Shower (Bathroom) wheelchair
5. Reclining back rigid frame sports chair
6. Power wheelchair
7. Transport wheelchair
8. Tilt in wheelchair
9. Pediatric wheelchair
10. Bariatric wheelchair

WHEELCHAIR FOR CUSTOMIZED FIT: ILLUSTRATIONS

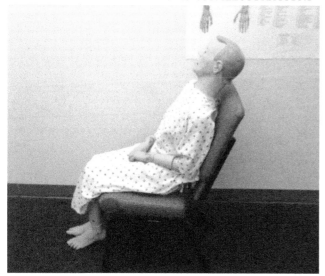

Figure 15.1 Patient in a chair

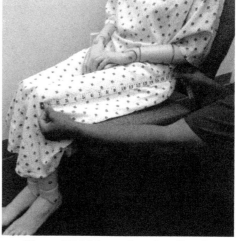

Figure 15.2 Measuring: Seat Depth

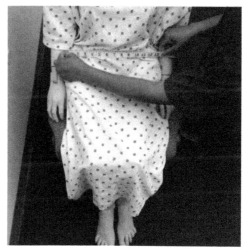

Figure 15.3 Measuring: Seat Width

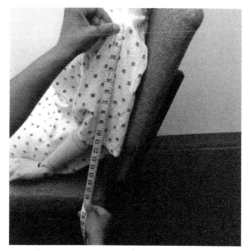

Figure 15.4 Measuring: Seat Height

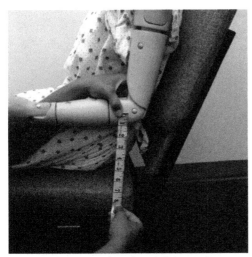

Figure 15.5 Measuring: Arm Rest

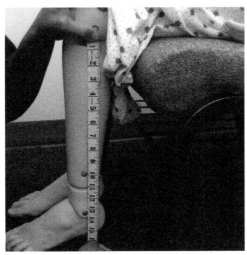

Figure 15.6 Measuring: Leg Length

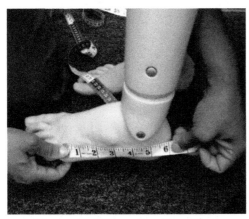

Figure 15.7 Measuring: Foot Plate

WHEELCHAIR MEASUREMENT FOR CUSTOMIZED FIT

COMPONENT	MEASUREMENTS
Seat height/leg length Figure 15.6	Measure from the patient's heel to the popliteal fold, add 2 inches to this measurement.
Seat depth Figure 15.2	Measure from the patient's posterior buttock area, along the lateral thigh, to the popliteal fold, then subtract approximately 2 inches to this measurement.
Seat width Figure 15.3	Measure the widest aspect of the user's buttocks, hips or thighs and add approximately 2 inches to this measurement.
Back height Figure 15.4	Measure from the seat of the chair to the axilla, subtract 4 inches to this measurement. If the cushion is to be used, add the thickness of the cushion to this measurement.
Armrest height Figure 15.5	Measure from the seat of the chair to the olecranon process with the patient's elbow flexed at 90 degrees, add approximately 1 inch to this measurement.

Table 15.1

Problems encountered due to improper measurements:

TOO NARROW SEAT:

- Becomes uncomfortable for the patient to sit.
- Difficult for patient to fit into the seat.
- The patient may develop pressure sores.

TOO WIDE SEAT:

- The patient may lean to one side.
- May promote scoliosis.
- May cause difficulty in propulsion.

TOO SHALLOW SEAT:

- Less area of contact.
- More pressure over soft tissues.
- Less support to feet & legs.
- Poor balance.

TOO DEEP SEAT:

- Restricted leg circulation.

- Extended leg / forward slide in the chair.
- Difficult propulsion.

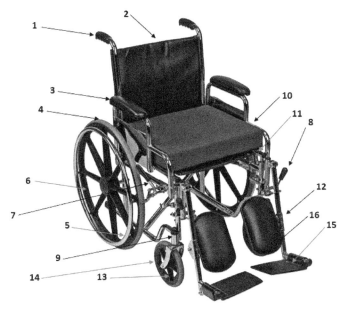

Figure 15.8

1. Push handle bracket tubes
2. Back rest
3. Arm rests
4. Pneumatic tires
5. Push rim
6. Wheel rim
7. Locks
8. Swing away release lever
9. Caster housing cover
10. Seat cushion
11. Seat sling
12. Swing away foot rest
13. Caster wheel
14. Caster tire
15. Foot rest
16. Leg rest

WHEELCHAIR: GOING UP A CURB

Front caster wheels are to be placed on the curb first, followed by propelling the large wheel forward till the complete wheelchair reaches the curb.

Note: wheelchair should face the curb while getting up on the curb.

WHEELCHAIR: GOING DOWN A CURB

Option 1. Large wheels should be placed on the edge of the curb, followed by moving the trunk and neck forward and stepping down the large wheels off the curb first, balance the wheelchair and finally bring the front caster wheels off the curb.

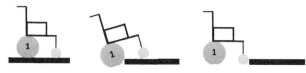

Fig. Option 1

Option 2. The patient can descend forward with caster wheels descending first, followed by the large wheels.

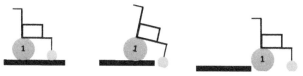

Fig. Option 2

Going up and down the curb needs practice and should be explained and demonstrated to the patient several times before it can actually be perform.

WHEELCHAIR: PERFORMING WHEELIE

1. Ask the patient to place hands posteriorly on the drive wheels.
2. Next instruct the patient to pull the drive wheels anteriorly with an abrupt force, while doing so the patients head and trunk should be flexed forwards to prevent the wheelchair from falling backward. This causes the wheelchair to go into a wheelie position (wheelchair on drive wheels only).

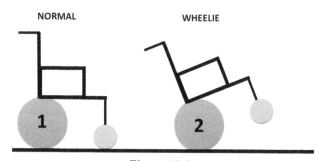

Figure 15.9

MUSCLES TO BE TRAINED FOR WHEELCHAIR MANEUVER

1. Elbow Flexors and Extensors
2. Shoulder Flexors and Extensors
3. Wrist Flexors
4. Phalangeal Flexors (Hand Grip Muscles)
5. Pectoralis Major (Chest)
6. Trunk Flexors

WHEELCHAIR MANEUVERS INCLUDE

1. Forward Pushing
2. Backward Pulling
3. Turning and Pivoting
4. Stopping
5. Tilting (Wheelie)

Note: Patients should be instructed to perform wheelchair pushups to prevent pressure sores.

CHAPTER 15
END OF CHAPTER REVIEW QUESTIONS

Question Set 1: Match the Following
10 points: 2 points each

Answer	Column 1		Column 2
	Seat height	a.	Measure from the patient's heel to the popliteal fold, add 2 inches to this measurement.
	Armrest height	b.	Measure from the patient's posterior buttock, along the lateral thigh, to the popliteal fold, then subtract approximately 2 inches to this measurement.
	Leg length	c.	Measure the widest aspect of the patient's buttocks, hips or thighs and add approximately 2 inches to this measurement.
	Seat depth	d.	Measure from the seat of the chair to the axilla, subtract 4 inches to this measurement.
	Seat width	e.	Measure from the seat of the chair to the olecranon process with the patient's elbow flexed at 90 degrees, add approximately 1 inch to this measurement.

Question Set 2: Essay Questions
30 points: 5 points each

1. List the parts of a wheelchair.
2. Explain the steps involved in performing a wheelie.
3. Explain in brief the procedure of going down a curb using a wheelchair.
4. Explain in brief the procedure of going up a curb using a wheelchair.
5. List the muscles of wheelchair maneuver.
6. What are the goals of wheelchair management?

SECTION 4
CHAPTER 16: PATIENT CARE SKILLS COMPETENCY SKILLS

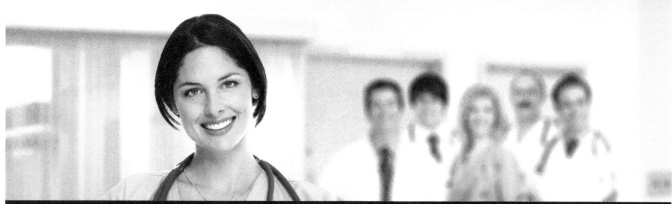

LEARNING OBJECTIVES
At the end of this chapter the student will be able to describe the following:

Competency Skills 1: Indirect Care (General Overview)
Competency Skills 2: Hand Washing
Competency Skills 3: For Giving a Bed Bath & Back Rubs
Competency Skills 4: Make an Occupied Bed
Competency Skills 5: Assist with Range of Motion Exercises
Competency Skills 6: Undressing and Dressing Patients
Competency Skills 7: Take/Record Height
Competency Skills 8: Take/Record Weight
Competency Skills 9: Assisting with Applying And Removing Prosthesis Devices
Competency Skills 10: Assisting with Applying Ace (Elastic) Bandages
Competency Skills 11: Assisting with Applying TED'S (Elastic Stockings)
Competency Skills 12: Assisting with Applying Binders
Competency Skills 13: Urine Output Measurement
Competency Skills 14: Collect / Test Urine Specimen
Competency Skills 15: Collecting a Stool Specimen
Competency Skills 16: Perineal Care (Female)
Competency Skills 17: Perineal Care (Male)
Competency Skills 18: Catheter Care (Female And Male)
Competency Skills 19: Gait Belt and Transfer Belt Use: Ambulation
Competency Skills 20: Lifting a Patient Using a Mechanical Lift (Hoyers)

Competency Skills 21: Positioning on Side (Turning Patient Towards You)
Competency Skills 22: Change Non-Sterile (Clean) Dressing
Competency Skills 23: Assisting Patients in using Bed Pan
Competency Skills 24: Feeding Patients
Competency Skills 25: Foot Care
Competency Skills 26: Denture Care
Competency Skills 27: Mouth Care
Competency Skills 28: Hand and Nail Care
Competency Skills 29: Hot Compresses Application
Competency Skills 30: Applying Cold Compresses
Competency Skills 31: Care of a Non-Infected Decubitus Ulcer
Competency Skills 32: Demonstrating a Skill to a Patient
Competency Skills 33: Teaching a Task or Skill

PATIENT CARE INTERVENTION: COMPETENCY CHECKLIST

COMPETENCY SKILLS 1: INDIRECT CARE (GENERAL OVERVIEW)		
PERFORM THE FOLLOWING	YES	NO
LISTED STEPS:-		

Indirect care are steps that are to be performed during every skill that is performed. The below-mentioned steps must be applied to all the competency skills.

1. Greet patients, address them by name and introduce self appropriately.

2. Explain the procedure to the patient before and during care.

3. Make sure to address patient's preferences if any.

4. Perform standard precautions and infection control measures, by washing hands and wearing gloves.

5. Ask the patient about comfort or needs during care or before the care is completed.

6. Promote, establish and maintain patient's rights, safety and comfort during care.

COMPETENCY SKILLS 2: HANDWASHING		
PERFORM THE FOLLOWING	YES	NO
LISTED STEPS:-		

1. Start by opening faucet and wetting hands, followed by applying soap to the hands.

2. Use appropriate frictional movements to evenly apply soap. Create lather and
   a. *clean hands from front to back,*
   b. *clean between fingers,*
   c. *clean around the nail cuticles,*
   d. *clean under the nails and*
   e. *clean the wrist.*
   Note: both hands must be clean.

3. The process of using a frictional movement on the above-listed areas (**a-e**) should be done for a minimum of **20 seconds** or as **recommended**.

4. Next rinse hands, between fingers and wrists washing off the soap that was applied.

5. Use a clean paper towel to dry hands (between palms, fingers, and wrists). Finally, dispose of the paper towel in an appropriate container.

6. The last step would be to turn off the faucet using a clean paper towel. Do not contaminate the hands by turning off the faucet with clean bare hands.

COMPETENCY SKILLS 3: FOR GIVING A BED BATH & BACK RUBS		
PERFORM THE FOLLOWING	YES	NO
LISTED STEPS:-		

1. Identify your patient and start by greeting the patient, followed by introducing yourself.

2. Explain the procedure to the patient prior to performing it.

3. Maintain patient privacy by pulling the curtains to cover the area.

4. Perform standard precautions and infection control measures by washing hands and wearing gloves.

5. Collect the equipment needed to perform the procedure.
   o Water: appropriate temperature (check temperature with bath thermometer: no more than 105°F)
   o Washcloth
   o Bed protector linen
   o Face towel
   o Bath towel
   o Soap and soap dish
   o Bath blanket
   o Laundry bag or hamper
   o Bath basin
   o Lotion and/or powder
   o Bath thermometer

6. Position the patient in an appropriate manner, avoid placing the patient on the extreme edges of the bed. A safe position should always be maintained.

7. Protect bed linens prior to starting the procedure. Double check to see if the bed is not wet after the procedure.

8. Start by cleaning the face and outer aspect of the eyes. Rinse and dry the area before moving to another part of the body for performing the bed bath. Remember to use non-soap water for face and eyes.

9. Clean the neck, arms, underarms (axilla), hands, chest, and abdominal area with washcloth containing soap water. Rinse the above parts using another clean cloth.

10. Dry the neck, arm, hand, chest, abdominal area with dry cloth.

11. Change patient's position to expose back. Once exposed clean and rinse using a washcloth.

12. Dry the back using a dry cloth.

13. Warm lotion by placing the bottle in warm water container or by rubbing the lotion between the palms of your hand.

14. Apply lotion to the back area gently and in a circular manner.

15. If advised, provide back rubs in a circular manner while performing step 14.

16. Maintain patient modesty at all times.

230

17. Dress the patient with clean clothes or gown.

18. Collect and place soiled sheets into an appropriate bag or container, dispose of the trash in an appropriate container. Rinse and dry the basin used for the procedure followed by placing it in a designated area.

19. Patient's preference must be taken into consideration.

20. Check to see if the patient needs are addressed, also check to see if the patient is comfortable. This step should be performed before and during the procedure.

21. Know the patient's safety and patient's rights during care.

22. Before leaving the patient, make sure to place the call light or other call signal devices within the patient's reach.

COMPETENCY SKILLS 4: MAKE AN OCCUPIED BED		
PERFORM THE FOLLOWING	**YES**	**NO**
LISTED STEPS:-		

1. Identify your patient and start by greeting the patient, followed by introducing yourself.

2. Explain the procedure to the patient prior to performing it.

3. Maintain patient privacy by pulling the curtains to cover the area.

4. Perform standard precautions and infection control measures, by washing hands and wearing gloves.

5. Collect the equipment needed to perform the procedure:
   a. Mattress pad (if needed)
   b. Bottom sheet
   c. Drawsheet/Plastic Drawsheet
   d. Top sheet
   e. Blanket and/or bedspread (as per requirement)
   f. Pillowcase(s)

6. Turn the patient to one side of the bed (Log or segmental rolling). Head and neck support should be maintained during the entire process using a pillow except for changing pillow covers.
   a. *Note:* Position the patient in an appropriate manner, avoid placing the patient to the extreme edges of the bed. A safe position should always be maintained. Side rails on one side should be raised (follow your facility policy).

7. Untuck the bottom sheet from the head side to the foot side of the mattress. Replace the bottom sheet with a **CLEAN BOTTOM SHEET**. Repeat step 6 & Step 7 for the other side.

8. If using a
   a. Fitted Sheet: tuck or secure the bottom of the sheet to the mattress of the bed from all four sides.
   b. Flat Sheet: tuck the sheet into the head side of the mattress, followed by the sides of the mattress and finally the foot side of the mattress.

9. Care must be taken to avoid any folds in the bottom sheet.

10. While performing the procedure and turning the patient to either side of the bed to replace the bottom sheet, make sure that the skin does not rub against the bottom sheet. Avoid pulling of the bottom sheet.

11. Place a drawsheet onto the bottom sheet and tuck it under the mattress on both sides.

12. Next step would be to change the top sheet and replace it with a clean top sheet. *Note*: while tucking the top sheet avoid tucking it into the sides of the mattress, but instead should just be tucked into the foot side of the mattress. Ensure that the top sheet is loose and will allow appropriate foot and toe movement.

13. Top sheet should extend from the foot side of the bed to the shoulder level of the patient.

14. Change pillow cover/s.

15. Collect and place soiled sheets into an appropriate bag or container, dispose of the trash in an appropriate container.

16. Patient's preference must be taken into consideration.

17. Check to see if the patient needs are addressed, also check to see if the patient is comfortable. This step should be performed before and during the procedure.

18. Know the patient's safety and patient's rights during care.

19. Before leaving the patient, make sure to place the call light or other call signal device within the patient's reach.

COMPETENCY SKILLS 5: ASSIST WITH RANGE OF MOTION EXERCISES		
PERFORM THE FOLLOWING	YES	NO
LISTED STEPS:-		

1. Identify your patient and start by greeting the patient, followed by introducing yourself.

2. Explain the procedure to the patient prior to performing it.

3. Maintain patient privacy by pulling the curtains to cover the area.

4. Position patient in an appropriate position.

5. Select joint on which the range of motion is to be performed

    a. Exercise the shoulder: *(Recommended Joint Movements)*

    b. Exercise the elbow: *(Recommended Joint Movements)*

    c. Exercise the forearm: *(Recommended Joint Movements)*

    d. Exercise the wrist: *(Recommended Joint Movements)*

    e. Exercise the thumb: *(Recommended Joint Movements)*

    f. Exercise the fingers: *(Recommended Joint Movements)*

    g. Exercise the hip: *(Recommended Joint Movements)*

    h. Exercise the knee: *(Recommended Joint Movements)*

   i. Exercise the ankle: *(Recommended Joint Movements)*

   j. Exercise the foot: *(Recommended Joint Movements)*

   k. Exercise the toes: *(Recommended Joint Movements)*

6. Prevent restrictions if any for the joint to move through the range of motion.

7. Identify the side on which the procedure is to be performed.

8. Stabilize and support body parts as deemed necessary.

9. Perform range of motion slowly and gently, avoid sudden jerky and twisting movements.

10. Check to see if there is any discomfort felt by the patient during the procedure.

11. An appropriate number of repetitions are to be performed (**5-6 times**). Make sure to return joint and body part to its natural position after the range of motion is performed.

12. Return top linens to the proper position.

13. Wash hands.

14. Document the following:

   a) The date and time of the exercise.

   b) The joint/s on which ROM is performed.

   c) Any complaints of pain during and after performing ROM.

   d) A number of times the exercises were performed (repetition).

15. Collect and place soiled sheets into an appropriate bag or container dispose of the trash in an appropriate container (if necessary).

16. Patient's preference must be taken into consideration.

17. Check to see if the patient needs are addressed, also check to see if the patient is comfortable. This step should be performed before and during the procedure.

18. Know the patient's safety and patient's rights during care.

19. Before leaving the patient, make sure to place the call light or other call signal device within the patient's reach.

COMPETENCY SKILLS 6: UNDRESSING AND DRESSING PATIENTS		
PERFORM THE FOLLOWING	**YES**	**NO**
LISTED STEPS:-		

1. Identify your patient and start by greeting the patient, followed by introducing yourself.

2. Explain the procedure to the patient prior to performing it.

3. Maintain patient privacy by pulling the curtains to cover the area.

4. Perform standard precautions and infection control measures by washing hands and wearing gloves.

5. Ask the patient about the type of clothing they would like to wear (check your facility policy).

6. Gather the clothing required.

7. Assist patient as needed to complete undressing and dressing. Remove the clothing/gown from the **UNAFFECTED SIDE FIRST**. Make a tunnel of the sleeves and pass the arm through one end of it so that the sleeves are completely off.

8. Keep the patient covered at all times during the procedure.

9. Remove clothes and place it in the laundry hamper.

10. Dress the patient from the **AFFECTED SIDE FIRST**.
    Note: Affected side should be supported during dressing and undressing.

11. Dress the patient by gently sliding the hand of the patient into the sleeve and grasping it from the other end, align the sleeve appropriately.

12. Secure the clothing appropriately in place.

13. If "IV" is in place, the same procedure is to be performed.
    a. To undress, unaffected side is undressed first followed by the "IV side".
    b. To dress, "IV" side is dressed first followed by unaffected side.
        i. Never change the "IV" position. Follow facility policy or recommended guidelines.

14. Collect and place soiled sheets into an appropriate bag or container, dispose of the trash in an appropriate container.

15. Patient's preference must be taken into consideration.

16. Check to see if the patient needs are addressed, also check to see if the patient is comfortable. This step should be performed before and during the procedure.

17. Know the patient's safety and patient's rights during care.

18. Before leaving the patient, make sure to place the call light or other call signal device within the patient's reach.

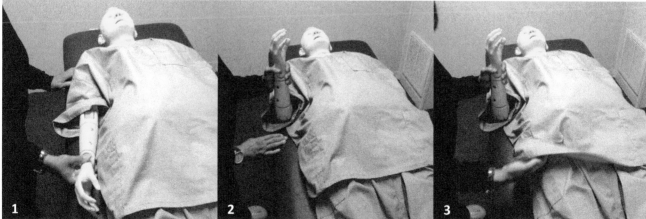

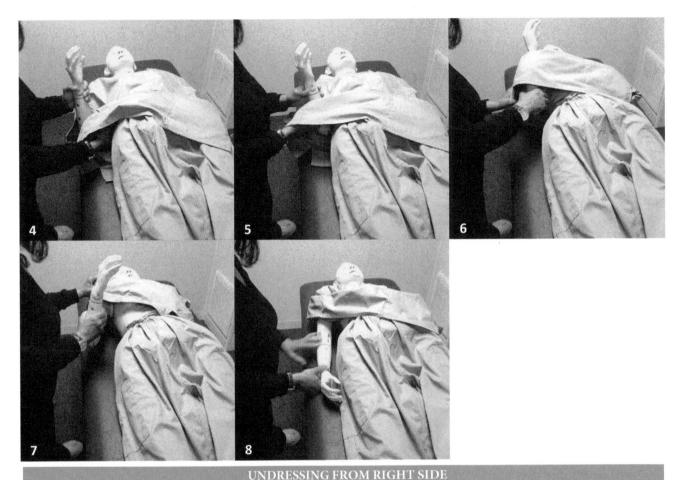

UNDRESSING FROM RIGHT SIDE

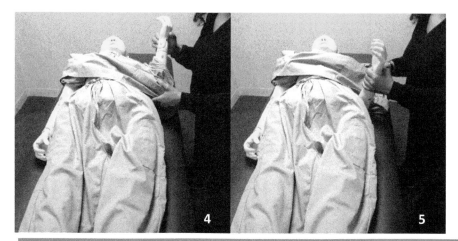

UNDRESSING FROM LEFT SIDE

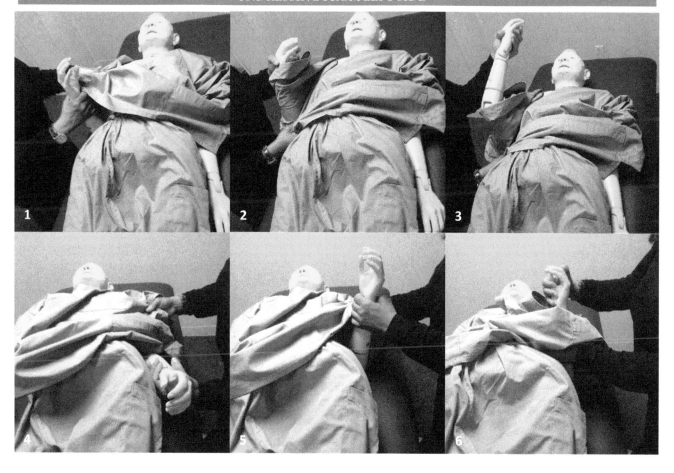

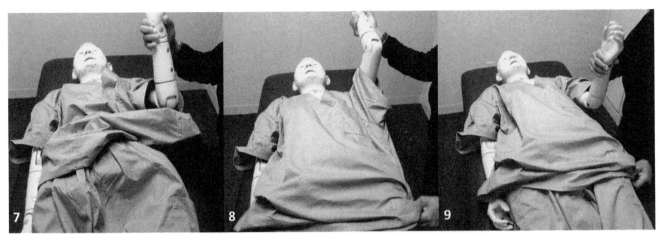

DRESSING (RIGHT SIDE AND LEFT SIDE)

COMPETENCY SKILLS 7: TAKE/RECORD HEIGHT		
PERFORM THE FOLLOWING	YES	NO
LISTED STEPS:-		

1. Identify your patient and start by greeting the patient, followed by introducing yourself.

2. Explain the procedure to the patient prior to performing it.

3. Perform standard precautions and infection control measures by washing hands and wearing gloves.

4. Gather equipment:

    a. Portable height measurement rod (height & weight scale)

    b. Paper towels

    c. Paper and pen

5. Place paper towel/s onto the scale platform on which the patient will stand.

6. Ask and assist the patient in removing shoes as required.

7. Raise the height measurement rod which is usually a part of the height and weight machine.

8. Have the patient stand on the scale platform, provide assistance as required.

9. Lower height measurement rod to a point where it touches the superior surface of the patient's head.

10. Record height on paper and assist the patient in getting off the scale.

11. Provide time for the patient to put on their shoes, provide assistance as required.

12. Patient must be comfortable throughout the procedure.

13. Wash hands and record height as per facility requirements. Dispose of paper towel in an appropriate container.

COMPETENCY SKILLS 8: TAKE/RECORD WEIGHT		
PERFORM THE FOLLOWING	**YES**	**NO**
LISTED STEPS:-		
1. Identify your patient and start by greeting the patient, followed by introducing yourself.		
2. Explain the procedure to the patient prior to performing it.		
3. Perform standard precautions and infection control measures by washing hands and wearing gloves.		
4. Gather equipment:		
a. Portable weight scale (height & weight scale)		
b. Paper towels		
c. Paper and pen		
5. Place paper towels on scale platform where the patient will stand.		
6. Ask and assist patient in removing shoes and other heavy clothing as required.		
7. Have the patient stand on the scale platform, provide assistance as required.		
8. Record weight on paper and assist the patient in getting off the scale.		
9. Provide time for the patient to put on their shoes, provide assistance as required.		
10. Patient must be comfortable throughout the procedure.		
11. Wash hands and record weight as per facility requirements. Dispose of paper towel in an appropriate container.		

COMPETENCY SKILLS 9: ASSISTING WITH APPLYING AND REMOVING PROSTHESIS OR ORTHOSIS		
PERFORM THE FOLLOWING	**YES**	**NO**
LISTED STEPS:-		
1. Identify your patient and start by greeting the patient, followed by introducing yourself.		
2. Explain the procedure to the patient prior to performing it.		
3. Maintain patient privacy by pulling the curtains to cover the area.		
4. Perform standard precautions and infection control measures by washing hands and wearing gloves.		
5. It may include but not limited to the following examples:-		
• Leg brace		
• Leg splints		
• Prosthetic limb		
• Eye prosthesis		
• Hearing device		

6. Make sure to provide skin care according to the facility policy.

7. Assistance must be provided for positioning and securing prosthesis or orthosis (device) as per facility policy.

8. Place soiled wraps into an appropriate container.

9. Any change in the appearance of the skin must be reported to the registered nurse or appropriate healthcare professional.

COMPETENCY SKILLS 10: ASSISTING WITH APPLYING ACE (ELASTIC) BANDAGES		
PERFORM THE FOLLOWING	YES	NO
LISTED STEPS:-		

1. Identify your patient and start by greeting the patient, followed by introducing yourself.

2. Explain the procedure to the patient prior to performing it.

3. Maintain patient privacy by pulling the curtains to cover the area.

4. Perform standard precautions and infection control measures by washing hands and wearing gloves.

5. Start collecting equipment required to perform the procedure:

   a. An ace bandage (elastic) determined by healthcare professional

   b. A clip, or tape

6. Position the patient in a comfortable position, expose the area on which the ace bandage is to be applied. Before putting on the ace bandage, make sure that the area is clean and dry.

7. Hold the bandage and start by applying it to the smallest area (extremity).

8. Cross it over the smallest area, leaving the distal most section of the part exposed. If bandaging foot, leave the toes. If bandaging wrist, leave the fingers.

9. Make a circular turn over this smallest area; next cross a circle over the first circle. Overlap the spirals turning them in an upward direction. **Note:** each turn made should overlap 2/3rd of the previous turns.

10. Maintain even pressure while applying the bandage. The application should be wrinkle free.

11. Once done, tape or pin the tail of the bandage to hold the bandage in place.

12. Check to see the distal part (human body) for color change, or if the part feels cold or if the patient complains of pain, tingling or numbness. Report the healthcare professional (nurse) at the earliest.

13. End the procedure by removing gloves and washing hands.

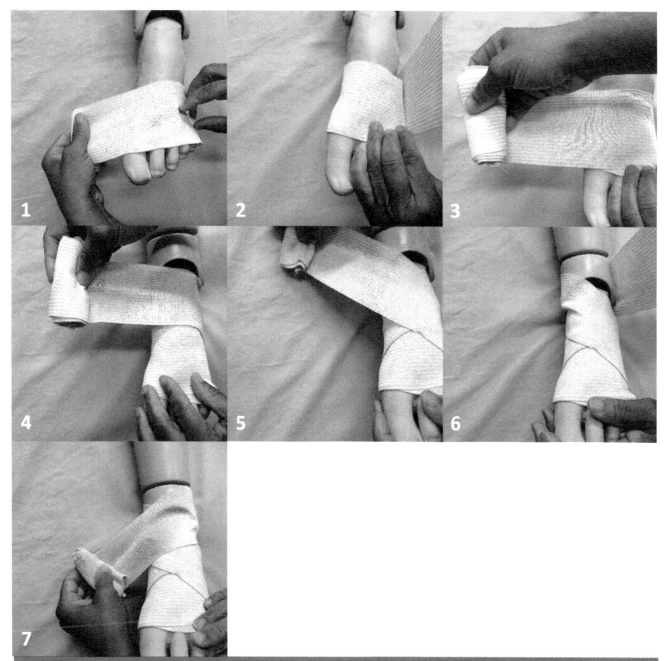

ACE BANDAGE APPLICATION		
COMPETENCY SKILLS 11: ASSISTING WITH APPLYING TED's (ELASTIC STOCKINGS)		
PERFORM THE FOLLOWING	YES	NO
LISTED STEPS:-		
1. Identify your patient and start by greeting the patient, followed by introducing yourself.		
2. Explain the procedure to the patient prior to performing it.		
3. Maintain patient privacy by pulling the curtains to cover the area.		

4. Perform standard precautions and infection control measures by washing hands and wearing gloves.

5. Start collecting equipment required to perform the procedure:

    a. Elastic stocking determined by healthcare professional.

6. Position the patient in a comfortable position, expose the area on which the stocking is to be applied. Before putting on the stocking, make sure that the area is clean and dry.

7. Gather stockings.

8. Start the application process by supporting the patient's foot at heel. The foot is the first part that is inserted into the stocking followed by the ankle, lower leg, and other parts as per the extent of the requirement.

9. Gently pull the stocking over the leg. Do the same for the other leg.

10. Check for the proper fit of the stocking. It should be comfortable and not be left too tight.

11. Check to see for color change, or if the part feels cold or if the patient complains of pain, tingling or numbness. Remove the stockings and report the healthcare professional (nurse) at the earliest.

12. Finally end the procedure by removing gloves and washing hands followed by recording the procedure as per facility requirements.

COMPETENCY SKILLS 12: ASSISTING WITH APPLYING BINDERS		
PERFORM THE FOLLOWING	YES	NO
LISTED STEPS:-		

1. Identify your patient and start by greeting the patient, followed by introducing yourself.

2. Explain the procedure to the patient prior to performing it.

3. Maintain patient privacy by pulling the curtains to cover the area.

4. Perform standard precautions and infection control measures by washing hands and wearing gloves.

5. Start collecting equipment required to perform the procedure:

    a. Binders: determined by healthcare professional

6. Position the patient in a comfortable position.

7. Apply the binder to the body part such that the pressure is evenly distributed over the entire area of application. Maintain patient body alignment while performing the application process.

8. Binder should not be loose or too tight (Wrinkle free, pain-free and should be in the right position/location). Avoid application over the site of pain (incision sites).

9. Binders should be changed if they become moist or soiled.

10. If the patient does not want to have the binder put on them, respect the patient's decision and report the healthcare professional (nurse) about the patient's refusal to wear the binder.

11. The last step would be to remove gloves and wash hands, followed by recording the procedure as per facility requirements.

COMPETENCY SKILLS 13: URINE OUTPUT MEASUREMENT		
PERFORM THE FOLLOWING	YES	NO
LISTED STEPS:-		

1. Identify your patient and start by greeting the patient, followed by introducing yourself.

2. Explain the procedure to the patient prior to performing it.

3. Maintain patient privacy by pulling the curtains to cover the area.

4. Perform standard precautions and infection control measures by washing hands and wearing gloves.

5. Transfer the entire urine from the bed pan or drainage bag into the measurement container.
   a. If using a bed pan, directly pour the entire urine carefully into the measuring container. This should be done over the toilet.
   b. If using drainage bag, open the drainage clamp and empty the entire urine into the measuring container. Make sure the drainage tubes are not getting contaminated. Once the entire urine is poured into the container, close the drainage clamp.

6. Read the level of urine output, while keeping the measuring container on a flat surface. The reading should be done at "EYE LEVEL".

7. After measuring the urine, discard it into the toilet. Rinse and dry the container and place it in the designated area as per facility policy.

8. Remove gloves and wash hands.

9. Record output in cc or ml (amount).

10. Record the output of urine content of the container within +/- 50 ml/cc or 25 ml/cc of evaluators or nurse's measurement.

11. Record the output of urine and the time the measurements were taken.

COMPETENCY SKILLS 14: COLLECT / TEST URINE SPECIMEN		
PERFORM THE FOLLOWING	**YES**	**NO**
LISTED STEPS:-		
1. Identify your patient and start by greeting the patient, followed by introducing yourself.		
2. Explain the procedure to the patient prior to performing it.		
3. Maintain patient privacy by pulling the curtains to cover the area.		
4. Perform standard precautions and infection control measures by washing hands and wearing gloves.		
5. Collect equipment:		
a. Clean bedpan, urinal, or specimen pan		
b. Specimen container and lid		
c. Label		
d. Urine container with lid		
e. Dip-stick		
6. A label with patient's name and information should be labeled onto the container.		
7. Inform the patient to clean the perineal area before voiding the sample into the container.		
8. Place a lid on specimen container once received from the patient.		
9. Clean specimen pan or bedpan, if used during the collection procedure.		
10. Collected specimen:		
a. If sending it to a lab, label and store it as per recommended guidelines		
b. If performing a dip-stick test:-		
i. Remove reagent strip from bottle and dip it into urine specimen.		
ii. Remove strip from urine after 2 seconds as per manufacturer instructions.		
iii. Gently tap the edges of the strip against the specimen container.		
iv. Compare strip with the color chart on the bottle for results.		
v. Discard urine specimen and container.		
vi. Clean equipment.		
11. Remove and discard gloves and wash hands.		
12. Record and report results according to facility policy.		

COMPETENCY SKILLS 15: COLLECTING A STOOL SPECIMEN		
PERFORM THE FOLLOWING	**YES**	**NO**
LISTED STEPS:-		
1. Identify your patient and start by greeting the patient, followed by introducing yourself.		
2. Explain the procedure to the patient prior to performing it.		
3. Maintain patient privacy by pulling the curtains to cover the area.		
4. Perform standard precautions and infection control measures by washing hands and wearing gloves.		
5. Collect equipment:		
a. Bedpan and cover		
b. Urinal		
c. Tongue blade		
d. Specimen pan		
e. Toilet tissue		
f. Specimen container and lid		
g. Label		
6. A label with patient's name and information should be labeled on the container.		
7. Position patient on bedpan or commode. If the patient is able to use the commode place the specimen pan in the toilet, under the toilet seat.		
8. Instruct the patient that he/she should not discard any toilet papers into the bedpan or specimen pan.		
9. Remove gloves, wash hands and give patient privacy.		
10. Leave call light or call bell within patient's reach.		
11. Return to the room when patient requests.		
12. Wash hands and put on gloves.		
13. Use a tongue blade to collect feces from the bedpan or specimen pan and transfer it into the specimen container.		
14. Specimen container should be covered with the lid.		
a. *Precaution: do not touch the inside of the lid.*		
15. Bedpan or specimen pan must be emptied, cleaned, and disinfected. Provide assistance to patient with hand washing. Provide paper towel/s or wipes to dry their hands.		
16. Remove and discard gloves and wash hands. Assure your patient is comfortable.		
17. Pack the specimen container appropriately as per facility policy and send it to the laboratory.		
18. Report and record observations to nurse according to the facility policy.		

COMPETENCY SKILLS 16: PERINEAL CARE (FEMALE)		
PERFORM THE FOLLOWING	**YES**	**NO**
LISTED STEPS:-		

1. Identify your patient and start by greeting the patient, followed by introducing yourself.

2. Explain the procedure to the patient prior to performing it.

3. Maintain patient privacy by pulling the curtains to cover the area.

4. Perform standard precautions and infection control measures by washing hands and wearing gloves.

5. Start collecting equipment required to perform the procedure:

   a. Washable (bath) blanket

   b. Disposable gloves

   c. Bed protector

   d. Washcloth (cotton balls) (100 - 105 degrees F). Use a bath thermometer to check the water temperature.

   e. Disposable bag

   f. Bedpan and cover

   g. Liquid soap or soap dish with soap

   h. Basin with warm water

   i. Towel

6. Collect the water of appropriate temperature. Check the temperature of the water using a bath thermometer.

7. Start by placing all the required equipment on the table.

8. Raise the bed to an appropriate level for proper body mechanics (if required).

9. If the underpad is soiled, make sure to replace them prior to pericare.

10. Position the patient in supine position (on their back). The under pad should be positioned in such a way that the appropriate area over it is covered. Help patient in flexing their knees and spreading their legs (hip joint abduction).

11. Draping should be done for the patient by covering the upper and the lower body parts while exposing only the area of pericare.

12. A washcloth is immersed in water. Soap is then applied to the wet washcloth.

13. Using the wet washcloth, wash:
    a. Each side of the labia (front to back stroke).
    b. Skin folds between the perineal area and the thigh (front to back stroke).
    c. Skin folds between the perineal area and the buttock (front to back stroke).

14. Using another wash cloth, rinse:
    a. Each side of the labia (front to back stroke).
    b. Skin folds between the perineal area and the thigh (front to back stroke).

    c.   Skin folds between the perineal area and the buttock (front to back stroke).

15. Using another wash cloth, dry:
    a.   Each side of the labia (front to back stroke).
    b.   Skin folds between the perineal area and the thigh (front to back stroke).
    c.   Skin folds between the perineal area and the buttock (front to back stroke).

16. The next step would be to lower the patient's leg and turn the patient to one side. Turn to the side away from you. Using a washcloth with soap, stroke the rectal area from front to back. Next step would be to rinse the area in the same pattern followed by drying the area.

17. Once done have the patient dressed appropriately and make sure that the patient is in a comfortable position. Assure patients safety.

18. Discard all soiled linen in hamper and dispose of trash in an appropriate container.

19. Rinse and dry basin. Place it in the designated area as per facility policy. Note: clean and store equipment as required by the facility policy.

20. Remove gloves and discard them in an appropriate container.

21. Wash hands appropriately.

22. Record and report date, time, and observations according to the facility policy.

COMPETENCY SKILLS 17: PERINEAL CARE (MALE)

PERFORM THE FOLLOWING	YES	NO
LISTED STEPS:-		

1. Identify your patient and start by greeting the patient, followed by introducing yourself.

2. Explain the procedure to the patient prior to performing it.

3. Maintain patient privacy by pulling the curtains to cover the area.

4. Perform standard precautions and infection control measures, by washing hands and wearing gloves.

5. Start collecting equipment required to perform the procedure:
    a.   Washable (bath) blanket
    b.   Disposable gloves
    c.   Bed protector
    d.   Washcloth (cotton balls) (100 - 105 degrees F). Use a bath thermometer to check the water temperature.
    e.   Disposable bag
    f.   Bedpan and cover
    g.   Liquid soap or soap dish with soap
    h.   Basin with warm water

   i. Towel

6. Collect the water of appropriate temperature. Check the temperature of the water using a bath thermometer.

7. Start by placing all the required equipment on the table.

8. Raise the bed to an appropriate level for proper body mechanics (if required).

9. If the underpad is soiled, make sure to replace them prior to pericare.

10. Position the patient in the supine position (on their back). The under pad should be positioned in such a way that the appropriate area over it is covered.

11. Draping should be done for the patient by covering the upper and the lower body parts while exposing only the area of pericare.

12. A washcloth is immersed in water. Soap is then applied to the wet washcloth.

13. If the patient is uncircumcised, retract the foreskin by grasping the penis.

14. Clean tip of the penis in a circular motion (*concentric circles: inside to outside circle*). Starting at urethral opening and moving outward while cleaning. Discard washcloth used.

15. Rinse the area using another washcloth. Make sure to return the retracted foreskin to its normal position (for uncircumcised penis).

16. Next clean shaft of the penis with firm up to down strokes. Rinse the same area.

17. Help patient in flexing their knees and spreading their legs (hip joint abduction).

18. Clean scrotum appropriately, then rinse it well. Dry penis and scrotum.

19. The next step would be to lower the patient's leg and turn the patient to one side. Turn to the side away from you. Using a washcloth with soap; stroke the rectal area from front to back. Next step would be to rinse the area in the same pattern followed by drying the area.

20. Once done have the patient dressed appropriately and make sure that the patient is in a comfortable position. Assure patients safety.

21. Discard all soiled linen in hamper and dispose of trash in an appropriate container.

22. Rinse and dry basin. Place it in the designated area as per facility policy. Note: clean and store equipment as required by the facility policy.

23. Remove gloves and discard them in an appropriate container.

24. Wash hands appropriately.

25. Record and report date, time and observations according to facility policy.

COMPETENCY SKILLS 18: CATHETER CARE (FEMALE AND MALE)

PERFORM THE FOLLOWING	YES	NO
LISTED STEPS:-		

1. Identify your patient and start by greeting the patient, followed by introducing yourself.

2. Explain the procedure to the patient prior to performing it.

3. Maintain patient privacy by pulling the curtains to cover the area.

4. Perform standard precautions and infection control measures by washing hands and wearing gloves.

5. Collect equipment:

   a. Washable (bath) blanket

   b. Disposable gloves

   c. Bed protector

   d. Washcloth (cotton balls) (100 - 105 degrees F). Use a bath thermometer to check the water temperature.

   e. Disposable bag

   f. Bedpan and cover

   g. Liquid soap or soap dish with soap

   h. Basin with warm water

   i. Towel

   j. Washcloth

   k. Plastic bag

   l. Paper towels

6. Place underpad beneath the patient's buttocks and upper thigh. Remove the under pad after the procedure is complete.

7. Collect the water of appropriate temperature. Check the temperature of the water using a bath thermometer.

8. Start by placing all the required equipment on the table.

9. Raise the bed to an appropriate level for proper body mechanics (if required).

10. Position the patient in the supine position (on their back). The under pad should be positioned in such a way that the appropriate area over it is covered.

11. Draping should be done for the patient by covering the upper and the lower body parts while exposing only the area of pericare.

12. A washcloth is immersed in water. Soap is then applied to the wet washcloth.

13. For female patients:

   a. Clean the catheter tubes proximal to distal.

   b. Clean the labia on each side from front to back.

14. For male patients:

   a. Clean the catheter tubes proximal to distal.

   b. If the patient is uncircumcised, retract the foreskin by grasping the penis.

c. Clean tip of the penis in a circular motion (*concentric circles: inside to outside circle*). Starting at urethral opening and moving outward while cleaning. Discarded washcloth used.

d. Rinse the area using another washcloth. Make sure to return the retracted foreskin to its normal position (for uncircumcised penis).

e. Next clean shaft of the penis with firm up to down strokes. Rinse the same area.

f. Help patient in flexing the knees and spreading legs.

g. Clean scrotum appropriately, then rinse it well. Dry penis and scrotum.

15. The next step would be to lower the patient's leg and turn the patient to one side. Turn to the side away from you. Using a washcloth with soap; stroke the rectal area from front to back, Next step would be to rinse the area in the same pattern followed by drying the area.

16. Once done have the patient dressed appropriately and make sure that the patient is in a comfortable position. Assure patient's safety.

17. Check for catheter tubing's; there should be no obstruction or kinking in the tubes. The catheter tubes or drainage bag should not touch the floor. The drainage bag should be at a lower level than the urinary bladder.

18. Discard all soiled linen in hamper and dispose of trash in an appropriate container.

19. Rinse and dry basin. Place it in the designated area as per facility policy. Note: clean and store equipment as required by the facility policy.

20. Remove gloves and discard them in an appropriate container.

21. Wash hands appropriately.

22. Record and report date, time, and observations according to the facility policy.

COMPETENCY SKILLS 19: GAIT BELT OR TRANSFER BELT USE: AMBULATION		
PERFORM THE FOLLOWING	**YES**	**NO**
LISTED STEPS:-		

1. Identify your patient and start by greeting the patient, followed by introducing yourself.

2. Explain the procedure to the patient prior to performing it.

3. Perform standard precautions and infection control measures, by washing hands and wearing gloves.

4. Maintain your body mechanics during the entire length of the process.

5. Select an appropriate size gait belt/transfer belt.

6. Check to see the patient's initial or starting position.

    • In bed, provide assistance to change the patient's position from supine to sitting.

    • In chair, bring the patient to an appropriate position (sitting).

7. Secure the gait belt around the patient's waist. The gait belt should never be secured tightly, as this may cause discomfort to the patient. The best way to ensure that the gait belt is not secured tightly would be by inserting two fingers to check for the fit.
    Note: on a female patient, ensure that the gait belt is at the waist level and not at the breast level.

8. Once the above step of securing the gait belt is complete, give directions to the patient before making them stand up from a sitting position.

9. Grasp the gait belt at either end while assisting the patient to a standing position.

10. Ask patient, if he or she is comfortable while in standing position.

11. Stand on the side and slightly behind the patient.

12. Have the patient walk, hold gait belt while the patient is walking.

13. Ask if the patient is comfortable while walking.

14. Have the patient walk several steps.

15. Have the patient stand near a chair, with the back of the knee facing the seat of the chair. Assist the patient to sit.

16. Safely and gently remove the gait belt from the patient's waist. Avoid pulling of the gait belt while removing it.

17. Have the patient sit in the chair, with the hip against the back of the chair. Position the patient comfortably and safely in the chair.

18. Remove gloves (if applicable) and wash hands.

19. Document time of transfer (and/or ambulation) and patient's response to the procedure.

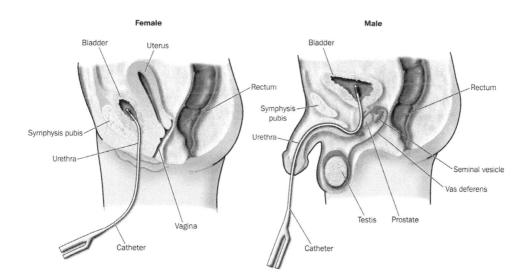

Skill 18: Catheter (Female and Male)

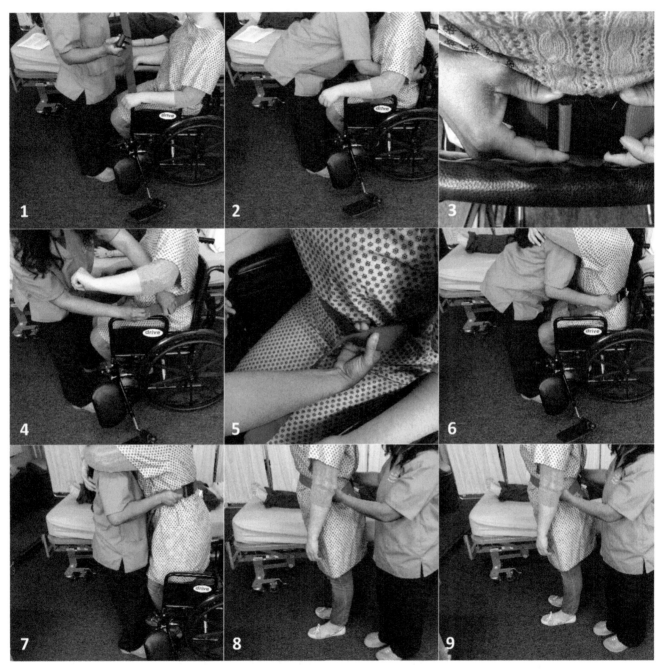

USING GAIT BELT

COMPETENCY SKILLS 20: LIFTING A PATIENT USING A MECHANICAL LIFT (HOYERS)		
PERFORM THE FOLLOWING	YES	NO
LISTED STEPS:-		
1. Identify your patient and start by greeting the patient, followed by introducing yourself.		
2. Explain the procedure to the patient prior to performing it.		

3. Perform standard precautions and infection control measures by washing hands and wearing gloves.

4. Maintain your body mechanics during the entire length of the process.

5. Follow manufacturer's instructions for transferring the patient.

6. Assemble equipment and obtain assistance from a coworker to help you with lifting and transferring of the patient using a mechanical lift. Check equipment for any damage or broken parts prior to starting the transfer.

7. If transferring to a wheelchair, place the wheelchair right angled to the bed near the foot of the bed facing the head of the bed. Make sure to lock the wheels.

8. Elevate bed to a comfortable height and lock wheels. Next turn the patient.

9. Position the sling(s) of the mechanical lift beneath the patient's shoulder, thighs, and buttocks. Roll the patient back onto the sling and position it properly under shoulders and hips.

10. Position the lift frame over the bed and secure the sling to the mechanical lift frame.

11. Slowly lift the patient using the hydraulic control available in the mechanical lift.

12. Slowly turn the lift and position it over the chair or wheelchair.

13. Slowly lower the patient into chair or wheelchair, release straps from patients body parts and move the mechanical lift away from the patient.

14. Provide patient with call signal in reach.

15. Wash hands.

16. Reverse the process to return the patient to his/her bed.

17. Record and report date, time and any abnormal observations according to the facility policy.

COMPETENCY SKILLS 21: POSITIONING ON SIDE (Turning Patient Towards You)		
PERFORM THE FOLLOWING	YES	NO
LISTED STEPS:-		

1. Identify your patient and start by greeting the patient, followed by introducing yourself.

2. Explain the procedure to the patient prior to performing it.

3. Maintain patient privacy by pulling the curtains to cover the area.

4. Perform standard precautions and infection control measures, by washing hands and wearing gloves.

5. Position the bed flat. Check for precautions.
Note: - in some scenarios, the patient's head of the bed should not be lowered than a certain angle. Ensure to know these precautions prior to making the bed flat.

6. Once the bed is flat, raise the rails on one side and assist the patient to turn (onto the side of the bed where the rails are raised). To turn the patient (turning to left side) starting with patient in supine position:

    a. Slightly bend the knee and cross the right leg over the left leg.

    b. Cross the right arm across the patient's chest, with elbow flexed.

    c. Place your hand on patient's right shoulder and anchor another hand on hip.

    d. Finally, roll the patient towards the left side.

7. For comfort, check to see that a pillow supports the patient's head and chin.

8. Once the patient is turned to the side, place a positioning device or a pillow behind the patient's back. This ensures the support required to maintain the position.

9. Place the positioning device or pillow under patient's upper knee. The upper knee must be flexed or bent and should be on top and in front of the lower leg.

10. Place the lower arm onto the side and in front, so that patient is not lying on it.

11. Place a positioning device or pillow, under the upper arm.

12. Remove gloves (if applicable) and wash hands.

13. Document time, position change, and patient's response to procedure.

COMPETENCY SKILLS 22: CHANGE NON-STERILE (CLEAN) DRESSING		
PERFORM THE FOLLOWING	YES	NO
LISTED STEPS:-		

1. Identify your patient and start by greeting the patient, followed by introducing yourself.

2. Explain the procedure to the patient prior to performing it.

3. Maintain patient privacy by pulling the curtains to cover the area.

4. Perform standard precautions and infection control measures by washing hands and wearing gloves.

5. Collect equipment:

    a. 4x4 gauze pads

    b. Non-allergenic tape

    c. Disposable plastic bag

    d. Hydrogen peroxide or cleaning agent (as recommended)

    e. Disposable gloves

    f. Notepad and pen

    g. Antibiotic ointment

6. Maintain appropriate body mechanics during the procedure.

7. Position the patient comfortably and expose the area that is to be dressed.

8. Open a gauze pad without touching it, next, open a bottle of cleaning solution and ointment if required.

9. Don gloves.

10. From the previous dressing: Gently remove tapes and dressing. If it does not come off easily, try pouring a solution to loosen the dressing. Remember: dressing can be very painful when removed, this process must be done gently and with great precision.

11. Discard used dressing in the appropriate container.

12. Damp clean gauze with a solution (recommended as per the healthcare professional).

13. Clean the area from center to the periphery. The gauze pad used must be discarded into an appropriate bag.

14. If an ointment will be used, apply it on the gauze pad. Place the gauze pad on the wound followed by tapping the gauze appropriately.

15. Remove gloves and discard in appropriate container.

16. Wash hands.

17. Document date, time and observations of the wound.

COMPETENCY SKILLS 23: ASSISTING PATIENTS IN USING BED PAN		
PERFORM THE FOLLOWING	**YES**	**NO**
LISTED STEPS:-		

1. Identify your patient and start by greeting the patient, followed by introducing yourself.

2. Explain the procedure to the patient prior to performing it.

3. Maintain patient privacy by pulling the curtains to cover the area.

4. Perform standard precautions and infection control measures by washing hands and wearing gloves.

5. Collect equipment:

   a. Water: Appropriate temperature (check temperature with bath thermometer: no more than 105°F).

   b. Washcloth

   c. Bed protector linen

   d. Face towel

   e. Bath towel

   f. Soap and soap dish

   g. Bath blanket

   h. Laundry bag or hamper

   i. Bath basin

j.   Lotion and/or powder

k.   Bath thermometer

6.   Collect water in the basin.

7.   Start by placing a protective pad on top of the bottom sheet. Main areas are to be covered, which includes the buttocks and upper thigh.

8.   Select an appropriate size bed pan to fit the patient's need.

9.   Place the bedpan using the following techniques:

    a.   Have the patient turn to one side, place bed pan and turn the patient onto the bedpan or

    b.   Have the patient lift hips off the bed and place the bedpan. Then have patient slowly lower hips onto the bedpan.

10.   The head of the bed must be raised after the bedpan is placed or positioned under the patient's hip.

11.   Instruct the patient to call when finished. Leave a call light within the patient's reach.

12.   Before leaving the patient, the following items must be placed within the patient's reach:

    a.   Wipes

    b.   Tissue or toilet papers

13.   Depart from the patient and discard the gloves.

14.   Return when the patient has finished using the bedpan and don new gloves.

15.   Removing the bed pan should be done by lowering the head of the bed and either turning the patient to one side or asking the patient to raise the hips. Provide assistance as required.

16.   Empty the bedpan as advised.

17.   Provide patient with hand wipes and dry paper towels.

18.   Discard any used hand wipes and other materials, if any. Bedpan should be rinsed and stored in the designated area as per facility requirements.

19.   Remove gloves and discard them.

COMPETENCY SKILLS 24: FEEDING PATIENTS		
PERFORM THE FOLLOWING	**YES**	**NO**
LISTED STEPS:-		

1.   Identify your patient and start by greeting the patient, followed by introducing yourself.

2.   Explain the procedure to the patient prior to performing it.

3.   Have the patient sit while feeding (45°-90° angle preferred).

	YES	NO
4. Have the patient wash their hands using a damp washcloth, paper towel, or hand wipes before feeding.		
5. Protect patient's clothes before feeding.		
6. Place the food tray in a position where the patient can see it.		
7. Use a spoon to feed.		
8. Check to match the patient's food tray with patient's diet.		
9. Explain the types of foods that are available. Offer moderate size bites.		
10. Provide liquid and solid food.		
11. Alternate liquid and solid foods, while asking the patient for their preference.		
12. Appropriate time should be given to the patient to chew and swallow the food before the next bite is given.		
13. Once done, clean patients mouth and hands with wipes.		
14. Record the amount of fluid intake, within 25% of the nurse's measurement.		
15. Record the amount of food intake, within 25% of nurse's measurement.		

COMPETENCY SKILLS 25: FOOT CARE		
PERFORM THE FOLLOWING	YES	NO
LISTED STEPS:-		
1. Identify your patient and start by greeting the patient, followed by introducing yourself.		
2. Explain the procedure to the patient prior to performing it.		
3. Maintain patient privacy by pulling the curtains to cover the area.		
4. Perform standard precautions and infection control measures by washing hands and wearing gloves.		
5. Collect equipment.		
6. Collect warm water in a basin. Check the temperature of the water (95°F-110°F). Use a bath thermometer to check the temperature of the water in the basin.		
7. The patient should be in a comfortable position.		
8. Water filled basin is placed on a protective sheet.		
9. Place patient's foot in the basin and soak.		
10. Apply soap to a washcloth. Lift patient's foot out once soaked.		
11. Wash the foot entirely and between toes.		
12. Rinse the foot entirely and between toes.		
13. Dry the foot entirely and between toes.		
14. Apply warm lotion. Lotion can be warmed by placing the bottle of lotion in hot water or by rubbing the lotion between the palms of your hand.		
15. Apply lotion on the foot. Excess lotion, if applied, should be wiped off.		

16. A sock is put on the foot. Barefoot should not be placed on the floor.

17. Support the lower extremity throughout the procedure.

18. Discard all soiled linen in hamper and dispose of trash in an appropriate container.

19. Rinse and dry basin. Place it in the designated area as per facility policy.

20. Remove gloves and discard them in an appropriate container.

COMPETENCY SKILLS 26: DENTURE CARE		
PERFORM THE FOLLOWING	YES	NO
LISTED STEPS:-		

1. Identify your patient and start by greeting the patient, followed by introducing yourself.

2. Explain the procedure to the patient prior to performing it.

3. Maintain patient privacy by pulling the curtains to cover the area.

4. Perform standard precautions and infection control measures, by washing hands and wearing gloves.

5. Collect equipment:

    a. Toothbrush

    b. Toothpaste

    c. Emesis basin

    d. Denture cup

    e. Paper towel

6. Start by collecting equipment.

7. Wear gloves.

8. Line the sink with paper towels or wash clothes and/or fill the sink with water. These steps are performed to avoid damage of dentures, in case they are dropped.

9. Remove dentures from denture cup.

10. Prevent contamination of dentures.

11. Use cold water for denture care.

12. Toothpaste must be applied to the toothbrush, followed by brushing all the possible surfaces of the dentures (upper, lower, inner and outer).

13. Rinse denture with cold water, removing toothpaste.

14. Fill denture cup with cool water and place clean denture in the cup.

15. Place denture cup in an appropriate location (within patient's reach).

16. Provide mouth care (upper and lower gums) using appropriate supplies. Make sure to protect patient's clothes while providing mouth care.

17. Have the patient rinse their mouth in an emesis basin or disposable cups.

18. The patient mouth should be left clean and dry.

	YES	NO
19. Rinse toothbrush and place it in an appropriate container.		
20. Remove the paper towels or wash clothes used to line the sink and discard it into a suitable container.		
21. Drain the sink.		
22. Remove and dispose gloves and wash hands.		
COMPETENCY SKILLS 27: MOUTH CARE		
PERFORM THE FOLLOWING	YES	NO
LISTED STEPS:-		
1. Identify your patient and start by greeting the patient, followed by introducing yourself.		
2. Explain the procedure to the patient prior to performing it.		
3. Maintain patient privacy by pulling the curtains to cover the area.		
4. Perform standard precautions and infection control measures, by washing hands and wearing gloves.		
5. Collect equipment:		
a. Toothbrush		
b. Toothpaste		
c. Emesis basin		
d. Paper towel or wash cloths		
6. Patient should be in an upright position 60° – 90° angle for brushing teeth.		
7. Wear gloves and drape patient with appropriate protective cover to avoid soiling of patient's clothes.		
8. Moisten toothbrush and apply toothpaste.		
9. Gently brush the upper and lower teeth (inside and outside).		
10. Have the patient rinse their mouth in an emesis basin or disposable cup(s).		
11. Clean and dry patient's mouth and chin.		
12. Remove protection covers. Rinse and place toothbrush into an appropriate container.		
13. Rinse/dry basin and place it in a designated area as per facility policy.		
14. Discard disposables in an appropriate container.		
15. Dry any area on the bed that was soiled or wet during mouth care.		
16. Remove gloves and dispose them in an appropriate container followed by performing hand hygiene or hand wash.		

COMPETENCY SKILLS 28: HAND AND NAIL CARE		
PERFORM THE FOLLOWING	**YES**	**NO**
LISTED STEPS:-		
1. Identify your patient and start by greeting the patient, followed by introducing yourself.		
2. Explain the procedure to the patient prior to performing it.		
3. Maintain patient privacy by pulling the curtains to cover the area.		
4. Perform standard precautions and infection control measures, by washing hands and wearing gloves.		
5. Collect equipment:		
a. Basin		
b. Washcloth		
c. Soap		
d. Orange stick		
e. Lotion		
6. Collect warm water in a basin. Check the temperature of the water (95°F-110°F). Use a bath thermometer to check the temperature of the water in the basin.		
7. Have the patient immerse their hand and finger in the basin. Support the patient arm while doing so.		
8. Clean hands, nails (underneath nails), and fingers (between fingers).		
9. Remove hands from the basin and place it on a clean dry towel.		
10. Use an orange stick to clean underneath the nails, make sure to clean the orange stick before using it on another nail.		
11. Dry the following areas: hands, underneath nails and between fingers.		
12. Shape the nails (if required).		
13. Apply lotion to hands, remove access lotion using a paper towel.		
14. Rinse/dry basin and place it in a designated area as per facility policy.		
15. Discard disposables in appropriate container.		
16. Remove gloves and dispose them in an appropriate container followed by performing hand hygiene or hand wash.		

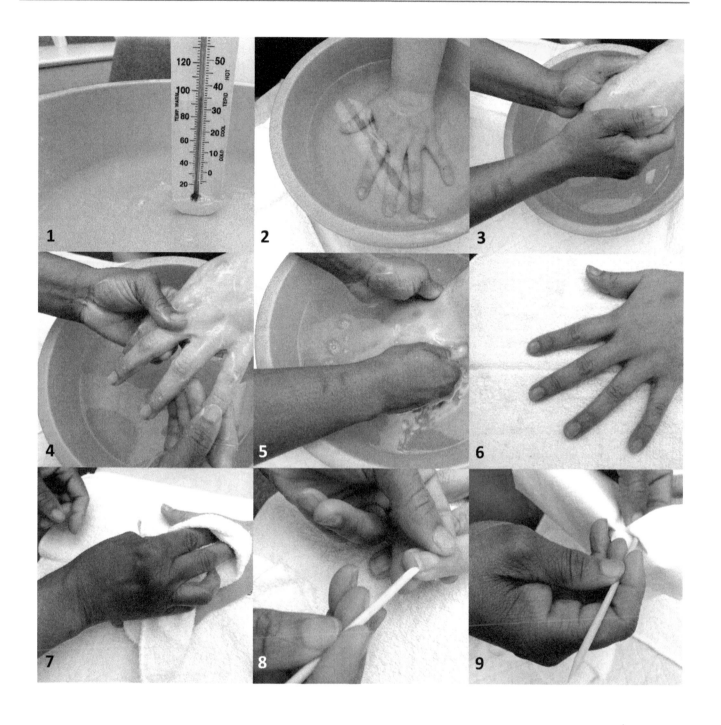

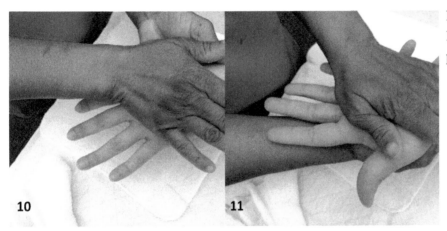

10   11

HAND AND NAIL CARE
Illustration for educational
purposes only.

COMPETENCY SKILLS 29: HOT COMPRESSES APPLICATION		
PERFORM THE FOLLOWING	YES	NO
LISTED STEPS:-		

Before starting the procedure make sure to check that the patient's plan does include a hot compress. Double check to see if you or a licensed healthcare professional will be performing it. If you are responsible for performing this procedure, then proceed as follows:

1. Identify your patient and start by greeting the patient, followed by introducing yourself.

2. Explain the procedure to the patient prior to performing it.

3. Maintain patient privacy by pulling the curtains to cover the area.

4. Perform standard precautions and infection control measures by washing hands and wearing gloves.

5. Collect equipment:

    i. Basin

    ii. Plastic wrap

    iii. Ties, tape or rolled gauze

    iv. Bath towel

    v. Waterproof bed protector

    vi. Small towel, washcloth or gauze

6. Place waterproof bed protector sheet under the body part receiving the compressed pack.

7. Fill a basin with one-half to two-thirds full with hot water.

8. Place compress in the hot water present in the basin.

9. Wring out the compress.

10. Observe and note any type of skin changes, prior to placing the compress.

	YES	NO

11. Apply the compress to specified area. Make sure to note the time of application.

12. Next, step would be to immediately cover the compress with a plastic wrap. Followed by covering it with the bath towel.

13. Secure the towel in place.

14. Give the patient a call light or bell. Make sure that this is within patients reach.

15. Check the area frequently every 3-5 minutes. Check for any changes in the skin after application of compress, also make sure to ask your patient if he/she is comfortable with the application. If the patient complains of any discomfort immediately remove the compress. Report this to the appropriate healthcare provider (nurse).

16. If the compress temperature drops, change the compress.

17. Compress should be removed after recommended duration. The area on which the compress was placed should be dried using a dry towel unless in some situation where contraindicated.

18. Clean and store equipment in an appropriate location as per the facility policy.

19. Remove gloves and wash hands appropriately.

20. Finally, document and report the following:
    a. Time,
    b. Site and
    c. Length of the application

COMPETENCY SKILLS 30: APPLYING COLD COMPRESSES

PERFORM THE FOLLOWING	YES	NO

LISTED STEPS:-

Before starting the procedure make sure to check that the patient's plan does include a cold compress. Double check to see if you or a licensed healthcare professional will be performing it. If you are responsible for performing this procedure then proceed as follows:

1. Identify your patient and start by greeting the patient, followed by introducing yourself.

2. Explain the procedure to the patient prior to performing it.

3. Maintain patient privacy by pulling the curtains to cover the area.

4. Perform standard precautions and infection control measures, by washing hands and wearing gloves.

5. Collect equipment:
    a. Large basin with ice
    b. Small basin with cold water
    c. Gauze squares, washcloths or towels
    d. Waterproof pad
    e. Bath towel

6. Place waterproof bed protector sheet under the body part receiving the compress pack.

7. Place small basin with cold water into a large basin with ice.

8. Place compress in the small basin.

9. Wring out the compress.

10. Observe and note any type of skin changes, prior to placing the compress.

11. Apply compress to specified area. Make sure to note the time of application.

12. Check the area frequently every 3-5 minutes. Check for any changes in the skin after application of compress, also make sure to ask your patient if he/she is comfortable with the application. If the patient complains of any discomfort immediately remove the compress. Report this to the appropriate healthcare provider (nurse).

13. If the compress temperature rises, change the compress.

14. Compress should be removed after recommended duration. The area on which the compress was placed should be dried using a dry towel unless in some situation where contraindicated.

15. Clean and store equipment in an appropriate location as per the facility policy.

16. Remove gloves and wash hands appropriately.

17. Finally, document and report the following:
    a. Time,
    b. Site and
    c. The length of the application.

COMPETENCY SKILLS 31: CARE OF AN NON-INFECTED DECUBITUS ULCER		
PERFORM THE FOLLOWING	YES	NO
LISTED STEPS:-		

1. Wash hands.

2. Collect equipment:
    a. Clean wash basin with warm water
    b. 4x4 gauze pads
    c. Skin cleansing agent
    d. Disposable gloves
    e. Towel or bed protector pad
    f. Plastic trash bag
    a. Heat lamp (if ordered)

3. Wear gloves (for cleaning).

4. Wash, disinfect and rinse basin well. Fill with warm water. Remove cleaning gloves.

5. Explain procedure to the patient.

6. Wash hands.

7. Open the prepackaged 4x4 gauze and place it in water (warm). This must be done without touching the gauze with hands or any objects.

8. Wear gloves.

9. Place a bed protector pad underneath the area of the body about to be cleansed.

10. Expose the non-infected ulcerated area.

11. Remove gauze previously placed in water (step 7), and gently cleanse the affected area starting from the center of the ulcer and washed outwardly.

OR

12. Place the area to be cleansed in the basin of water and use clean gauze to wipe affected area.

13. Next, **dry affected** area with clean gauze.

14. Inspect area for further skin breakdown and/or drainage.

15. Place a clean dressing over the affected area and/or as ordered by the plan of care

16. Position patient comfortably and safely so that the affected area is not under physical pressure.

17. Remove gloves and wash hands.

18. Document the following at procedure completion; date, time, observations and patient's response to procedure if any or applicable. Report observations to nurse.

COMPETENCY SKILLS 32: DEMONSTRATING A SKILL TO A PATIENT		
PERFORM THE FOLLOWING	**YES**	**NO**
LISTED STEPS:-		

1. Identify the task or skill selection as per plan.

2. Let the patient know that you will be demonstrating the skill or task.

3. Inform the patient that he/she will be required to observe the task while it is demonstrated.

4. Perform the task and explain each step of the task.

5. Check with the patient to see if he/she has any questions or concerns.

6. Ask the patient whether he/she would like to participate in learning the task or skill. Motivating the patient during this procedure may be required.

COMPETENCY SKILLS 33: TEACHING A TASK OR SKILL		
PERFORM THE FOLLOWING	**YES**	**NO**
LISTED STEPS:-		
1. Identify the task or skill to be performed as per plan.		
2. Check to see if the patient is ready for the task or skill to be performed. Decrease the number of distractions present where the task or skill is to be performed.		
3. **Caregiver:** Explain and/or demonstrate the skill or task (parts or whole).		
4. **Patient:** • First, the patient should be asked to "**EXPLAIN**" the steps in the proper sequence. • Next, the patient should be asked to "**PERFORM**" the steps in the proper sequence.		
5. Steps properly explained and performed should be praised (positive feedback as this helps in learning), while on the other hand the improper steps or steps that were skipped should be reminded and corrected.		
6. Finally, review and discuss the task or skill with the patient to see if there is any concern, or are there any areas which the patient needs more assistance with.		
7. Perform the task several times with the patient while giving appropriate feedbacks.		

SECTION 5: SPECIAL TOPICS PART I
Topic 1: Postural Imbalance

PATIENT CARE INTERVENTION: BODY POSTURE

Body mechanics is the correct use of muscles and joints to efficiently and safely perform an activity without application of undue pressure or strain on the muscles and joints.

Center of Gravity (COG)

- It is considered the "**balance point of the body**".
- Center of gravity shifts as the human body assumes different positions.
- When the center of gravity is low, the body is considered in a state of equilibrium, for example sitting and kneeling lowers the center of gravity and also increase the stability.
- When the center of gravity is high, the body is considered in a state of less equilibrium, for example running and jogging causes an upward shift of the center of gravity and therefore decreases the stability.

Two main factors that affect the center of gravity are

1. Base of support

- The wide base of support increases the possibility of maintaining balance. (Example: standing with feet apart)
- The narrow base of support decreases the possibility of maintaining balance. (Example: standing with feet close to each other)

2. Line of Gravity (aka gravity line):

It is an imaginary line vertically passing through the center of gravity down towards and within the base of support.

Line of gravity: from head to ankle

I. Head: gravity line falls anterior to the atlantooccipital joint.

II. Trunk: gravity line passes through the bodies of the lumbar and cervical vertebrae

III. Hip: gravity line varies with sway:
   a. When it passes through the joint, no external force is required.
   b. When it passes posterior to the joint, hip flexors comes into play.
   c. When it passes anterior to the joint, the hip extensors comes into play.

IV. Knee: gravity line is anterior to the joint.

V. Ankle: gravity line is anterior to the joint.

PAIN SYNDROMES RELATED TO POOR POSTURE

CROSS SYNDROME

UPPER CROSS SYNDROME:

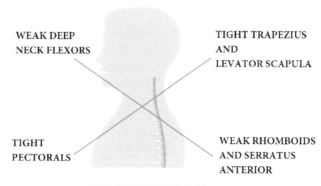

WEAK DEEP NECK FLEXORS

TIGHT TRAPEZIUS AND LEVATOR SCAPULA

TIGHT PECTORALS

WEAK RHOMBOIDS AND SERRATUS ANTERIOR

UPPER CROSS SYNDROME

Figure S.1

LOWER CROSS SYNDROME

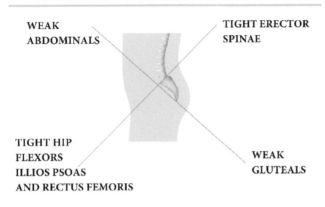

WEAK ABDOMINALS

TIGHT ERECTOR SPINAE

TIGHT HIP FLEXORS ILLIOS PSOAS AND RECTUS FEMORIS

WEAK GLUTEALS

LOWER CROSS SYNDROME

Figure S.2

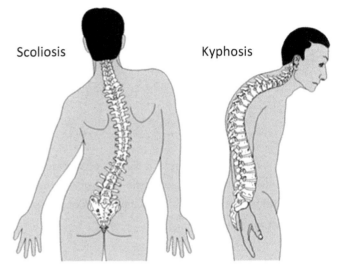

Scoliosis

Kyphosis

Figure S.3

CORRECT STANDING POSTURE:

- Body weight over both feet.
- Knees straight (not locked).
- Mild inward curve in the lower back.
- Shoulders back and relaxed.
- Chest held slightly up and forward.
- Top of head is oriented towards the ceiling, chin tucked in slightly, ears directly in line with shoulders.

CORRECT SITTING POSTURE:

- Feet are flat on the floor.
- Knees and hips bent at a 90-degree angle.
- The low back curve is supported by the chair or lumbar support.
- Upper and middle back must also be supported by the chair.
- Shoulder, chest and head positions are the same as standing.

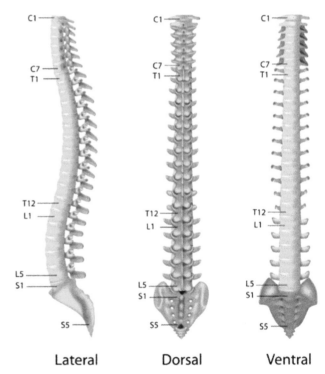

Lateral   Dorsal   Ventral

Figure S.4 Vertebral Column

COMMON POOR POSTURES

FAULTY POSTURE	CHARACTERISTICS	MUSCLE IMBALANCES
Lordosis	I. Increased lumbosacral angle II. Increased lumbar lordosis III. Increased anterior pelvic tilt IV. Increased hip flexion	I. Tight: hip flexors & lumbar extensor muscles II. Weak: abdominals
Relaxed	I. Pelvic shifted anteriorly II. Thoracic shifted posteriorly III. Hip extension IV. Flexion of thorax & upper lumbar spine	I. Tight: upper abdominals, intercostals, hip extensors, and lower lumbar extensor muscles II. Weak: lower abdominals, extensor muscles of lower thoracic & hip flexors
Flat low back	I. Decreased lumbosacral joint II. Decreased lumbar lordosis III. Hip extension IV. Posterior pelvic tilt	I. Tight: trunk flexors & hip extensors II. Weak: lumbar extensors & hip flexors
Rounded back or increased kyphosis	I. Increased kyphosis II. Protracted scapulae III. Forward head	I. Tight: anterior thorax muscles, upper extremity muscles originating on the thorax, cervical spine & head muscles attached to the scapula II. Weak: thoracic erector spinae & scapula retractors
Flat upper back	I. Decreased in thoracic curve II. Depressed scapulae III. Depressed clavicle IV. Flat neck posture	I. Tight: erector spinae & scapular retractors II. Weak: scapular protractor & intercostals muscles of anterior thorax
Forward head	I. Increased flexion of lower cervical & upper thoracic regions II. Increased extension of the occiput on 1st cervical vertebrae III. Increased extension of upper cervical vertebrae IV. Possible temporomandibular joint dysfunction	I. Tight: levator scapulae, sternocleidomastoid muscle, scalene, suboccipital muscles II. Weak: throat muscles, lower cervical, upper thoracic erector spinae muscles

Table S.1

SECTION 5: SPECIAL TOPICS PART I
Topic 2: Confusion & Dementia

Confusion can cause the inability to think quickly in order to make a decision. It may occur as a result of certain conditions, diseases, infections, loss of vision, loss of hearing, medication, and brain injury. Acute confusion (delirium) occurs suddenly and is usually temporary.

Delirium is a severe form of confusion with decreased awareness of one's environment and change in brain function.

Dementia is a term used to describe a decline in the mental ability (loss of cognitive function) of a person which is severe enough to interfere with routine personal, occupational and other activities. A person suffering from alzheimer's disease may have dementia. The condition occurs as a result of brain cell damage.

As per alzheimer's association, alzheimer's disease accounts for 60 to 80 percent of dementia cases.

Some other facts by alzheimer's association are:

- It is a progressive disease; its symptoms worsen over time.
- Dementia in early stages is mild and in the later stage is severe.

Stages of Alzheimer's disease as per alzheimer's association

Stage 1: No impairment: No signs or memory loss.

Stage 2: Very mild decline: Feeling of memory lapses, like forgetting familiar words or the location of daily routine elements.

Stage 3: Mild decline: Others notice the difficulty the person is facing. The person forgets the proper words or names, have problems remembering names, misplacing valuables and have trouble planning.

Stage 4: Moderate decline: Forgets recent events, the complex task becomes difficult.

Stage 5: Moderately severe decline: Identifying time of day, week and day problems. Having difficulty remembering their own address and phone number.

Stage 6: Severe decline: Personality and behavioral changes. Needs help with daily life activities. Remembers their own name. Have trouble remembering the name of family members.

Stage 7: Very severe decline: Ability to respond decline severely. Needs help with the majority of daily life activities.

Assisting patients who have memory loss, confusion or understanding problems:-

1. **Care plan**: know your patient care plan and proceed as recommended.
2. **Entering patient's room**: knock the door, address patients by their name.
3. **Introduction**: always introduce yourself.
4. **Identify**: always identify the patient.
5. **Behavior**: be respectful and kind to the patient.
6. **Communication**: try to keep the conversation simple, clear and short.
7. **Instructions**: address the patient in a respectful manner and repeat instructions as required.
8. **Listen**: do not talk when the patient is talking, listen to them first, give response by speaking slowly using simple words, and make sure to pronounce your words appropriately and accurately.
9. **Sensitive**: some patients many have mood changes. Do not be aggressive or agitated with such mood changes. Try to be in a neutral mood. If a patient is frustrated, give them time to calm down, and once calm, proceed and perform task slowly and appropriately.
10. **Offer options**: Make sure to provide options as this makes it easy to make decisions. Numerous options can make the patient confused and agitated.
11. **Corrections**: if a patient is wrong about what time of the day it is or what day is it, gently and respectfully let them know the correct details. Remind patient about the time and date of the day. Use of large sized calendars and clocks are recommended.
12. **Assistance**: appropriately assist the patient as required.
13. **Environment**: keep area bright and lighted with minimum to no noise or distractors.

14. **Fall prevention**: keep patients area clean and free from clutter that can cause fall(s). Check for any liquid on the floor. If present, immediately clean it. Provide patients with special slippers (non-skid). Provide the patient with an appropriate device to call for help.

15. **Sleep cycle**: have the patient rest at regular intervals.

16. **Feeding needs**: if required, assist the patient with feeding.

17. **Feedbacks**: provide patients with feedback, encourage the patient when they perform an activity successfully.

18. **Stress**: relaxation techniques must be practiced as per recommended facility policy.

19. **Needs**: ensure that all needs of the patients are met.

20. **Familiarity**: place similar objects in the close vicinity.

21. **Task performance**: perform the task in steps rather than as a whole.

22. **Visual cues**: provide visual cues appropriately.

SECTION 5: SPECIAL TOPICS PART I
Special Topic 3: Nutrition & Meal

NUTRITION
CARBOHYDRATE

The main function of carbohydrate in the human body is to:

- Provide energy for contracting muscles
- Acting as a fuel for the central nervous system
- Help enable fat metabolism
- Prevents utilization of protein for energy

Carbohydrate is considered a preferred source of energy for human body functions.

The two main forms of carbohydrates are:

Simple: small molecules and have small structures. They are broken down and absorbed easily by the digestive system. Provides rapid energy which lasts for short duration.

Examples: sugars, syrups, candy, lactose and honey.

Complex: large molecules and have large structures. They are slowly broken down and absorbed by the digestive system. Provides energy at a slow rate, which lasts for longer duration.

Examples: cereals, bread, pasta, potatoes, rice, whole grain, vegetables and in many fruits.

PROTEIN

Protein is made up of amino acids and is formed by a complex structure molecule. The body takes longer to break down proteins due to its complex structure. This is the reason why protein is a long-lasting source of energy. It is required to maintain the function of growth.

Examples: chicken, eggs, soy, fish and beef.

FAT

It is composed of fatty acid and glycerol. It also acts as a source of energy (an energy reserve). Fats also help in synthesizing hormones. It is required for optimal health. Another important role of fat is that it helps the body absorb vitamins.

Examples: butter and cream.

VITAMINS

Two types are water soluble and fat soluble. They can either be a macronutrient or micronutrient. They have numerous functions in the body. The water soluble vitamins travel through the blood stream and is used when required, while the body excretes the rest of it. The fat soluble vitamins remain in the body for a longer duration or till the body requires them.

Examples of both vitamins include: Vitamin A, B, C, D, and E.

MINERALS

Minerals are required for numerous functions within the human body. They are mainly two types macro-mineral and micro-mineral. There are various minerals found in the human body, and each has their own function(s).

Few functions of minerals are:

1) Act as a catalyst for body functions.
2) Maintain PH balance within the body.
3) Helps in the regulation of tissue growth.
4) Maintains nerve conduction.

Examples: calcium, iron, magnesium, chloride, potassium, zinc, iodine and phosphorus.

WATER

Functions to transport oxygen and nutrients from one location to another. It also helps in maintaining body temperature and in lubrication of joints and moistening of tissues such as eyes, mouth, and nose,

Dehydration

Can cause an increase in heart rate while trying to compensate for decreased blood supply to the organs. Some signs of dehydration are muscle cramps, dizziness, and fatigue.

Causes:

- Lower fluid intake.
- Excessive sweating.
- Improper replacement of fluids after activities.
- Weather conditions.

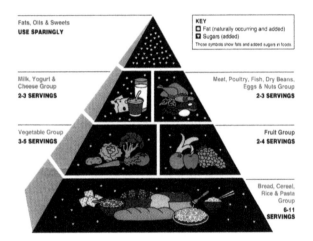

Figure S.5 Food Guide Pyramid

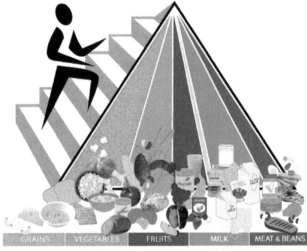

Figure S.6 My Pyramid

The U.S. Department of Agriculture (**USDA**) developed the Food Guide Pyramid to promote healthy eating practices later in response to new scientific information about nutrition, health, and new technology. A support tool "MyPyramid" was developed. My Pyramid replaces the Food Guide Pyramid. MyPyramid is basically a more personalized component that allows individual plans based on age, gender and activity level.

Build a healthy plate:-

Before you eat, think about what goes on your plate or in your cup or bowl. Foods like vegetables, fruits, whole grains, low-fat dairy products, and lean protein foods contain the nutrients you need without too many calories. Try some of these options.

- Make half your plate fruits and vegetables.
- Switch to skim or 1% milk.
- Make at least half your grains whole.
- Vary your protein food choices.

Cut back on foods high in solid fats, added sugars, and salt:-

Many people eat foods with too much of solid fats, added sugars, and salt (sodium). Added sugars and fats load foods with extra calories you do not need. Too much sodium may increase your blood pressure.

- Choose foods and drinks with little or no added sugars.
- Look out for salt (sodium) in foods you buy - it all adds up.
- Eat fewer foods that are high in solid fats.

Eat the right amount of calories for you:-

Everyone has a personal calorie limit. Staying within yours can help you get to or maintain a healthy weight. People who are successful at managing their weight have found ways to keep track of how much they eat in a day, even if they do not count every calorie.

- Enjoy your food, but eat less.
- Cook more often at home, you are in control of what's in your food.
- When eating out, choose lower calorie menu options.
- Write down what you eat to keep track of how much you eat.

Be physically active your way:-

Pick activities that you like and start by doing what you can, at least 10 minutes at a time. Every bit adds up, and the health benefits increase as you spend more time being active.

The food group recommendations of the pyramid are as follows:

The Grains

Includes all foods made from wheat, rice, oats, cornmeal, barley, such as bread, pasta, oatmeal and breakfast cereals.

What counts as a serving?

In general, 1 slice bread; 1 cup ready-to-eat cereal; 1/2 cup cooked rice, pasta, or cooked cereal.

The Vegetables

Includes all fresh, frozen, canned, and dried vegetables and vegetable juices.

What counts as a serving?

In general, 1 cup raw or cooked vegetables or vegetable juice; 2 cups raw leafy greens; 1 medium baked potato.

The Fruits

Includes all fresh, frozen, canned, dried fruits and fruit juices.

What counts as a serving?

In general, 1 cup fruit or 100% fruit juice; 1/2 cup dried fruit; 1 small apple; 1 medium pear; 1 large banana, orange, and peach

The Milk

Includes all fluid milk products or milk-containing foods that retain their calcium content, such as yogurt and cheese. Foods made from milk that have little to no calcium, such as cream cheese, cream, and butter, are not part of the Milk Group.

What counts as a serving?

In general, 1 cup milk or yogurt; 1 1/2 ounces natural cheese; 2 ounces processed cheese; 2 cups cottage cheese. Choose fat-free or low-fat foods to cut down on calories and fat.

The Meat & Beans

Includes lean meat, poultry, fish, egg, dry beans, nuts and seeds.

What counts as a serving?

In general, 1-ounce lean meat, poultry, fish; 1 egg; 1 tablespoon peanut butter; 1/4 cup cooked dry beans; 1/4 cup tofu; 1/2 ounce nuts or seeds.

SERVING FOOD

Serving food to geriatric patients is crucial, as the requirement for certain vitamins, minerals and proteins increases. Individuals having pressure ulcers may need an increased intake of protein, minerals and vitamins intake as this helps to decrease healing time. Some individuals may lose weight as a result of improper diet which may lead to weakness and illness. Also, as age advances, the digestive system mobility decreases. This calls for an increase in fiber intake to prevent constipation.

REQUIREMENT OF ASSISTANCE WHILE FEEDING

Mainly 3 types of individuals

Type 1: Needs Complete Assistance
Type 2: Needs Partial Assistance
Type 3: Needs No Assistance

Dysphagia

A condition in which an individual has difficulty swallowing food. Follow the plan recommended by your facility for such individuals.

Special Aids

Some individuals may need special aids for eating or drinking. These aids should be provided to them for the ease of independent feeding.

RESTORATIVE DINING PROGRAM

A restorative dining program helps patients to increase their independence during meals, while getting a complete diet. Restorative feeding programs use the skills of nursing, occupational therapy, speech therapy, a dietitian and others during dining. Residents in restorative feeding programs may:

- Get cues, or reminders, to eat.

- Have a plate guard to hold the food on the plate. Plate guards are safe for patients who are only able to use one hand or have weak hands.
- Use placemats that stop plates and cups from moving across the table.
- Drink fluids with a cup or glass that has a weight on the bottom to prevent it from tipping and spilling, a special handle so the patient can hold it, a built in straw or a spill-proof lid so that the liquid does not spill.
- Eat well with special forks, knives and spoons with special handles that can help in eating with little or no help.
- Have plates that have sections or high sides so that the food stays on the dish.
- Use protective clothing items to keep patients clothes free of food and fluids in order to maintain patient's dignity.

Technicians and assistants along with the healthcare professionals should always be present in a restorative dining room to direct the patient as needed to help them increase their independence with meals.

SERVING FOOD TO THE PATIENT

Precautions

1. The patient should be in a comfortable position.
2. Oral hygiene should be followed appropriately.
3. Promote independence.
4. Maintain appropriate room temperature. Hot food must be served hot and cold food must be served cold.
5. Food should be served fresh.
6. Always follow agency policy.

Reference:
USDA's Center for Nutrition Policy and Promotion
http://www.ers.usda.gov

SECTION 5:
SPECIAL TOPICS PART I
Special Topic 4:
Measurement of Intake and Output

MEASUREMENT OF INTAKE AND OUTPUT
PURPOSE

An intake and output (**I&O**) measurement may be ordered by a nurse or a doctor. Every fluid that the person drinks is called an **INTAKE**. This fluid enters the body and is absorbed by the body as per its requirements. The fluid that leaves the body is called the **OUTPUT**. Output includes urine, vomitus, diarrhea, and wound drainage. All kinds of oral fluids and foods that are melted at room temperature are measured and recorded. Nurse measures and records intravenous (IV) fluids and tube feedings. I&O records are used to evaluate fluid balance and kidney function. I&O measurements are also required when the patient has special fluid orders. The unit used to measure the intake and output is milliliters (mL). Following conversions are important to remember

1 ounce (oz.) equals 30 mL
1 pint is about 500 mL.
1 quart is about 1,000 mL.

Always familiarize yourself with the sizes of the serving bowls, dishes, cups, pitchers, glasses, and other containers used. A container used for measuring fluid is called a **graduate**. It is used to measure fluids, urine, vomitus, and drainage from suction. It is marked in ounces and milliliters. Hold the measuring device (graduate) on a flat surface at an **eye level** to read the amount of content.

An I&O record is usually available at the bedside within the patients I&O record card or sheet. Record the input in the input column and output in the output column. The sum of all the totals is performed at the end of the shift or as recommended. All the totals added are recorded in the patient's chart.

SECTION 5:
SPECIAL TOPICS PART I
Special Topic 5:
Ostomy and its Care

OSTOMY AND ITS CARE

A surgical opening created for the purpose of discharging body wastes. The protruding part that is created outside the body is called a stoma, which is the end of the ureter, small or large intestines.

Colostomy

Surgery performed to draw one end of the large intestine or colon through the incision in the anterior abdominal wall by creating an opening (stoma) in the anterior abdominal wall, followed by suturing it in place. This is done to allow the stool from the large intestine or colon to flow out through this opening into a bag or pouch. It may be **temporary** or **permanent**. It may further be defined by the section of the colon involved:

1. *Temporary Colostomy*
2. *Permanent Colostomy*
3. *Sigmoid Colostomy*
4. *Descending Colostomy*
5. *Transverse Colostomy*
6. *Loop Colostomy*
7. *Ascending Colostomy*

Ileostomy

Surgery performed to draw one end of the ileum (Small intestine) through the incision in the abdominal wall by creating an opening (stoma). This is done to allow the stool from the ileum (Small intestine) to flow out through this opening into a bag or pouch.

Urostomy

Surgery performed to create an opening (stoma) for the urinary system to allow the urine to flow directly outside the body in a urostomy pouch or bag.

OSTOMY CARE COMPETENCY CHECKLIST

Steps to be performed:

1. Identify your patient and start by greeting the patient and introducing yourself.
2. Explain the procedure to the patient.
3. Maintain patient privacy by pulling the curtains to cover the area.
4. Perform standard precautions and infection control measures, by washing hands.
5. Collect equipment:
Bed protector and blanket, ostomy bag and belt/appliance, toilet paper or gauze squares, towels, basin with warm water, soap or cleansing solution, clean dry washcloth, lotion as advised, disposable bags and gloves.
6. Position the patient appropriately. Avoid placing the patient towards the extreme edges of the bed. A safe position should always be maintained. Bed must be raised to an appropriate level comfortable to perform the procedure, followed by raising the head of the bed.
7. Protect bed linens prior to starting the procedure. Double check to see if the bed is not soiled after the procedure. Drape the patient appropriately to expose the ostomy area only.
8. Don PPE (GLOVES)
9. Remove the ostomy pouch or bag and place it in a recommended bag. Check for the amount, odor, color and characteristics of the ostomy pouch or bag contents.
10. Clean the skin around the stoma gently using a paper towel or gauze.
11. Wash the area away from the stoma in one direction using a washcloth containing soap water.
12. Using a dry towel, dry the area and apply lotion or cream, as recommended.
13. Apply an ostomy bag (clean) to the patient. Make sure that the bottom clamp of the bag is locked and not open.
14. Collect and place soiled sheets into the hamper, dispose the trash in an appropriate container. Rinse and dry the basin used for the procedure followed by placing it in a designated area.
15. Remove gloves and wash hands.
16. Lower patient's bed.
17. Any changes in the color of the stoma should be reported.
18. Patient's preference must be taken into consideration.
19. The patient should be comfortable before and during the procedure.
20. Know your patient's safety and rights during care.
21. Before leaving the patient, make sure to place the call light or other call signal device within the patient's reach.
22. Document the procedure.

SECTION 5: SPECIAL TOPICS PART I
Special Topic 6: Draping Techniques

DRAPING PATIENTS:

1. It provides exposure and access to areas which are required to be seen visually while performing patient care skills.
2. It provides modesty for patients by protecting other areas of the body.
3. It helps in keeping the body temperature balanced.
4. It provides protection of patient's clothing.

PRIOR TO DRAPING:

1. Patient must be informed about the procedure that will be performed.
2. Always explain the procedure to your patient.
3. Gain consent from the patient prior to performing the technique.
4. Give rationale to the patient about exposing the area.
5. Provide patient privacy by pulling curtains.
6. Maintain patient modesty prior, during and after the procedure.

DURING DRAPING:

1. Drape using an appropriate size clean cloth.
2. Draping should not restrict any joint movement.
3. Draping should be secured to avoid undue exposure of body parts.
4. Expose only the area that is required for the procedure.

DRAPING TYPES:

1. UPPER BODY COVER

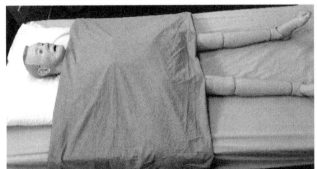

Figure S.8

2. LOWER BODY COVER

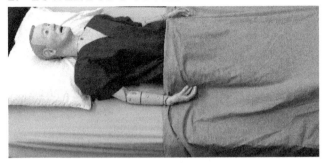

Figure S.9

3. LEFT SIDE BODY COVER

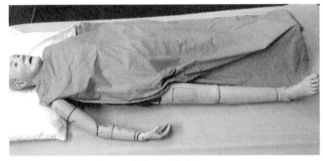

Figure S.10

4. PERICARE DRAPING

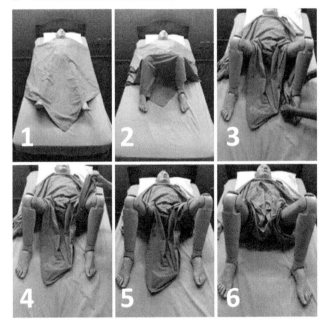

Figure S.10a

SECTION 5
END OF SECTION REVIEW QUESTIONS

Question Set 1: Essay Questions
45 points: 5 points each

1. Explain center of gravity.
2. Explain, in brief, the difference between confusion and dementia.
3. Explain the stages of alzheimer's disease.
4. List some strategies in dealing with a patient with memory loss, confusion or understanding problems.
5. Explain in brief about restorative dining program.
6. Explain in brief about nutrition and meal for patient care.
7. Explain in brief about the measurement of intake and output.
8. List and explain different types of ostomy.
9. Explain the importance of draping technique.

Question Set 2: True or False
6 points: 3 points each

1. The center of gravity is the balancing point of the body.
   Answer: True or False
2. Colostomy is the surgery performed to draw one end of the ileum (Small intestine) through the incision in the abdominal wall by creating an opening (stoma). This is done to allow the stool from the ileum (Small intestine) to flow out through this opening into a bag or pouch.
   Answer: True or False

Question Set 3: Match the Following
9 points 3 point each

Answer	Column 1	Column 2
	Ileostomy	Surgery performed to create an opening (stoma) for the urinary system to allow the urine to flow directly outside the body in a pouch or bag.
		Is the surgery performed to draw one end of the ileum
	Colostomy	(Small intestine) through the incision in the abdominal wall by creating an opening (stoma). This is done to allow the stool from the ileum (Small intestine) to flow out through this opening into a bag or pouch.
	Urostomy	Surgery performed to draw one end of the large intestine or colon through the incision in the anterior abdominal wall by creating an opening (stoma) in the anterior abdominal wall, followed by suturing it in place. This is done to allow the stool from the large intestine or colon to flow out through this opening into a bag or pouch.

Question Set 4: Multiple Choice
6 points: 3 points each

1) Which of the following component is not a part of the correct standing posture:
   a) Body weight over the middle of your feet.
   b) Knees bend.
   c) Mild inward curve in lower back.
   d) Shoulders back and relaxed.
   e) Chest held slightly up and forward.
   f) Top of head is oriented towards the ceiling, chin tucked in slightly, ears directly in line with shoulders.
2) Which of the following component is not a part of the correct sitting posture:
   a) Feet are flat on the floor.
   b) Knees and hips bent at a 45-degree angle.
   c) The low back curve is supported by the chair or lumbar support.
   d) Upper and middle back must also be supported by the chair.
   e) Shoulder, chest, and head positions are the same as in standing.

SECTION 6: SPECIAL TOPICS PART II
Special Topic 7: Aphasia & Types

APHASIA

A disorder that affects a person's ability to communicate due to an injury sustained on the part of the brain that processes language. Most commonly seen in older adults with stroke.

Language processing becomes difficult

- Decreased ability to comprehend words,
- Decreased ability to use words and
- Decline in ability to speak words.

BROCA'S APHASIA (Expressive Aphasia)

This is a type of aphasia in which the person is unable to say what he/she wants to say. It is also called expressive or nonfluent aphasia. Expressing one's self becomes difficult. Patients with this type of aphasia are frustrated.
Patients with this conditions are:

- *Able to say basic words.*
- *Have difficulty forming complete sentences.*

WERNICKE'S APHASIA (Receptive Aphasia)

This is a type of aphasia in which the person is unable to understand spoken or written language. Patient is unaware of the fact that the words spoken are not correct. This severely affects the patient's ability to comprehend words or spoken language, but can speak words.

GLOBAL APHASIA

This type of aphasia is a combination of problems. The problems associated with this type of aphasia are

- Person is unable to say what he/she wants to say.
- Expressing one's self becomes difficult.

- Person is unable to understand language spoken or written. Patient is unaware of the fact that the words spoken are not correct

It is a widespread impairment and also the most severe form.

PRIMARY PROGRESSIVE APHASIA

A disorder which causes degenerative changes in the brain leading to aphasia over the period of time. It progresses slowly over time, hence known as progressive aphasia.

MIXED NONFLUENT APHASIA

This is considered a severe form of **Broca's Aphasia**. In this type of aphasia, the speech is sparse and effortful. Understanding is limited, and the patient may not be able to read or write beyond a certain level.

ANOMIC APHASIA

Anomia can be defined as an inability of an individual to recall names of objects, places, and people. Anomic aphasia deals with word finding problems and is considered a least severe form.

Strategies to communicate with aphasic patients:

1) Before starting your communication with the patient, make sure you have his or her attention. Make eye contact with the patient.
2) While instructing the patient, break down the instructions into parts.
3) Distractions like loud noise should be minimized or eliminated during communication.
4) If the patient is unable to understand you, do not shout at the patient. Be patient and explain it again.
5) Simplify your communication by using short and easy to understand statements.
6) Avoid giving too many options as this may cause confusion.
7) Allow the patient to speak and give them time to respond after you are done speaking to them.

8) Incorporate use of hand gestures, drawings and writings into your communication skills as required to communicate with the patient (aphasic).

9) Do not overload them with thoughts, involve them in normal activities.

10) During communication, try taking a pause after several words as required according to the severity of the condition and comprehension level of the patient.

11) Use keywords in your sentences.

12) Pay attention to the facial expression of the patient.

SECTION 6: SPECIAL TOPICS PART II

Special Topic 8:

CPR, AED & Abdominal Thrust

Cardiopulmonary Resuscitation (CPR)

Competency Skills for performing CPR.

1. Call for help first.

2. Kneel on the victim's side and check for responsiveness from the victim. If unresponsive, place the victim onto their back. The surface should be flat.

3. For Compression: - Place the heel of your hand on the victim's chest. The location would be the center of the chest. Now place your other hand over your first hand and interlock or intertwine your fingers (fig S.11). Once this position is attained, start giving compressions. Compressions should be hard and fast, the depth of the compression should be 2 inches (5cm) but not more than 2.4 inches. While you are delivering the compressions, keep counting them. Once you reach a count of 30 compressions, proceed toward the airway. The rate of compressions should be 100 to 120 compressions per minute. Avoid leaning on the victim's chest when delivering compressions, since leaning on the victim's chest would not allow the chest to recoil. Note: for Infants the depth of compression is 1.5 inches, and for children, the depth of compression is 2inches.

4. For Airway: - Tilt the victim's head back and lift the chin to open the airway passage. Using your forefinger and thumb, close the victim's nose.

5. For Breaths:- Next, step would be to deliver the breaths, this can be done by taking in a normal breath and covering victim's mouth with your mouth in order to completely seal the area to prevent the escape of air. Once done, give 2 breaths and while doing so check to see if the victim's chest rises and falls.

6. Again deliver 30 compressions followed by 2 breaths. Continue the cycle until medical help arrives.

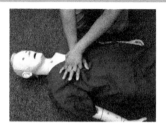

Chest Compressions
Figure S.11

Automated External Defibrillator

Competency Skills for Using AED

1. Turn on the AED device.
2. Select the correct size pads to be used on the victim.
3. Attach the AED pads onto the victim's chest as illustrated on the AED machine unit.

• The victim's chest should be bare and dry. Remove the covering on the adhesive side of the AED pads. Using the illustration on the package, attach them firmly to the chest. ***Please note***: *it is extremely important to place pads correctly. One pad is placed on the victim's upper right chest area while the other is on the lower left chest area. Thick chest hair must be removed before placing the adhesive pad to have adequate contact.*

4. Allow the AED device to analyze the current heart rhythm of the victim.

• Several AED devices automatically analyze the heart rhythm, while other AED devices will prompt the rescuer to activate an analyze button. Make sure no one is in contact with the victim while the heart rhythm is being analyzed.

• If the AED indicates "shock", continue to step 5.

- If the AED indicates that the victim is not in need of a shock, check pulse again. If there is absence of pulse, proceed to attempt CPR for one minute and analyze again. Continue sequence every minute until the help arrives.

5. When the AED gives a verbal command for shock advised, press the shock button.

Some precautions while applying AED:

1. If the victim is covered with water or in water, move the victim away from water. Wipe away water from the victim's chest and then apply pads. For example: victim near a swimming pool or covered in sweat.

2. If the victim has a pacemaker, ensure that the application of pads is atleast 1 inch away from the pacemaker.

3. If the victim has hair on the chest:

a. Firmly press down on the skin.

b. If the AED cannot detect the pads applied, remove the pads and retrieve razor from the AED Kit and shave the designated area of use.

c. Apply a new set of pads on the recently shaved victim's chest and continue the procedure.

PUTTING ON A SLING

Steps in making a sling

1. Get a piece of cloth (square in shape) and fold it in half diagonally, shaping it into a triangle.

2. Using this triangular piece of cloth, have the patient bend the elbow (assistance should be provided as required).

3. Place the triangular end of the cloth pointing towards the elbow.

4. With the other two ends:-

a. One end passes underneath the elbow and behind the neck passing over the opposite shoulder.

b. Other end passes over the elbow and behind the neck passing over the same shoulder.

c. Both the end meet behind the neck, which is then tied together.

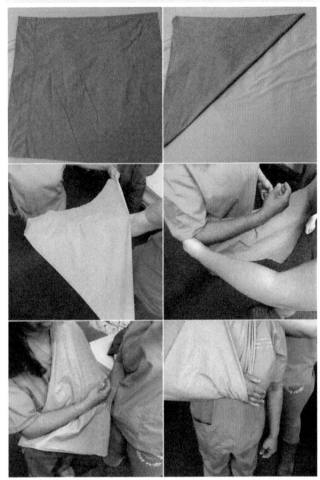

Figure S.12 Putting on a Sling

ABDOMINAL THRUSTS

STEPS

Competency skills for delivering abdominal thrust:-

1. Position yourself appropriately behind the victim who is choking.

2. Place arms around the victim's waist.

3. Make a fist just above the navel, thumb side into the victim.

4. Grab the fist with the other hand and push inward and upward, in one swift motion.

5. Repeat step 4, until the object is expelled.

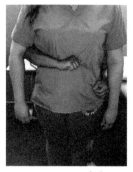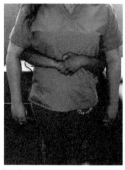

Abdominal Thrust

Figure S.13

SECTION 6: SPECIAL TOPICS PART II

Special Topic 9: Patient Defense Mechanism

Primitive Defense Mechanisms

1. DENIAL

A phase in which the individual does not accept reality or facts and tries to deny the events that have happened in the past.

2. REGRESSION

A reversal to a former or earlier stages of development. For example: acting childish.

3. ACTING OUT

Expressing one's self with an extreme behavior as one feels that he or she cannot express themselves otherwise.

4. DISSOCIATION

In this type of defense mechanism, the individual disconnects from their thoughts, feelings, memories or sense of identity.

5. COMPARTMENTALIZATION

In this type of defense mechanism there is:
- The existence of conflicting ideas that exists at the same time. The individual does not acknowledge the existence of the conflicting ideas creating a compartment, thereby separating values in each compartment.
- The individual may have negative and positive ideas, and keeps them separate from each other.
- May have **several identities** instead of **an identity**.

6. PROJECTION

In this type of defense mechanism,
- The individual puts their own feelings and undesired thoughts onto other people.
- The individual in projection denies the existence of negative qualities that they may have and ascribes such qualities (negative) on others.
- For example: Mr. X does not trust his friend, but will feel that his friend does not trust him.

7. REACTION FORMATION

In this type of defense mechanism the individual does the opposite of what they feel or think. For example: Mr. Y does not like Mr. X's new car, but will admire it in Mr. X's presence.

8. REPRESSION

In this type of defense mechanism the individual blocks the unwanted or unaccepted feelings, memories and thoughts. The blocking occurs unconsciously. For example; an adult went through child abuse as a child. When the child grows into an adult and is asked about the child abuse, the adult may not remember any instance of child abuse.

9. DISPLACEMENT

In this type of defense mechanism, the individual diverts the thoughts and feelings of one person or object onto a less threatening person or object. For example: "Z" slams the door on his way out of the classroom, after his teacher scolded him. In this example, the door is the weaker object.

10. INTELLECTUALIZATION

In this type of defense mechanism, an individual is confronted by an unwanted situation. The individual then engages in abstract thinking rather than facing the situation. For example; a person is told about his terminal medical condition and rather than showing his emotions towards the situation he/she starts asking questions about available treatment options.

11. RATIONALIZATION

In this type of defense mechanism the individual makes excuses or gives rationale or logical explanations in order to avoid the truth. For example; "I would have scored higher in the exam, but the exam was tough". The fact is that the individual was under-prepared and therefore could not achieve high scores.

12. UNDOING

In this type of defense mechanism the individual tries to undo the unwanted behavior or thoughts.
For example: Mr. X is excessively praising his wife after having insulted her.

13. SUBLIMATION

In this type of defense mechanism the individual transforms the unacceptable thoughts and emotions into less harmful or more acceptable ones. It is considered as one of the most constructive defense mechanisms. For example: a person is angry about something and starts exercising.

14. COMPENSATION

In this type of defense mechanism the individual tries to compensate the areas of weakness with their strengths. For example; a person may say "I may not be able to do this, but i can definitely do that".

15. ASSERTIVENESS

In this type of defense mechanism the individual expresses themselves effectively and non-aggressively while respecting the rights of others.

SECTION 6:
SPECIAL TOPICS PART II
Special Topic 10:
Admission, Discharge & Transfer

ADMISSIONS, DISCHARGE, AND TRANSFER
ADMISSION
This sets the patient's entry into a health care facility.
DISCHARGE
This sets the patient's release from a health care facility.
TRANSFER
This sets the patient from one unit to another unit, or from hospital to another nursing unit, or from one health care facility to another health care facility.

Assistants and technicians play a major role in patients or residents admission, discharge and transfer procedure. It takes time for the patient to acclimate to the surroundings when admitted into the healthcare facility. This accommodation period can be shorter if the technician and assistants make the patient environment pleasant by using the right communication skills and fulfill the needs as applicable. This is the first time the assistant and/or technician encounters the patient or resident. Communication at this point of contact is crucial. Techniques and procedures performed should always be performed within the scope of practice for your chosen profession. Every facility has their own policy and procedure plan for admitting, transferring and discharging patients.

I. ADMISSION PROCESS FOR PATIENTS OR RESIDENTS

A. PREPARING THE ROOM

The room should be prepared prior to the resident's or patient's arrival, as this provides a feeling of comfort. The room should be well lighted and ventilated. Remember, it is not easy to acclimate in a new setting. Make sure that the room is clean. The bed is made neatly, check to see if all the supplies are available. Have an admission kit ready.

Admission kit includes:
1. Basin
2. Emesis basin and urinals (male/female)
3. Pitcher (water)
4. Glass (drinking water)
5. Toothpaste
6. Soap, lotion, napkins and towels
7. Comb.
8. Overbed trapeze (If applicable)

B. ARRIVAL

On patient or resident arrival make sure to:-
- Note the time of arrival,
- Also keep a note of the condition,
- Check to see if the patient or resident requires use of assistive devices,
- Make attempts to check for patient's level of consciousness and the state in which the arrival occurs,
- Check for any attachments patient may have, such as a catheter bag, ostomy pouch or anything that can be seen visually.

C. GREETING

Start by introducing yourself with your credentials. This process should be done in a pleasant manner. The process should be at a speed that the patient or resident does not feel that it all happened in a rush. If possible try introducing the new patients or residents to the other patients or residents in the room.

D. FAMILIARIZATION

Most of the patients admitted to the healthcare facility are nervous. This may be due to the new environment that they are entering into or a fear of being in the hospital. Help patients or residents adjust to the healthcare facility. Explain the patient about healthcare policy that the facility might want the patient to know and familiarize with. A short tour of the facility if required must be provided to the patient, just to familiarize with the environment. Let the patient know about their rights. Show the patients or residents on how to operate certain equipment like operating a call bell, controlling the bed and operating a television. Explain the patient or resident about the breakfast, lunch and dinner time. Show the storage space to the patient, and let the patient know that his or her belongings can be kept in the designated storage space. Depending on the facility policy, a list of the patients or residents belongings should be prepared by the assistants and/or technicians and signed by the patient or resident or their family members.

E. GETTING READY

Pull the screen for patient privacy and ask the patient to change to either more comfortable gown (facility) or clothes from home as required by the facility policy. Most facility would require the technicians and assistants to record the vital signs within their scope of practice and fill out a short questionnaire which may include any allergies the patient has or any condition that he or she may be aware of at the time of admission. Once done, have the patient sit in the chair or lay on the bed as to their preference. Offer to raise the head of the bed for a comfortable sitting position on the bed. Check the supervisor (nurse) instructions if the side rails are to be raised. Place the call bell within the patient's reach.

F. RECORD

As per admission policy of your facility, record all the data and complete the admission checklist appropriately.

SUMMARY OF ADMISSION PROCEDURE:
1. Prepare the room.
2. Wash your hands.

3. Introduce yourself.
4. Explain the procedure to the patient or resident.
5. Provide privacy to the patient or resident to change his or her clothes.
6. Record vital signs, height, and weight, in some cases, specimen collections may also be required.
7. Introduce the patient to other patients.
8. Show the storage space for keeping their (patient or resident) belongings.
9. Show the bathroom and its use, as per facility policy.
10. Place call light within patient's or resident's reach.
11. Wash your hands.
12. Document the encounter and record the assessments.

II. TRANSFERRING THE PATIENT OR RESIDENT

A. TRANSFER REASONS

Few reasons for the transfer:
1. Change in the health status that might require a more specialized treatment or observation.
2. Change of room due to equipment failure (bed).
3. Change at patient's or resident's request.
4. Change at physician's request.
5. Change at medical staff's request.

B. PROCESS
1. Inform the patient about the transfer.
2. All the patient's or resident's items should be collected carefully. Double check the storage area to see if all the patient or resident items have been collected.
3. Some equipment may also be transferred along with the patient or resident. Follow instructions from the supervisors.
4. Patient's or resident's transfer must be recorded on the patient's or resident's record or chart. The details may include the location of the transfer, time of transfer, patient's reaction towards transfer and the rationale for transferring the patient.

C. TRANSFER LOCATION PREPARATION

As discussed in the admission procedure about preparing the room, the same should be done while transferring the patient from one room to another.

SUMMARY OF TRANSFER PROCEDURE:
1. Wash your hands.
2. Identify yourself and your patient.
3. Inform and explain the procedure to the patient.
4. Collect patient belongings.
5. Assist patient to transfer.
6. After transfer, have the patient comfortably situated.
7. Show the storage area and place all personal belongings appropriately.
8. Introduce the patient to other patients.
9. Give time to accommodate.
10. Record vital signs, height and weight if required.
11. Place call light within patient's or resident's reach.
12. Wash your hands.
13. Document the encounter and record the other assessments.

III. DISCHARGING THE PATIENT OR RESIDENT

In this stage, the patient or resident is discharged from the facility. The assistant or technician may assist the patient or resident in packing his or her belongings. Make sure that all the patient's or resident's belongings are packed. Check the storage area. Give patient or resident the privacy they require to change their clothes since they are getting discharged. Offer assistance as required. Always try and promote independence. Know your patients or residents condition at discharge. Any questions aroused by the patient should be addressed and answered within your scope of practice. If this is not within your scope of practice, inform the supervisor about the questions patient or resident addressed. These questions can be directly addressed and answered to the patient by the supervisor (nurse or appropriate healthcare providers). The healthcare team does discharge planning. A physician writes the discharge plan; nurses make sure that the discharge plan is written by the physician and will start taking the appropriate steps to initiate the discharge procedure. Patient or resident may be asked to follow recommended guidelines as a part of patient education; this is given by the physician or the nurse during the discharge process. A written copy of the instructions may also be provided to the patient. In some cases, a follow-up visit may be required, which may be addressed during the discharge process. Informing the family about the discharge is important since they may also have to make some arrangements to take the patient or resident home.

1. Double check that the discharge has been officially ordered.
2. Wash your hands.
3. Identify yourself and your patient or resident.
4. Explain the procedure to the patient or resident.
5. Make sure to follow the discharge checklist appropriately.
6. Provide privacy to the patient or resident to change his or her clothes.
7. Collect patient belonging.
8. Answer questions within the scope of your practice.
9. Help patient or resident as per assistance required during discharge.
10. Wash your hands.
11. Document the patient or resident encounter, which may include the time of discharge, assistance required during discharge, vital signs (if recorded) at discharge, and document any other details of the patients or residents as required.
12. Lastly, clean the patient or resident room and make it ready for the next patient or resident admission or transfer.

SECTION 6: SPECIAL TOPICS PART II
Special Topic 11: Activities of Daily Living

What are the Activities of Daily Living (ADLs)?
The Activities of Daily Living are basic activities performed by an individual on a daily (regular, everyday) basis necessary for living independently within their home or within the community.

5 basic categories of activities of daily living are:

1. **Transferring:** this includes the ability of the patient or resident to moving oneself from seated to standing and getting in and out of bed.
2. **Maintaining Continence:** this includes the ability of the patient or resident to use the restroom (mental or physical).

3. **Dressing:** this includes the ability of the patient or resident to appropriate clothing decisions and physically dress oneself.
4. **Personal hygiene:** this includes the ability of the patient or resident to bathing, grooming and oral care.
5. **Eating:** this includes the ability of the patient or resident to feed oneself but not necessarily to prepare food.

The patient's or resident's ability to perform or not perform the activities with partial or complete dependence serves as a comparative measure of their independence.

What are the Instrumental Activities of Daily Living (IADLs)?
IADLs activities are crucial for an individual in order to be independent.

The IADLs include:

1. *Ability to perform basic communication skills.*
2. *Ability to perform transportation (driving using public transportation).*
3. *Ability to prepare a meal.*
4. *Ability to shop or make purchases.*
5. *Ability to perform housework.*
6. *Ability to manage their medications, like taking the appropriate dosage at the right time(s) as recommended.*
7. *Ability to manage personal finances.*

Why are ADLs and IADLs important?

A patients or residents ability to perform the ADLs and IADLs is crucial, not only to determine the level of assistance they may need but also for the type of services they make require.

FOUR STEPS OF ADL PERFORMANCE
Step 1:
Choose an activity.
Step 2:
Have the patient perform the selected activity.
Step 3:
Analysis the functional deficit, check to see if a joint, muscle or other structures are involved.
Step: 4

<table>
<tr><td>

Post-analysis plan
Based on involvement of:
1. Joint
2. Muscle
3. Other Structures

Note: post analysis plan are to be performed by an appropriate healthcare professional.

</td></tr>
</table>

Precautions:

1. Do not over perform the activities.
2. Do not cross the painful range threshold while performing range of motion.
3. Do not cause discomfort to the patient while performing the therapeutic exercise.
4. Know your patient's health condition status prior to performing any technique(s).
5. Understand the functional limitation that the patient may have.

ACTIVITIES OF ADL

1. Feeding
2. Dressing
3. Grooming
4. Toileting
5. Transferring
6. Counting object
7. Moving objects
8. Making bed
9. Change bed sheet
10. Cleaning floor
11. Cleaning table
12. Picking up coin
13. Opening bag
14. Opening door
15. Wearing shoes
16. Wearing socks
17. Lifting objects
18. Folding clothes
19. Unwrapping
20. Overhead activity
21. Reaching out activity
22. Balancing activity
23. Walking
24. Jogging
25. Running
26. Clapping
27. Side-lying reach
28. Prone reach
29. Supine reach
30. Supine to stand

Types of Hand Grips

Power Grip: requires power and appropriate finger flexor symmetry.

TYPES OF POWER GRIPS:-

- cylindrical grip (holding a bottle by its belly)
- spherical grip (holding a tennis ball)
- hook grip (holding carrying bags)
- lateral prehension (grasping)

Precision Grip: this grip is used for performing skilled activities.

TYPES OF PRECISION GRIPS:-

- palmar prehension (holding a pencil to write)
- tip-to-tip (holding a coin tip to tip between fingers)
- lateral prehension (holding a card)

SPECIAL AIDS REQUIRED FOR ACTIVITIES OF DAILY LIVING (ADL)

Button hook

This is a special aid used for individuals who have difficulty unbuttoning or buttoning clothes they wear.

The parts of a button hook consist of a handle and a wire loop. Slide the wire loop through the button hole and have the button sit within the wire loop. Next pull back the wire loop with the button into the buttonhole which causes the buttoning.

Zipper pull

This is a special aid used for individuals who have difficulty zipping or unzipping clothes they wear.

The parts of a zipper pull consist of an extended handle and a hook. The hook is connected through the zipper hole. This makes it easy to pull the zipper.

Handwriting aid

This is a special aid used for individuals who have difficulty with precision grips. The difficulty may enable the individual to write using a pen or pencil. To ease this, a foam gripper is put on the pen or pencil which makes the surface larger and easy to hold. The foam gripper can be used on any similar objects with which the individual might have trouble holding. For example, spoons, toothbrush, etc.

Key holder

This is a special aid used for individuals who have difficulty with precision grips and lacks hand strength.

Parts of the key holder consists of a handle on the back end and a key holder on the front end. The key is attached to the front end. The individual grips the handle to lock the key into the lock and turn the handle clockwise or counter-clockwise to either lock or unlock.

Bath mitt

A type of special aid worn over the hand. It covers to the extent of the wrist. Individual holds the soap and puts on the mitt; the mitt also functions as a washcloth. It is usually used for individuals having difficulty in holding soap.

Rocker knife

It is utilized by individuals having difficulty using a regular knife to cut food. The rocker knife is a special aid with an enlarged handle and a curved blade. The individual using this must do so by gripping the handle and cutting the food with the curve blade, using a rocking movement.

Doorknob extenders

A special aid used for opening door knobs or other knobs as recommended by the manufacturer. The knob extender provides an extended handle that provides a large surface area to grip and manipulate while opening the door.

Bottle Opener

A special aid that sits on top of the bottle cap or jar and minimum strength is required to turn. This turning causes the jar or the bottle to open.

Loop scissors or Easy Grip Scissors

A special aid that assist individuals in cutting an object that they are unable to cut using a regular scissor due to the requirement of its complex grip. The loop scissors require a squeezing movement to cut the object and make it easy for an individual to use it.

Long Straw

If an individual is unable to drink water using the glass by lifting it, a long straw is used to assist in drinking water.

Gripping Utensils

A set of special aid utensils that consist of a tablespoon, tea spoon, rocker knife and fork. The heads of all the utensils may be angled to make it easier for the individual to eat without having to bend the wrist joint. The gripping part of the utensils are large, making it easy to hold.

Reacher

A special aid that helps an individual reach and grasp an object from a distance. The reacher has a trigger handle on the back end and a gripper clip on the front end. Using the trigger handle, the individual can cause the gripper end to open and close. This movement of opening and closing of the gripper end can help grasp the object from a distance.

Table/Chair Riser and Toilet Seat Riser

A special aid used to raise the height of the table or chair as per requirements for fitting the individual's need. The risers are placed underneath the legs of the tables or chairs to raise the height.

The toilet seat riser is also a type of riser with the same function of increasing the height of the toilet seat so that the individual can sit at a higher level. This may help the individual in standing up easily since it is easier to stand up from a higher surface than from a lower surface.

Universal cuff

A special aid that looks like a band and can be wrapped around the individual's hand. It is used to grip a pencil, pen, utensil, toothbrush, etc. The reason it is called universal cuff is that it can be used to manipulate various objects.

Elastic shoe laces

Converts the laced shoe into a slip-on shoe.

Long handle comb

Makes is easy to comb hairs using minimum reach.

Sock aid

A special aid used to put on a sock. Put on the sock on the front end of the sock aid. Place the foot into the sock aid. Using the gripping ropes on the back end, pull the sock aid towards you. This motion will cause the sock to cover your foot and ankle.

Leg Lifter

Used by individuals that require assistance in lifting their legs from the floor and placing it at a higher surface. Leg Lifter's **front end** consist of a **foot loop,** whereas the **back end** consist of the **grip**. The individual places the foot into the front end loop and pulls the leg lifter unit using the back end grip to direct the placement of the leg as desired.

Toilet aids

Some of the toilet aids are grab bars on walls, rails on the bath tub, folding shower bench, hand-held shower, non-slip mats and toilet tissue aid.

SECTION 6
END OF SECTION REVIEW QUESTIONS

Question Set 1: Essay Questions
100 points

1. What is aphasia? **5 points**
2. List and explain different types of aphasia's. **5 points**
3. List the steps involved in performing CPR. **5 points**
4. List the steps involved in performing AED. **5 points**
5. How to put on a sling? **5 points**
6. How to deliver abdominal thrust for choking patient? **5 points**
7. Explain different types of primitive defense mechanisms. **2 points each**
   a. Denial
   b. Regression
   c. Acting out
   d. Dissociation
   e. Compartmentalization
   f. Projection
   g. Reaction formation
   h. Repression
   i. Displacement

   j. Intellectualization
   k. Rationalization
   l. Undoing
   m. Sublimation
   n. Compensation
   o. Assertiveness
8. Explain the process of admission, discharge and transfer. **5 points**
9. Explain about ADL and its importance. **5 points**
10. Explain IADL and its importance. **5 points**
11. What are the 4 steps of performing ADL? **5 points**
12. Explain in brief about special aids. **1 point each**
    1) Button hook
    2) Zipper pull
    3) Handwriting aids
    4) Key holder
    5) Bath mitt
    6) Rocker knife
    7) Doorknob extenders
    8) Bottle opener
    9) Loop scissors
    10) Long straw
    11) Gripping utensils
    12) Reacher
    13) Table/Chair Risers
    14) Universal cuff
    15) Elastic Shoe Lace
    16) Long Handle Comb
    17) Sock Aid
    18) Leg Lifter
    19) Toilet Aids
    20) Toilet Seat Risers

SECTION 7: SPECIAL TOPICS PART III
Special Topic 12: Levels of Need

According to Maslow, there are five levels of needs:-

1. Biological and Physiological Needs

Basic things required for biological and physiological needs such as air, food, drink (water), shelter, warmth, sex, sleep, and breathing. If the biological and physiological needs are not met the human body may not continue to function.

2. Safety Needs

After the biological and physiological needs are met, the next stage of the levels of need is the safety needs; this makes us feel secure to live our life.
Examples would be; security, law and order, stability, freedom from fear and protection from certain elements
Real life examples; securing your job, getting insurance (life), saving earning for future and being healthy.

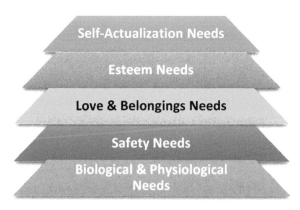

Figure S.14 LEVELS OF NEED

3. Love and Belonging Needs

After biological/physiological and safety needs are met, the next stage of human needs are the love and belonging needs. This involves emotions and feelings. It makes us feel that we need love and care. Humans need to feel the love and belonging, at the same time, we need acceptance from other individuals. The absence of this may lead to unconscious stress for example; depression, a sense of loneliness or not being accepted.
Examples of love and belonging needs would be: friendship, intimacy, affection and love, family, friends, romantic relationships.

4. Esteem Needs

After the love and belonging needs are met, the next stage of human needs are the self-esteem needs. Humans have a need for self-respect and self-esteem. The absence of this may lead to an inferiority complex. Humans usually get involved in a task which gives them a sense of accomplishment. There are two types of esteem

- High
- Low

Example would be: achievement, mastery, independence, status, dominance, prestige, self-respect, and respect from others.

5. Self-Actualization Needs

This is the final stage of human needs as per the levels of need. In this stage, the individual realizes the potential he or she has, which is then achieved by self-fulfillment. The individual explores himself to the fullest potential and talents which is a drive or a need that is present in every individual.

SECTION 7: SPECIAL TOPICS PART III

Special Topic 13: Aging and Its Changes

AGING

Aging is a gradual and a continuous process that takes place during one's lifetime. During this process, the bodily function tends to decline, and physical changes are visible.

THREE TYPES OF AGING:

Chronological aging: based on time. It is usually counted in years. For example; Mr. Jones is 64 years old. This number "64" is considered the chronological age.

Biological aging: based on biological changes that take place in the human body. This can occur at an early age.

Psychological aging: based on thoughts. Aging in this type is characterized on the basis of the individual's thoughts.

Theories of aging

Cellular level aging

Each cell has its own function in the human body, as age advances, the function of the cells decline. In order for new cells to develop, the old cells are destroyed by the body via a process called apoptosis. Apoptosis is the process of programmed cell death (PCD).

Telomere Shortening Aging Theory

The cell divides and gives rise to another set of cells. According to the telomere shortening aging theory, the cells divide to a stage after which the cells can no longer divide due to shortening in size. As per this theory, older adults have a short telomere; this keeps becoming shorter after which the division of the cell becomes difficult.

Cross-Linkage Theory

Protein molecules stick to each other forming a cross-linkage. This cross-linking is rare in young individuals and increases in older individuals, the increase in the number of cross-linkage causes stiffness. The stiffness causes a decrease in the function of the tissue. It is also said that the glucose if remains in the blood stream can activate cross-linking of protein molecule, and this leads to the stiffening of the tissue and eventually to decline in the function of that tissue.

Changes in human body as a result of aging

Sensory Changes
HEARING

- Loss of hearing.
- Decline in hearing capacity.
- Hearing high pitch sounds becomes difficult.

Strategies to deal with: hearing problems

✓ Try speaking clearly and in a tone that the individual can understand.
✓ Speak slowly, do not speak in a loud voice.
✓ Have his or her attention before starting communication.
✓ Eye contact is necessary.
✓ Eliminate distractors like television, radio or other people speaking.
✓ If the individual does not understand the complete sentence, break it down into parts.
✓ Use of hand gestures may help.
✓ You may have to repeat certain words while communicating.

Sensory Changes
VISION

- Cornea becomes less sensitive.
- Pupils decrease in size.
- Lens becomes less flexible and slightly cloudy.
- The eye muscles become weak.
- Vision gradually declines.
- Decrease in the vitreous humor.
- Reduction in peripheral vision and loss of near vision
- Need for brighter light for clear vision.
- Problems in color perception.

Strategies to deal with: vision problems

- Have the individual in a well-lighted room, but not with too much brightness.

- Avoid glares to come in direct contact with the individual's area of vision.
- Provide dim light for night time, to prevent fall of these individuals.
- Areas like staircases should be well lighted.
- Appropriate light should be available while performing activities which need precision.
- Edges of the stairs should have contrasting colors.
- Do not expose eyes directly to sunlight.

Sensory Changes
TASTE AND SMELL

- Taste and smell (thickening of nose lining) ability decreases.
- Decrease in function of taste buds.
- Mouth usually remains dry to decrease in function of saliva producing tissues.
- Decrease in recognizing food taste.
- Receding of gums.
- Tooth decay and cavities increases.

Strategies to deal with: taste and smell problems

- ✓ Have appropriate nutritious diet as recommended.
- ✓ Offer foods that the individual likes the most.
- ✓ Provide taste enhancer like seasonings.

Sensory Changes
TOUCH

- Skin becomes thin and loses elasticity resulting in dryness and wrinkles due to loss of collagen.
- Skin is more prone to injuries.
- Individual is less tolerant to cold climate.
- Difficulty in differentiating between hot and cold, resulting in injury to the skin.
- Decrease in nerve endings, resulting in decrease sensitivity to pressure, pain and temperature.
- Decrease in the functioning of sweat glands.
- Decrease in exposure to sunlight results in vitamin D deficiency.

Strategies to deal with: touch problems

- ✓ Exposure to extreme temperatures should be avoided. Extreme heat can cause burns, and extreme cold can cause frost bites.
- ✓ Minimize drying of skin by applying light lotion.

- ✓ Skin should be dried appropriately after having a bath.
- ✓ Maintain hydration.
- ✓ Check for temperature prior to having bath using a bath thermometer.
- ✓ Skin should be inspected at intervals.
- ✓ While communicating try using touches appropriately.

Changes in bones, joints and muscles
Changes in bones

- Density of bone decreases.
- Bone becomes weak and more prone to fracture.
- Hormonal changes affect the bones in women post menopause, leading to osteoporosis.
- Bone loses calcium and minerals.
- Changes in bone structure.

Changes in muscle

- Reduction in muscle fibers.
- Disuse atrophy (muscle wasting).
- Muscle tone decreases.
- Muscle contraction becomes weaker which leads to decrease muscle strength.
- Reduction in fast twitch muscles.

Changes in joints

- Joint movements become stiffer.
- Decrease in the volume of lubricating fluid.
- Thinning of joint cartilage.
- Shortening of ligaments.
- Decrease elasticity of ligaments resulting in joint stiffness.

Strategies to deal with: bones, joints, and muscular problems:

- ✓ Exercise should regularly be performed as per recommendation from a physician.
- ✓ Well balanced diet.
- ✓ Preventing fall.

Changes in digestion

- Decreased bowel movements.
- Dehydration.
- Decrease esophageal movement.
- Stomach loses elasticity.
- Decrease intolerance of dairy products.
- Swallowing difficulty.

- Heartburn and gastro-esophageal reflux disease (GERD).
- Absorption capacity of small intestine decreases.
- Stomach contents take a long time to pass through the large intestine, which may result in constipation.

Strategies to deal with: digestion problems

- ✓ Regular exercises as advised.
- ✓ Well balanced diet.
- ✓ Proper hydration.

Changes in circulation

- Blood vessels tend to lose elasticity causing increase in blood pressure.
- Circulation becomes slow.
- Slight increase in heart size.
- Hypertrophy of heart muscles may occur.
- Deposition of aging pigment lipofuscin.
- Slight valve thickening.
- Change in heart rate.
- Orthostatic hypotension.
- Decrease in blood volume.
- If an individual has impaired circulation, this may lead to pressure ulcers.

Strategies to deal with: circulation problems

- ✓ Frequent change in position to prevent pressure sore.
- ✓ Feet on a footstool when sitting if foot unable to reach the floor.
- ✓ Follow the recommended guidelines as prescribed by the physician.

SECTION 7: SPECIAL TOPICS PART III

Special Topic 14: End of Life Care

WHAT IS END OF LIFE CARE?

End of life care can be described as comfort and needs provided to an individual who will be dying due to advanced illness or near to death. Minimizing or preventing the suffering is the goal of the end of life care.

End of life care includes comfort and needs like:

- Physical
- Mental and Emotional
- Spiritual
- Social
- Financial
- Practical

PHYSICAL COMFORT

1. If the pain is severe, report this to your supervisor.
2. Patient's room should be quiet and clean.
3. Communicate with them.
4. Keep the patient clean and dry.
5. If the patient is experiencing breathing problems while in the supine position, have the head of the bed raised.
6. If the patient has dry skin, apply lotion since dry skin can cause irritation.
7. Change patient position more frequently, since staying in one position for a long time may lead to a pressure ulcer.
8. Mouth and face care should be performed. Have patient drink a small quantity of water.
9. Help patient with feeding.
10. Check to see if the patient is comfortable with the room temperature.
11. Avoid patient from performing tiring activities.

MENTAL AND EMOTIONAL COMFORT

1. Communicating with patient and letting them express their concerns can cause mental relief to patients.
2. Have a light bell within patients reach.
3. If the patient calls, try to attend them as soon as possible and take care of their needs.
4. Let the patient speak to people they wish to talk, for example; their family member(s).
5. Any unusual signs that are observed about the patient should be reported to the supervisor.

SPIRITUAL COMFORT

1. If the patient needs spiritual support, respect their decision.
2. Provide patient with sufficient time to practice their religious beliefs.

3. Let the patient pray and read their religious books.
4. If the patient would like to see a religious representative, inform the nurse.

Remember: This is an END OF LIFE CARE individual, special care should be taken.

SOCIAL NEEDS

1. If the patient has a visitor, let them meet the patient.
2. Allow patient to become socially active at their will.
3. Do not stop patient from talking to their family and friends. A patient is at an end of life care and may want to speak to them, inorder to fulfill his or her own needs.

FINANCIAL NEEDS

1. If a patient expresses financial matters that he or she needs to take care of, inform the nurse.
2. The patient may be introduced to a social worker, who then can help the patient further.

SECTION 7: SPECIAL TOPICS PART III
Special Topic 15: Fall In Elderly

WHAT IS A FALL?

It can be described as a sudden change of position which is unintentional, resulting the person in reaching a lower level (ground). A fall can occur anywhere, for example; home, workplace, on a street, while performing a recreational or non-recreational activity, etc.

FACTORS CAUSING A FALL

- Loss of balance or coordination
- Accident
- Dizziness or fainting or hypotension
- Muscle weakness
- Joint problems
- Sudden shock
- Vision problems
- Cognition problems
- Balance problems
- Medication

- Feet problem
- Confusion
- Slow reaction time
- History of fall
- Living by themselves (without caregiver(s) or family members)
- Using assistive devices
- Shuffling gait (short steps)
- Decrease range of motion
- Alcohol (consumption)
- Environmental hazards
  - ✓ Loose rugs
  - ✓ Object on floor
  - ✓ Wet floor
  - ✓ Poor light.
  - ✓ Cords in walking areas
  - ✓ Uneven floor or walking surface
  - ✓ Wet Bathroom

FEW THINGS THAT CAN OCCUR AS A RESULT OF A FALL

- Fracture
- Bruise
- Ligament sprain
- Muscle tear
- Head injury
- Shock
- Dehydration

PREVENTION OF FALL IN ELDERLY

1. **Exercise and Physical Activity**
   - ✓ Brisk walking.
   - ✓ Light resistance training for leg muscles.
   - ✓ Balance and coordination exercises.
   - ✓ Control movements when getting up and sitting down.
   - ✓ While walking with the patient, never rush the patient as this may cause the patient to lose balance. Slow and controlled walking is advised.

2. **Modifying Environment**
   - ✓ The environment should be free of unwanted objects (clutter free) throughout the walking path (area of walking).

✓ The environment should have minimal hurdles.
✓ Uneven floors within the house should be fixed.
✓ Stairs should have a contrast color edge and background.
✓ A grab bar should be installed near the toilet seat and bath tubs.
✓ A bath seat should be used, while bathing.
✓ In a healthcare facility, the call light should be within patients reach.
✓ Patient should not be left on the edge of the bed.

3. **Using of Hip Protectors**
   ✓ Instruct and educate the patient in use of hip protectors.

4. **Maintaining Safe Floor**
   ✓ The floor should be well lit with light.
   ✓ Increase the number of lights.
   ✓ Motion sensitive lights can be used.
   ✓ The floor should be dry.
   ✓ The floor should have a non-slip surface.
   ✓ Sitting surfaces should be stable and at an appropriate height for the individual to sit.
   ✓ Use of a chair with armrest is preferred.
   ✓ Elevated toilet seat.
   ✓ Railings should be available for all types of staircases.

5. **Providing Gait Training**
   ✓ Instruct patient in effective gait walking.

6. **Proper use of Assistive Devices**
   As per instructions instruct the patient in performing:
   ✓ 2 point gait
   ✓ 3 point gait
   ✓ 4 point gait
   ✓ Swing through gait
   ✓ Swing to gait

7. **Education Programs for Staff**
   ✓ Educate staff members about how to prevent a fall.

8. **Vision Checkup**
   ✓ If glasses are prescribed, wear them. This may help in preventing falls.

9. **Appropriate Footwear**
   ✓ Non-slip footwear.
   ✓ Proper size.
   ✓ Proper foot support.

10. **Fall Screening**
    ✓ Recommended fall screening must be used.

SECTION 7: SPECIAL TOPICS PART III
Special Topic 16: Relaxation Exercises

Relaxation exercises are performed to relief the level of anxiety and stress. For many years it has been used as a tool for stress management.

POINTS TO CONSIDER
- ✓ **Frequency**: Practice these exercises more frequently.
- ✓ **Environment**: Environment selected should have least to no distraction.
- ✓ **Position**: Choose a comfortable position.
- ✓ **Form**: Different types of exercises should be performed.

RELAXATION EXERCISES
Types of relaxation techniques

1. Guided Imagery
Guided Imagery is a relaxation technique that involves guiding an individual to a particular environment. An environment in which the individual forgets about his current stressful situation and concentrates more on the guided imagery instructions. In this technique, the individual mentally follows a guided script, for example; a tape or audio that is pre-recorded for the use of this particular technique.

2. Visualization
Visualization is a relaxation technique that involves forming a mental image of something that the person has experienced in the past.

The technique may start by closing your eyes and creating an imagery picture of your past experiences.

3. Controlled Breathing Exercises

Controlled deep breathing is performed when the air is inhaled through the nose, but exhaled through the mouth. In this type of exercise, the deep breathing pattern is used.

Steps in performing controlled breathing exercise are as follows:
1. Choose a comfortable posture (sit straight).
2. Place one hand on the stomach, and the other hand on the chest.
3. Breath in through your nose. When doing so, your stomach should rise (the hand on the stomach moves out). While the other hand should move slightly.
4. Next step should be breathing out. Do so while breathing out through your mouth pushing out (exhaling) as much air as possible. When doing so the hand on the stomach should move in, while the other hand should move only slightly.
5. After step 4, repeat the cycle.

4. Progressive Muscular Relaxation (PMR)

This technique of relaxation involves contracting and relaxing muscle groups along with deep breathing exercises.

Points to consider while performing PMR:
- ✓ Calm Environment,
- ✓ Loose Clothes,
- ✓ Comfortable Position,
- ✓ Proper Posture,
- ✓ Contracting should not be painful,
- ✓ Remove any eye lens if you wear one,
- ✓ Contraction should be above the normal level,
- ✓ Focus on tension created by contraction,
- ✓ Focus on relaxation after contraction,
- ✓ Performed from distal to proximal muscle groups.

Order of performing this technique is:
- ✓ Entire right foot only
- ✓ Entire left foot only
- ✓ Right calf muscles only
- ✓ Left calf muscles only
- ✓ Right thigh muscles only
- ✓ Left thigh muscles only
- ✓ Hips and buttocks muscles only
- ✓ Stomach muscles only
- ✓ Chest muscles only
- ✓ Back muscles only
- ✓ Right arm and hand muscles only
- ✓ Left arm and hand muscles only
- ✓ Neck and shoulder muscles only
- ✓ Face muscles only

1. *Contraction Phase & Inhalation:*

   Start the technique by slowly contracting the muscle and building tension, hold the contraction for recommended time. Take a deep breath while in the contraction phase.

2. *Relaxation Phase & Exhalation:*

   Next, exhale and relax the contracted muscle slowly. Focus on the feeling of relaxation.

3. *Once ready to shift your attention, start the same cycle in the order of muscle groups recommended.*

Note: Direction of muscle group contractions must be from distal to proximal.

Other techniques include:

- Hypnosis
- Massage
- Meditation
- Yoga
- Biofeedback
- Music and art therapy

SECTION 7
END OF SECTION REVIEW QUESTIONS

Question Set 1:
Essay Questions
50 points: 5 points each

1. Explain in brief about physiological and biological needs.
2. Explain in brief about safety needs.
3. Explain in brief about self-actualization needs.
4. Explain in brief about love and belongingness needs.
5. Explain about the following changes as a result of aging process.
   a) Vision
   b) Hearing
   c) Taste and smell
   d) Bones and muscles
   e) Digestion
   f) Circulation
6. Explain the needs of end of life care
   a) Physical comfort.
   b) Mental comfort.
   c) Spiritual comfort.
   d) Social needs.
   e) Financial needs.
7. List and explain in brief the causes of fall in elderly.
8. How to prevent fall in elderly?
9. List and explain relaxation techniques.
10. How to perform the progressive muscular relaxation technique of relaxation?

SECTION 8: SPECIAL TOPICS PART IV

Special Topic 17: Gait Belt and Its Uses

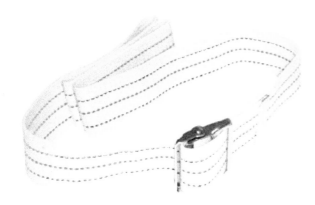

Figure S.15

A safety device that is utilized by the carer for:-

✓ Moving a patient from one place to another,

✓ Helping a patient walk or

✓ Lifting the patient from a seated position to standing position and vice versa.

A gait belt:-

✓ Prevents a patient from falling by providing support while walking.

✓ Makes it easy for a carer or person assisting to aid in the process of walking.

BODY MECHANICS WHILE USING GAIT BELT:

While using gait belt proper body mechanics should be used to protect the body from the back and other injuries. It involves lifting the patient from a seated position to standing and controlled lowering of patient from standing to sitting position and supporting the patient while walking.

Body mechanics while using gait belt for assisting a patient to stand from a sitting position:-

✓ Back should be straight.

✓ Knees should be bend (minimum to moderate as required). Note: Bend (flexions)

✓ Lift using your arm and leg muscles.

✓ Avoid using your back muscles.

Gait belt cannot be utilized for:

1. Patients with recent surgery

2. Pregnant female

3. Ostomy

4. If patient refuses its use

5. Pain

6. Declared unsafe for the patient

7. Should not be used as a restraint for patients

Steps in using a transfer or gait belt

1. Identify your patient and start by greeting the patient, followed by introducing yourself.

2. Explain the procedure to the patient prior to performing it.

3. Perform standard precautions and infection control measures, by washing hands and wearing gloves.

4. Maintain your body mechanics during the entire length of the process.

5. Select an appropriate size gait belt/transfer belt.

6. Check to see the patient's initial or starting position.
   - In bed, provide assistance to change the patient's position from supine to sitting.
   - In the chair, bring the patient to an appropriate position (sitting).

7. Secure the gait belt around the patient's waist. The gait belt should never be secured tightly, as this may cause discomfort to the patient. The best way to ensure that the gait belt is not secured tightly would be by inserting two fingers to check for the fit.

   Note: on a female patient, ensure that the gait belt is at the waist level and not at the breast level.

8. Once the above step of securing the gait belt is complete, give directions to the patient before making them stand up from a sitting position.

9. Grasp the gait belt at either end while assisting the patient to a standing position.

10. Ask patient, if he or she is comfortable while in standing position.

11. Stand on the side and slightly behind the patient.

12. Have the patient walk, hold gait belt while the patient is walking.

13. Ask if the patient is comfortable while walking.

14. Have the patient walk several steps.

15. Have the patient stand near a chair, with the back of the knee facing the seat of the chair. Assist the patient to sit.

16. Safely and gently remove the gait belt from the patient's waist. Avoid pulling of the gait belt while removing it.

17. Have the patient sit in the chair, with the hip against the back of the chair. Position the patient comfortably and safely in the chair.

18. Remove gloves (if applicable) and wash hands.

19. Document time of transfer (and/or ambulation) and patient's response to the procedure.

SECTION 8: SPECIAL TOPICS PART IV

Special Topic 18: Breathing Exercises

Breathing Exercises are performed by trained professionals which include respiratory therapist, physical therapist, nurses and other healthcare professionals. The Proper skill set is required to implement these techniques. Assistants, technicians, and aides can assist the professionals performing these techniques by preparing the patient and setting up the supplies required to perform these techniques.

Breathing exercises

1. Diaphragmatic Breathing
2. Segmental Breathing
3. Pursed-lip Breathing
4. Glossopharyngeal Breathing
5. Coughing and huffing
6. Incentive spirometer

DIAPHRAGMATIC BREATHING

A type of breathing exercise that can be performed in sitting, supine, and semi-fowler position. It can be either assisted or non-assisted.

Steps in performing assisted diaphragmatic breathing:

1. Greet the patient.

2. Introduce yourself and verify patient's identity.

3. Explain the procedure to the patient.

4. Select a comfortable (relaxed) position for the patient (sitting, supine or semi-fowler).

5. Caregiver's places hand on upper abdominal, just below the anterior costal margin.

6. The patient is instructed to perform deep inhalation via the nose, while doing so the chest and shoulders should be relaxed. A slight rise in the abdomen will occur.

7. The patient is then instructed to perform slow exhalation via the mouth.

8. The patient is instructed to practice the same. Getting hyperventilated during this procedure should be avoided.

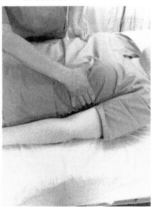 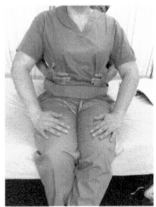

Supine Position   **Sitting Position**
DIAPHRAGMATIC BREATHING
Figure S.16

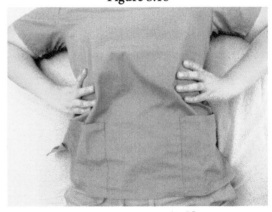

Supine Position (Self)
DIAPHRAGMATIC BREATHING
Figure S.17

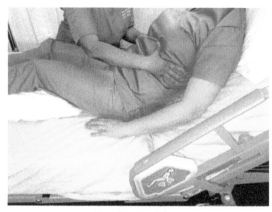

Fowler Position
DIAPHRAGMATIC BREATHING
Figure S.18

Steps in self-performing diaphragmatic breathing:

1. Select a comfortable (relaxed) position for the patient (sitting, supine or semi-fowler).
2. Place your hands on the upper abdomen, just below the anterior costal margin.
3. Perform deep inhalation via the nose, while doing so, the chest and shoulders should be relaxed. A slight rise in the abdomen will occur.
4. Perform slow exhalation via the mouth.

SEGMENTAL BREATHING

This is a type of breathing exercise performed using the same pattern used in diaphragmatic breathing.

It involves expansion of the localized area of the lung by placing the hand on the appropriate area of the chest as recommended for expansion. Some examples of localized areas include; apical, posterior basal and lateral basal. When placing hands on the localized area, the patient is instructed to concentrate on that specific location for the movement to occur during breathing. While the patient is exhaling, the hand placed on the area should provide slight pressure as recommended into the ribs using the palm of the hands. At the end of the expiration, when the patient is about to inhale, deliver a light and quick downward and inward stretch before the phase of inspiration begins.

PURSED LIP BREATHING

A type of breathing exercise in which the individual inhales through the nose and exhales using pursed lips.

While exhaling through pursed lips, avoid contracting abdominal muscles.

GLOSSOPHARYNGEAL BREATHING

It is considered to be a positive pressure breathing technique. The individual is instructed to perform a series of gulps of air to enter the lungs. Muscles of the mouth and pharynx are used to pull the air into the lungs. This is usually performed when the inspiratory muscles are weak.

Steps in performing glossopharyngeal breathing:

1. Instruct the patient to open the mouth and keep the tongue flat.
2. Slowly close the mouth and lips, have the tongue go back to its normal position. This closing of mouth with series of gulps will push the air further down towards the lung.
3. A series of gulps must be taken for sufficient amount of air to enter into the lungs.

HUFFING

It is a type of technique in which the mucus is forced to move upwards through the respiratory system.

Steps in performing huffing:

- Start by having the individual in a comfortable position.
- Breathing is performed using the diaphragm.
- Next step would be to hold the breath as recommended and breathe out forcefully.
- Start with a gentle huff and progress towards more forceful huff as recommended by the therapist.

COUGHING

It is a technique used to forcefully move the mucus upwards through the respiratory system using a high-speed expiration. It can cause shortness of breathing.

INCENTIVE SPIROMETRY

Steps in using incentive spirometer:

- Have the patient in a comfortable position.
- Ask the patient to exhale normally.
- Instruct the patient to place the mouthpiece of the device into their mouth, close the mouth by sealing the lips around the mouthpiece.
- Next instruct the patient to breathe in, while doing so, the indicator on the device will indicate the amount of air inspired.
- After breathing in, holding the breath may be recommended for at least 3 seconds, followed by breathing out.
- Repeat the cycle as recommended.

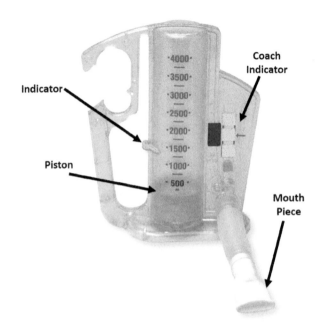

Figure S.19 Incentive Spirometer
Also known as Sustained Maximal Inspiration (SMI).

SECTION 8: SPECIAL TOPICS PART IV

Special Topic 19: Professions in Therapeutic Services

PROFESSIONS IN THERAPEUTIC SERVICES

1. Acupuncturist/Acupressurist
2. Allopathic Physician
3. Anesthesiologist Asst.
4. Art/Music/Dance Therapist
5. Athletic Trainer
6. Audiologist
7. CNA/LPN/RN
8. Chiropractor
9. Dental Asst./ Hygienist
10. Dental Lab Tech
11. Dentist
12. Dietician
13. Dietetic Tech/Asst.
14. Dosimetrist
15. EMT/Paramedic
16. Exercise Physiologist
17. Home Health Aide
18. Massage Therapist
19. Medical Assistant
20. Mortician
21. Occupational Therapist/ OT Asst.
22. Ophthalmic Medical Personnel
23. Optometrist
24. Orthodontist
25. Orthotist/ Prosthetist
26. Pharmacist/ Pharmacy Tech
27. Physical Therapist/ PT Assistant
28. Physician (MD/OD)
29. Physician Assistant
30. Psychologist
31. Recreation Therapist
32. Rehabilitation Counselors
33. Respiratory Therapist
34. Social Worker
35. Speech Language Pathologist
36. Surgical Technician
37. Therapist (Art, Dance/Movement, Drama, Horticulture, Music)
38. Veterinarian/ Vet Tech

PROFESSIONS IN DIAGNOSTIC SERVICES

1. Blood Bank Technologist
2. Cardiovascular Technologist
3. Clinical Lab Technician
4. CT Technologist
5. Cytogenetic Technologist
6. Cytotechnologist
7. Diagnostic Medical Sonographers
8. ECG Technician
9. EEG Technologist
10. Exercise Physiologist
11. Geneticist
12. Histotechnician
13. Histotechnologist
14. MRI Technologist
15. Mammographer
16. Medical Technologist/ Clinical Laboratory Scientist
17. Nuclear Medicine Technologist
18. Nutritionist
19. Pathologist
20. Pathology Assistant
21. Phlebotomist
22. PET Technologist
23. Radiologic Technologist/ Radiographer
24. Radiologist

SPECIALTY CARE

1. Anesthesiology; in reference to anesthesia.
2. Cardiology; in reference to cardiac or heart condition(s).
3. Dermatology; in reference to skin.
4. Endocrinology; in reference to hormones and metabolic disorder(s).
5. Gastroenterology; in reference to digestive system.
6. Hematology; in reference to blood related disorder(s).
7. Immunology; in reference to immune system.
8. Nephrology; in reference to kidney.
9. Neurology; in reference to nervous system.
10. Obstetrics/gynecology; in reference to pregnancy and female reproductive system.
11. Oncology; in reference to cancer.
12. Ophthalmology; in reference to eye.
13. Orthopedics; in reference to bone(s), joints and connective tissues (musculoskeletal system).
14. Otorhinolaryngology; in reference to ear, nose, and throat.
15. Rheumatology; in reference to rheumatism or joints, muscle(s) and ligament(s) disorders.
16. Urology; in reference to urinary tract (male and female) and male reproductive system.

HEALTHCARE PROFESSIONALS DESCRIPTION

Audiologist

Audiologists are health professionals that specialize in the science of hearing. They diagnose, treat, evaluate and manage hearing loss.

Physical therapists (PTs)

A healthcare professional involved in diagnosing and treating a condition that limits the ability of an individual to function. Physical therapist makes use of therapeutic techniques available within their scope of practice to treat the patient. Some goals of a physical therapist include restoring function, preventing disability and reducing pain.

Physical therapist assistants (PTAs)

Works under the direction and supervision of the physical therapist. They help the physical therapist in carrying out physical therapy services.

Physical therapy aides/technician[1]

Under close supervision of a physical therapist or physical therapy assistant, perform only delegated, selected, or routine tasks in specific situations. These duties include preparing the patient and the treatment area.

Rehabilitation Therapy Technician

Under close supervision of a physical therapist, physical therapy assistant, occupational therapist, assistant, or chiropractors.

Registered nurses (RNs)[1]

Provide and coordinate patient care, educate patients and the public about various health conditions, and provide advice and emotional support to patients and their family members.

Athletic Trainers and Exercise Physiologists[1]

Athletic trainers specialize in preventing, diagnosing, and treating muscle and bone injuries and illnesses. Exercise physiologists develop fitness and exercise programs that help patients recover from chronic diseases and improve cardiovascular function, body composition, and flexibility.

Chiropractors[1]

Chiropractors treat patients with health problems of the neuromusculoskeletal system, which includes nerves, bones, muscles, ligaments, and tendons. They use spinal adjustments, manipulation, and other techniques to manage patients' health concerns, such as back and neck pain.

Dentists[1]

Dentists diagnose and treat problems with a patient's teeth, gums, and related parts of the mouth. They provide advice and instruction on taking care of teeth and gums and on diet choices that affect oral health.

Dietitians and Nutritionists[1]

Dietitians and nutritionists are experts in food and nutrition. They advise people on what to eat in order to lead a healthy lifestyle or achieve a specific health-related goal.

EMTs and Paramedics[1]

Emergency medical technicians (EMTs) and paramedics care for the sick or injured in emergency medical settings. People's lives often depend on their quick reaction and competent care. EMTs and paramedics respond to emergency calls, performing medical services and transporting patients to medical facilities.

Home Health Aides[1]

Home health aides help people who are disabled, chronically ill, or cognitively impaired. They often help older adults who need assistance. In some states, home health aides may be able to give a patient medication or check the patient's vital signs under the direction of a nurse or other healthcare practitioner.

Licensed Practical and Licensed Vocational Nurses[1]

Licensed practical nurses (LPNs) and licensed vocational nurses (LVNs) provide basic nursing care. They work under the direction of registered nurses and doctors.

Medical Assistants[1]

Medical assistants complete administrative and clinical tasks in the offices of physicians, podiatrists, chiropractors, and other health practitioners. Their duties vary with the location, specialty, and size of the practice.

Nursing Assistants [1]

Nursing assistants help provide basic care for patients in hospitals and residents of long-term care facilities, such as nursing homes.

Occupational Therapists [1]

Occupational therapists treat injured, ill, or disabled patients through the therapeutic use of everyday activities. They help these patients develop, recover, and improve the skills needed for daily living and working.

Occupational Therapy Assistants and Aides [1]

Occupational therapy assistants and aides help patients develop, recover, and improve the skills needed for daily living and working. Occupational therapy assistants are directly involved in providing therapy to patients, while occupational therapy aides typically perform support activities. Both assistants and aides work under the direction of occupational therapists.

Orthotists and Prosthetists [1]

Orthotists and prosthetists, also called O&P professionals, design medical supportive devices and measure and fit patients for them. These devices include artificial limbs (arms, hands, legs, and feet), braces, and other medical or surgical devices.

Patient Care Technician/Assistant

Help provide basic care for patients in hospital and residents in long-term care facilities. Some patient care technicians or assistants also perform phlebotomy and electrocardiography in a hospital or other facilities.

Personal Care Aides [1]

Personal care aides help patients with self-care and everyday tasks and provide companionship.

Pharmacists [1]

Pharmacists dispense prescription medications to patients and offer expertise in the safe use of prescriptions. They also may provide advice on how to lead a healthy lifestyle, conduct health, and wellness screenings, provide immunizations, and oversee the medications given to patients.

Pharmacy Technicians [1]

Pharmacy technicians assist licensed pharmacists dispense prescription medication to customers or health professionals.

Phlebotomists [1]

Phlebotomists draw blood for tests, transfusions, research, or blood donations. Some explain their work to patients and provide assistance when patients have adverse reactions after their blood is drawn.

Physician Assistants [1]

Physician assistants, also known as PAs, practice medicine on a team under the supervision of physicians and surgeons. They are formally educated to examine patients, diagnose injuries and illnesses, and provide treatment.

Physicians and Surgeons [1]

Physicians and surgeons diagnose and treat injuries or illnesses. Physicians examine patients; take medical histories; prescribe medications; and order, perform, and interpret diagnostic tests. They counsel patients on diet, hygiene, and preventive healthcare. Surgeons operate on patients to treat injuries, such as broken bones; diseases, such as cancerous tumors; and deformities, such as cleft palates.

Podiatrists [1]

Podiatrists provide medical care for people with foot, ankle, and lower leg problems. They diagnose illnesses, treat injuries, and perform surgery involving the lower extremities.

Recreational Therapists [1]

Recreational therapists plan, direct, and coordinate recreation-based treatment programs for people with disabilities, injuries, or illnesses. Recreational therapists use a variety of modalities, including arts and crafts, drama, music, dance, sports, games, and community reintegration field trips to help maintain or improve a patient's physical, social, and emotional well-being.

Respiratory Therapists [1]

Respiratory therapists care for patients who have trouble breathing—for example, from a chronic respiratory disease, such as asthma or emphysema. Their patients range from premature infants with undeveloped lungs to elderly patients who have diseased lungs. They also provide emergency care to patients suffering from heart attacks, drowning, or shock.

Restorative Care Assistant or Aide

Restorative nursing care focuses on keeping residents as independent and physically active as possible.

The purpose is to encourage residents to perform as much of their own care as possible.

References:

1. Bureau of Labor Statistics, U.S. Department of Labor, Occupational Outlook Handbook.

SECTION 8: SPECIAL TOPICS PART IV
Special Topic 20: Psychological Disorders

PSYCHOLOGICAL DISORDERS
The Anxiety Disorders

Specific Phobia

Phobia means fear. The term specific phobia can be a fear of things or situations, for example, hydrophobia (fear of water).

Panic Disorder

A type of anxiety disorder that is characterized by panic attacks. It may be sudden in nature. The individual going through a panic disorder may have change in behavior during the attack, be out of control, and be exhausted after the attack subsides.

Post-traumatic Stress Disorder

A type of anxiety disorder, in which an individual is exposed to traumatic situations. Exposure to such events or situations causes emotional imbalance leading to stress. The person may get flashbacks, nightmares, experience difficulty sleeping and sometimes difficult to live a normal life. It is also known as **PTSD**.

Obsessive-Compulsive Disorder (OCD)

A type of anxiety disorder, in which unwanted thoughts, fears, ideas, etc. lead to a behavior. Obsessive – Compulsive is a combination of two main symptoms first **obsession** (thoughts, fears, feelings, etc.), second is **compulsion** (behavior as a result of the obsession).

Generalized Anxiety Disorder

A type of anxiety disorder in which a person is anxious and worried about numerous things and controlling such symptoms become difficult.

Somatoform Disorder

A mental disorder characterized by physical symptoms, which advocates physical injuries or illness. A person suffering from this disorder may have pain in a certain area of the body which will suggest the healthcare professional of an injury or condition that the person might be suffering from, but in reality, it is not the physical illness or condition that has led to this pain. A person suffering from this disorder may become frustrated as a result of the unexplained cause of pain.

Hypochondriasis

A person suffering from hypochondriasis has a belief that he or she has a serious medical condition, this belief develops as a result of misinterpreting symptoms they might experience.

Conversion Disorder (old name: Hysteria)

A condition in which the person suffers from symptoms that involve sensory and motor functions, whereas medical examination does not suggest any abnormalities.

Schizophrenia

A condition in which a person has an altered perception of what is real, this leads to the non-association with reality. There are several types of schizophrenia:

1. Paranoid Subtype
2. Disorganized Subtype
3. Catatonic Subtype
4. Undifferentiated Subtype

Hallucinations

A perception or sensation of stimulus that appears to be real to the person hallucinated, for example; a person may be able to see or hear something which another individual with him or her may not be able to see or hear. It involves the sensory organs of the human body for example eyes, nose, ears, tongue and skin.

Delusions

A belief which is firmly held by a person even though there is a presence of evidence to the contrary. For example delusion of grandeur: In this, the person may feel that he or she has the power to do certain things which others are incapable of doing, which in reality is not true.

Catatonia

The person may have resistance to movements, have waxy flexibility, retained grasp, aversion and other characteristics.

Bipolar Disorder (Manic-Depressive Disorder)

A person may experience symptoms which causes a shift in mood, energy and several other functions. It can involve a mood swing that ranges from depression characteristics to manic characteristics.

SECTION 8:
SPECIAL TOPICS PART IV
Special Topic 21: Personality Disorders

PERSONALITY DISORDERS

Antisocial Personality Disorder

Antisocial personality disorder is characterized by having no regards for right and wrong. People suffering from this disorder disregard or violate other people's rights.

Narcissistic Personality Disorder

Disorder in which a person has an excessive sense of grandiosity, lack of empathy, arrogance behavior, and a need to be admired.

Borderline Personality Disorder

A serious mental disorder in which the person experiences unstable mood, unstable behavior patterns, and sometimes unstable relationships.

SECTION 8: SPECIAL TOPICS PART IV
Special Topic 22: Death and Dying

Stages of Grief

Stage 1- Denial

In this stage, the person refuses to accept the reality of the situation. It is considered as a primitive defense mechanism. For example; a person learns about his diagnosis, but does not accept it.

2 - Anger

In this stage, the person after going through the denial stage shows his or her emotions in the form of anger. A person in this stage can get angry at themselves or with others (usually with people close to them).

3 - Bargaining

This is the 3rd stage, in which the person is now involved in bargaining to undo the situation or stop it from happening. The person starts negotiating. For example; a person who has a severe health condition will seek alternate treatments.

4 - Depression

In this stage, the person sinks into depression as a result of no hopes. It is more of an emotional stage. The individual feels depressed. The start of this stage usually indicates that the person is now accepting the reality.

5 - Acceptance

In this stage, the person accepts the reality and becomes ready to face it, as opposed to the first stage, in which the same individual was not accepting the reality or the facts. A person might show signs of emotional detachment.

The stages, popularly known by the acronym **DABDA**

Reference: Kübler-Ross E. On Death and Dying 1969 pub, Routledge, ISBN 0415040159

SECTION 8:
SPECIAL TOPICS PART IV
Special Topic 23: Restraints & Incident Reports

Restraints

An ideal restraint can be described as a safe and harm-free technique used to prevent the patient from hurting themselves. This is usually done by restricting their movement. The intensity of the restriction should be kept to a minimum. Restraint is not always required. There are ways in which a facility can keep the patient safe without using restraints.

Types of restraints

1. Physical Restraints
2. Chemical Restraints

Physical Restraints

Restraints can be used for various reasons, which may involve, preventing a person from moving, or prevent the person from accessing certain things. Restraint is applied with different material and equipment available today. Restraints are to be used only if they are ordered. Using them without an order may be considered false imprisonment. Some example of restraints are; hand mitts, jackets, bed rails, vest, etc. Remember, anything that prevents the person from moving can be considered a restraint. For example; tucking in the bed sheets tightly from over the bed to underneath the bed can also be considered a restraint if the patient is unable to move.

Chemical Restraints

Restraints in which medication are used to restraint a patient is considered a chemical restraint.

Note: The main reason for using a restraint is to protect the patient from harming themselves.

While on restraints

- Maintain patient's right to dignity by giving them privacy, while maintaining their safety and comfort.
- Make sure that the restraint is not painful or causing discomfort.
- Frequent monitoring of the patient is required. All observations should be documented while the patient is on restraint.

Assistants or Technicians involved in the application process of restraints should be well trained to do so. Avoid restraints to a movable object. Remember to perform within the scope of your practice, checking your state regulations and law regarding this is important.

Patients should be observed for any signs of injury while on restraint. If an injury occurs due to restraint, it should be reported.

Restraints should not be applied on:

- Open wounds
- Bruises
- Fractured bones
- On a recent surgery
- and more, check your facility policy on restraints.

Some reasons for using restraints;

- Preventing a patient from pulling on their intra-venous (IV) lines.
- Preventing a patient from a fall.
- Preventing a patient from harming themselves.
- If the patient is disoriented and not able to co-operate.

While on restraint, a patient may suffer from;

- Bruise
- Abrasion
- Depression
- Other problems

This may be as a result of:-

- Improper technique in the application of restraints.
- Inadequate observation while the patient is on restraint.
- Improper care delivered while the patient was on restraint.

INCIDENT REPORT

An incident is an unusual event or occurrence of an accident. An incident can occur during patient care.

The main purpose of the incident report is to document the details of the event or occurrence of an accident as soon as possible. For example; a patient falls while walking within the hospital, this accident may be reported on the incident report.

Check your healthcare facility policy on documenting incident report.

General information that may be required to fill the incident report may include but not limited to the following:

- Location and Name of the facility.
- Name of the person involved in the accident.
- Time of incident including AM or PM.
- Type of accident.

- Witness name(s).
- Description summary of the incident.
- Action taken for patient care.
- Other information as required by the facility.

SECTION 8: SPECIAL TOPICS PART IV
Special Topic 24: Urine Specimen Collection

Urine Specimen Types
Mid-Stream Clean Catch:

The patient should be educated about cleansing the urethral area.

MALE: Clean the penis in a circumcised penis. If uncircumcised then instruct the patient to retract the skin and clean the penis. While holding the retracted skin, void the first part (stream) of the urine in the toilet and then place the cup to collect the urine (mid-stream clean catch). On completion, place the lid on the container.

FEMALE: Hold the labia's apart and clean the labia on one side, from front to back, then on the other side of the labia from front to back. Finally, clean the center of the labia. While holding the labia apart void the first portion of the urine into the toilet and then place the cup to collect the urine (mid-stream clean catch). On completion, place the lid on the container.

Specimens after collection should be labeled correctly with the required information.

Timed Specimen (24 Hour Collection):

The patient is provided with a container to collect the urine for the next 24 hours and instructions are provided on when to start the 24 hour collection time and when to stop. Instruct the patient to avoid fecal contamination of the urine sample.

Procedure for collection:

The patient is asked to urinate the first-morning urine into the toilet and start the 24 hr. urine test. After urination, record the time and date. Continue collecting urine in the urine container for the next 24 hours.

First Morning Sample/First Voided Specimen:

This specimen is considered to be a specimen of choice for examination, due to the sample being concentrated in form. The sample is free of any dietary influences. Also urine stays in the bladder for a certain duration, which causes an increase in the cellular elements, if present. The patient is instructed to empty the bladder (pass urine) before bedtime and collect the first-morning sample (urine). This is a preferred collection for pregnancy, bacterial cultures, and microscopic analysis.

Random:

Most commonly used sample for urinalysis examination. The specimen can be collected at any time during the day from the patient. Random urine specimen can give inaccurate results depending on the patient's health. This type of urine sample has no guidelines for collection of specimen, but the patient is instructed to avoid contamination of the sample.

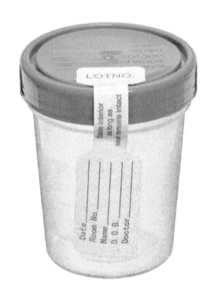

Figure: Urine Sample Container

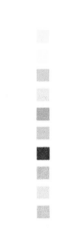

Figure: Urine Dip-Stick

AECA: Physical & Chemical Urinalysis Competency Check

Points to be awarded:	Performed	Not Performed
1. Assemble equipment and supplies.		
2. Verify physician's order.		
3. Wash hands/PPE (follow standard precautions).		
4. Greet the patient.		
5. Identify yourself (name & designation).		
6. Identify patient (full name & date of birth).		
7. Explain procedure to the patient.		
8. Instruct patient in specimen collection.		
9. Perform physical urinalysis.		
10. Perform chemical urinalysis.		
11. Dispose of contaminated supplies.		
12. Wash hands.		
13. Record results in patient's chart.		

Physical Recordings	Chemical Recordings

American Education Certification Association
AECA Competency Checklist
www.AECAcert.com

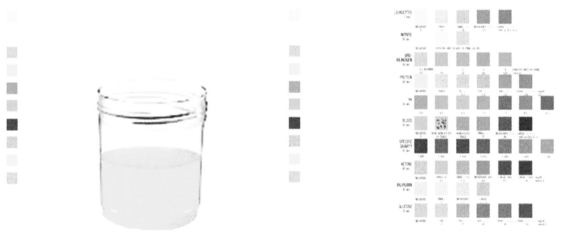

Test strip before dipping   Urine Sample   Test strip after dipping   Compare the test strip after dipping with the above chart

SECTION 8: SPECIAL TOPICS PART IV

Special Topic 25: Stool and Sputum Specimen Collection

FECAL SPECIMEN COLLECTION

3 TYPES OF FECAL TEST:

1. **Fecal occult blood test (FOBT)**

2. **Fecal immunochemical test (FIT), also called an immunochemical fecal occult blood test (iFOBT)**

3. **Stool DNA test (sDNA)**

Specimen collection methods:

✓ **Method 1:** Collection in a container.
✓ **Method 2:** Collection on a hemoccult card.

COLLECTION IN A CONTAINER:

- For accurate test results, collect the stool sample using a clean and dry container.
- Do not collect a sample if blood is visible in the stool or urine.
- Carefully read the specimen requirements for the procedure to be performed.
- Collect timed specimens in a pre-weighed container that is sealed.
- Next, measure the weight of the total sample.
- Mix contents of timed sample appropriately to obtain a homogeneous mixture.
- Remove the required amount of aliquot.
- Measure and record the total weight and collection time of

HEMOCCULT COLLECTION CARD

1
Patient Name: _____
Age:_____
Address:_____
Sample Collected Date:_____
Phone Number:_____
Physician Name:_____

A   **B**

2
Patient Name: _____
Age:_____
Address:_____
Sample Collected Date:_____
Phone Number:_____
Physician Name:_____

A   **B**

3
Patient Name: _____
Age:_____
Address:_____
Sample Collected Date:_____
Phone Number:_____
Physician Name:_____

A   **B**

the sample on both the sample container and the test requisition.

COLLECTION ON AN HEMOCCULT CARD:

- Patients should collect stool specimens from bowel movements on three different days and apply each specimen to a different card (three cards total). From each stool specimen, two samples should be collected from two different sections of each fecal specimen.
- Using the applicator provided with fecal specimen collection kit, collect a small amount of fecal sample. Open the front of the card. Apply a thin smear covering **Area A** of **Box 1**. Reuse the applicator to get a second

sample from a different section of the stool. Apply thin smear covering **Area B** of **Box 1**.

✓ Close the cover flap. Dispose of the applicator in a waste container.

✓ If 3 specimens have been requested, continue the same procedure on **Box 2** and finally **Box 3** on separate days.

SPUTUM COLLECTION:-

Step 1. Ask the patient to rinse the mouth with water.

Step 2. Breathe in and out three times.

Step 3. Cough and bring the mucous from the lungs up into the oral cavity.

Step 4. Open the container and transfer the sputum from the mouth into the container.

Step 5. Close the lid of the container and refrigerate until ready for transport to the lab.

SECTION 8:
SPECIAL TOPICS PART IV

Special Topic 26: Safety Data Sheet (SDS)

SAFETY DATA SHEETS (SDS) (formerly Material Safety Data Sheets or MSDSs)

The Hazard Communication Standard (HCS) requires that the chemical manufacturer, distributor, or importer provide Safety Data Sheets (SDSs) (formerly MSDSs or Material Safety Data Sheets) for each hazardous chemical to downstream users to communicate information on these hazards.

Safety Data Sheet (SDS) is a document that contains information on the potential hazards (health, fire, reactivity, and environmental) and how to work safely with the particular chemical product. The SDS includes information such as the properties of each chemical and its environmental health hazards, protective measures, and safety precautions for handling, storing, and transporting the chemical. It also contains information on the use, storage, handling, and emergency procedures all related to the hazards of the material. The SDS contains much more information about the material than the label. SDSs are prepared by the supplier or manufacturer of the material. It is intended to tell what the hazards of the product are, how to use the product safely, what to expect if the recommendations are not followed, what to do if accidents occur, how to recognize symptoms of over-exposure, and what to do if such incidents occur.

Reference:

https://www.osha.gov/Publications/OSHA3514.html

16 sections of the SDS	
Section 1	Identification
Section 2	Hazard(s) Identification
Section 3	Composition/Information on Ingredients
Section 4	First-Aid Measures
Section 5	Fire-Fighting Measures
Section 6	Accidental Release Measures
Section 7	Handling and Storage
Section 8	Exposure Controls/Personal Protection
Section 9	Physical and chemical properties
Section 10	Stability and Reactivity
Section 11	Toxicological Information
Section 12	Ecological Information (non-mandatory)
Section 13	Disposal Considerations (non-mandatory)
Section 14	Transport Information (non-mandatory)
Section 15	Regulatory Information (non-mandatory)
Section 16	Other Information

SECTION 8:
SPECIAL TOPICS PART IV

Special Topic 27: Postmortem Care

STEPS IN PERFORMING POST-MORTEM CARE

1. Wash your hands.
2. Collect the equipment and supplies required to perform the task.
3. Raise the bed.
4. Make sure that bed is flat.
5. Put on gloves.
6. Position the body in supine position.
7. Arms & legs straight.
8. Place a pillow under head and neck.
9. If the eyelids are open, gently close the eyes. If you are not able to do so, inform your supervisor.
10. Dentures should be placed in the mouth as per facility policy.
11. Place small towel under the chin to close the mouth.
12. Remove the jewelry as per the facility requirement, prepare a list of all jewelry removed and place it in a bag.
13. If tubes are present, ask the supervisor (nurse) to check if the tubes are to be removed.
14. Bath the body with water followed by drying the body using an appropriate size cloth or towel.
15. Wash soiled areas of the body, replace soiled dressing(s) with new dressing(s).
16. A new gown must be put on the body.
17. Groom the patient (body).
18. Attach an identification tag to the ankle or great toe.
19. All personal belongings should be placed in a bag and labeled with patient's name.
20. The room should be neat and clean.
21. Remove gloves & wash hand.
22. If the family is to view the body privately, provide them the privacy to do so, as recommended by facility policy.
23. Once done the body is transferred to the morgue room.
24. Wear gloves and place the body on the shroud or in a body bag.
    Shroud application technique:-
    a. *Fold the top of the shroud to cover the head. (See step 2 of shroud application)*
    b. *Fold the bottom of the shroud to cover the feet. (See step 3 of shroud application)*
    c. *Fold the sides of the shroud to cover the sides (left & right). (See step 4 & 5 of shroud application)*
    d. *Apply tape or securing pins to keep the shroud in place as per facility policy. (See step 5 of shroud application)*
25. One tag tied to right great toe and other on wrist. Tag the shroud with patient's identification as per facility policy.
26. Remove gloves and wash hands.
27. Follow facility policy for further instructions.

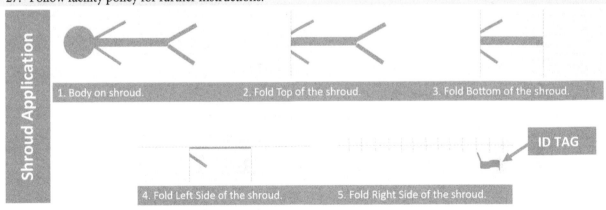

Shroud Application

1. Body on shroud. 2. Fold Top of the shroud. 3. Fold Bottom of the shroud.

ID TAG

4. Fold Left Side of the shroud. 5. Fold Right Side of the shroud.

SECTION 8:
SPECIAL TOPICS PART IV

Special Topic 28: Communication

WHAT IS COMMUNICATION?

Communication is an important tool used by all of us to share our feelings, messages, plans, requests, and thoughts. The main aim of communication is to relay message from one person to another person. Communication keeps us socially and occupationally involved.

Elements of Communication

- **Speaker**: the person sending the message.
- **Listener**: the person receiving the message.
- **Message**: the message being relayed.

Two main ways of communications are:

1. **Verbal (Spoken)**

   a. Verbal communication involves communication in the form of spoken words that deliver the message to another person.

      i. For example: Person A: "would you like to have your dinner", Person B: "Yes". This example involves a relay of message from **person A (speaker) to person B (listener)**, and a response is generated by person B.

2. **Non-verbal (Non-spoken)**

   a. Non-verbal communication involves communication in the form of a sign language, gestures (body language), written instructions, facial expressions, etc.

Note: communication is a crucial component of patient and healthcare professional relationship.

Some common examples of communications encountered by an assistant, technician and aide, would be as follows:

- Greeting a patient.
- Introducing yourself.
- Explaining the procedure.
- Seeking informed consent.
- Answer questions that is within the scope of your practice.
- Reporting to your supervisor.
- Gathering information for the patient.
- Talking to patient's family and more.

Communication with patients:-

- Respect your patients at all times. Address your patient in a respectful manner, call them by their first name. Do not address the patient by calling them "Honey", "Mama", "Grandma", "Grandpa", etc. For example, if your patient's name is "Z", address him by calling Mr. Z.

- Listen to the patient while he or she is speaking, and give feedback once they are done speaking or relaying their message. Do not interrupt their message.
- Be polite and stay calm, do not speak in a loud tone.
- Speak slowly and use simple words.
- If the patient is unable to understand the complete message, try breaking it down for them.
- Understand your patient's feelings.
- Use open-ended communication skills.
- If unable to clearly listen what the patient is trying to tell you, minimize the distractors.
- If unable to understand what the patient said, have he or she repeat it again. If you are still not sure, repeat what they said and ask them if this is correct.
- Avoid arguing with the patient.
- Have a positive body language while with the patient. For example; performing your task

quickly and exiting the room gives the patient an impression that you are not interested in what he or she wants to say.

- Observe patients for signs of pain or depression.

- If required, try including family members in patient communication as recommended by the facility policy.

- Instruct the patient about how to use the light bell or call bell to call you or other healthcare professional when a need arises.

SECTION 8

END OF SECTION REVIEW QUESTIONS

Question Set 1: Essay Questions
100 points

Question 1, 3, 5, 6, 7, 9-13 (50 Points 5 Points Each)
Question 2 (14 Points 2 Point Each)
Question 4 (30 Points 2 Point Each)
Question 8 (6 Points 2 Point Each)

1. What is gait belt? List its uses.
2. Explain in brief about:-
   a) *Diaphragmatic breathing*
   b) *Segmental breathing*
   c) *Pursed lip breathing*
   d) *Glossopharyngeal breathing*
   e) *Coughing*
   f) *Huffing*
   g) *Incentive spirometry*
3. List and explain 10 specialties of care.
4. Explain in brief about the following:-
   a) *Specific Phobia*
   b) *Panic Disorder*
   c) *Post-traumatic Stress Disorder*
   d) *Obsessive-Compulsive Disorder*
   e) *Generalized Anxiety Disorder*
   f) *Hypochondriasis*
   g) *Somatoform Disorder*

   h) *Conversion Disorder (old name: Hysteria)*
   i) *Hallucinations*
   j) *Delusions*
   k) *Catatonia*
   l) *Bipolar Disorder (Manic-Depressive Disorder)*
   m) *Antisocial Personality Disorder Symptoms*
   n) *Narcissistic Personality Disorder*
   o) *Borderline Personality Disorder Symptoms*
5. List and explain the five stages of grief (death and dying)?
6. Explain in brief about the types of restraints.
7. Explain in brief about the general information that may be required to fill an incident report.
8. Explain the different types of urine specimen collections:-
   a) Mid-stream

   b) Timed
   c) Random
9. Explain the procedure of fecal specimen collection.
10. List the 16 sections of safety data sheet (SDS).
11. List the steps required for post-mortem care.
12. What is communication? List the elements of communication.
13. List some strategies that should be used while communicating with patients.

CPSIA information can be obtained
at www.ICGtesting.com
Printed in the USA
BVOW07s1458031016

463480BV00023B/7/P